Posttraumatic Stress Disorder and Related Diseases in Combat Veterans

Elspeth Cameron Ritchie
Editor

Posttraumatic Stress Disorder and Related Diseases in Combat Veterans

Springer

Editor
Elspeth Cameron Ritchie
Department of Psychiatry
Uniformed Services University
of the Health Sciences
Bethesda, MD
USA

ISBN 978-3-319-22984-3 ISBN 978-3-319-22985-0 (eBook)
DOI 10.1007/978-3-319-22985-0

Library of Congress Control Number: 2015951824

Springer Cham Heidelberg New York Dordrecht London

Springer International Publishing AG Switzerland is part of Springer Science+Business Media (www.springer.com)

Foreword

Posttraumatic stress disorder (PTSD) is one of the most important health problems faced by service members, veterans, their families and their communities. One of us (HSK) recently assumed the role of chief consultant for mental health for the Department of Veterans Affairs (VA) after more than 30 years in the VA system as a clinician, researcher, teacher, and administrator with a primary focus on PTSD. The other (DMB) has, for many years, taught medical officers about PTSD, treated countless patients and conducted clinical trials of new treatments as professor of psychiatry at the Uniformed Services University of the Health Sciences (USUHS).

We are both well aware of the challenges and controversies surrounding the care of those who have experienced trauma during military service. We are both familiar with the current range of resources as well as the limitations of current approaches.

The concept of PTSD has faced its own challenges. Respected voices have called for PTSD to be reframed as an injury rather than a disorder. Some argue that the diagnosis is too broad while others believe that the diagnostic criteria are not yet fully inclusive. While there are advocates on all sides and pros and cons associated with any proposed change, we believe that it is the dialogue surrounding these controversies that is critically important. This new volume succeeds in taking that dialogue forward.

Many in VA and at the USUHS are calling out for a community-based approach to the management of PTSD and other trauma-related mental health problems. We do not believe that the responsibility for these thorny problems can or should lie solely in the hands of the Military Health System or VA (if only because so much of the care for service members and veterans actually takes place in community practices and depends on family and community support structures that are well beyond the scope of our respective agencies).

For these reasons, the treatment of the psychological effects of deployment must be a community issue with collaboration from across the Department of Defense, VA, and state and community systems. This requires the coordination of public and private clinicians, health systems, community leaders, and policy makers who share an understanding of the challenges faced by service members and their families during military service.

Sadly, with regard to the challenges of reintegration, it appears that our criminal justice system must also be part of the dialogue. Law enforcement personnel often find themselves in the role of "first responders" to domestic violence or public disturbances involving service members, veterans and/or their loved ones.

Their skill in approaching such incidents is a critical element of community response which may determine whether the outcome will be appropriate care, incarceration, or even death. In many cases the police are veterans themselves, but even these peers can benefit from crisis intervention training. Emergency medical responders, parole officers, public defenders, prosecutors and judges, all have important roles to play in a population health approach to PTSD.

As veterans of all ages make use of newly expanded GI Bill opportunities for education, the academic community is playing an expanding role in mitigating the burden of PTSD across the nation. It is critically important that admission officers, faculty, administrators, and campus health workers and campus police, recognize the challenges unique to veterans with PTSD, traumatic brain injury (TBI) or both. Awareness of key information and of effective, available treatment resources promotes retention in educational programs and increases the future productivity of these veterans, their families, and their communities.

Much of this volume focuses on innovative approaches to the treatment of PTSD. Although both the VA and the Military Health Systems fully embrace evidence-based treatment, both institutions recognize that present approaches are neither sufficient nor are they always what military members or veterans want. We agree that the virtue of the nontraditional approaches described in this volume (and others currently under development) must be further explored and discussed.

While we are by no means frequent collaborators, we are old friends who first met through COL (ret) Elspeth Cameron "Cam" Ritchie. Having both known Cam for many years, we were by no means surprised when she "threw us together" to craft this foreword. Nor were we disappointed!

As has been her practice for decades, Cam has collected a highly eclectic, highly qualified assortment of clinicians, scientists, academicians, and thought leaders to create a unique and useful product. Many of these contributors might never have had the opportunity to work together were it not for Dr. Ritchie. Service members, veterans, their families, and the public and private programs which serve them stand to gain significantly from this well-orchestrated collaboration.

We have only touched on a few key elements within and beyond the traditional clinical environment that play (and must continue to play) an important role in the care and reintegration of our nation's combat veterans. In doing so, we are simply expounding Dr. Ritchie's vision of a population health approach to deployment mental health.

In many ways, her approach is the natural extension of core concepts of combat stress doctrine established by the US Military as early as World War I but its further elaboration now benefits from Cam's unique ability to bring people and conversations together. We thank her and her coauthors for taking this important next step in an evolving and essential national dialogue.

David M. Benedek MD
Harold S. Kudler MD

Preface

Since 9/11, 2001 approximately 2.7 US million service members have served in the wars in Afghanistan and Iraq. PTSD and traumatic brain injuries (TBI) have been called as the "signature wounds" of war. Approximately a quarter of service members deployed to war have PTSD. The psychological injuries of war, PTSD, moral injury, and related conditions, lead to other issues with employment and intimate relationships.

There are conventional, evidence-based therapies that are effective—if the service member or veteran is able to tolerate the treatments. As numerous chapters in this volume demonstrate, many cannot tolerate either pharmacotherapy or talking exposure-based therapies. For example, the treatment of PTSD involves medications that often have sexual side effects, which causes many to cease their use. In addition, service members often do not want to talk over and over about their combat experience, so may reject the treatments which involve reliving the traumas.

However, the clinicians in the military and veteran's health-care systems are innovative. They have experimented with alternative ways to engage veterans. These include mindfulness, art therapy, stellate ganglion block, training service dogs, virtual reality, and more. All these and others are highlighted in this book. Not yet subjected to rigorous research, in many cases, these treatments are not yet officially approved in evidence-based guidelines or by the Food and Drug Administration.

PTSD from these wars seldom exists alone in our recent combat veterans. For example, the bomb blast has been the "signature weapon" of these conflicts. Service members wear helmets and body armor, which covers their torsos. Thus blasts primarily affect the lower exposed areas of the body, including the extremities and pelvic region. Numerous service members have lost a leg, and many have lost both legs and/or arms. In some cases they have lost part or all of their genitalia. The bomb blast or other weapons may also burn and scar faces and hands.

Pain from these injuries and subsequent surgeries is a constant theme. Pain has a host of consequences, including impacting sleep and decreasing sexual desire. Narcotics used to treat pain make sexual performance problematic. Too many start on prescription pain medications, and then become addicted to opioids. Overuse of alcohol is another constant problem.

In combat, TBI is commonly caused by blasts, gunshot wounds, and motor-vehicle events. The effects of TBI vary according to severity and location, but include cognitive difficulties, such as forgetfulness, irritability, and impulsivity. In addition the injury may damage the pituitary gland, which in turn affects the endocrine system and the levels of the sexual hormones, testosterone and estrogen. Other medications used for treatment of pain and TBI cause a myriad of issues, such as weight gain, ejaculatory delay, and sedation.

Less well known is the impact of toxic exposures on mental and physical health. All wars are environmentally dirty. Agent Orange is the best known toxic agent from Vietnam. The cause of "Desert Storm syndrome" is still unknown, but is generally believed to be from a combination of exposure to burning petroleum, nerve agents, particulate sand, and psychological stress. Antimalarial agents, used in Iraq and Afghanistan, cause a host of neuropsychiatric effects. Sexual assault is another type of toxic exposure.

This book is an edited collection from many authors. It is designed primarily for a medical audience, but should be accessible to service members and their families who are looking for information on the treatment of PTSD.

The purpose of this volume is several folds. We want to encourage medical personnel to: (1) understand and discuss combat-related mental and physical health issues with their patients; (2) know how to evaluate and treat PTSD, along with related physical injury, pain, and disability; (3) learn how to mitigate the sexual side-effects of medications commonly used for TBI, PTSD, and pain; and (4) be able to keep their patients engaged and in treatment.

The target medical audience includes all providers who treat injured service members and veterans, including primary care providers, psychiatrists, psychologists, social workers, physical and occupational therapists, nurses, and others. The volume should be useful for all those who treat PTSD, not just military service members, as PTSD is a major issue in the civilian population. The volume is not written from the perspective of advocates. But we hope that those who advocate for veterans will draw lessons from these pages.

There are real human stories here. However, to protect patient privacy, details have been changed or stories blended in together. So the reader should consider these as composite cases, with teaching points emphasized, rather than identifiable actual patients.

I was delighted when Springer asked me to do this PTSD casebook. It is time for the entire therapeutic community to learn more about these alternative ways of connecting to combat veterans, who have given so much for their country, the USA and their allies.

Col. (ret.), Prof. Elspeth Cameron Ritchie MD, MPH

Disclaimer

The views and opinions expressed in this book are those of the authors and do not necessarily reflect the official policy or position of any agency of the US government.

Contents

Contributors

Miguel M. Alampay Medical Corps United States Navy, Walter Reed National Military Medical Center, Bethesda, MD, USA

Stephanie Alley Southern California Institute for Research and Education, Long Beach VA Medical Center, Long Beach, CA, USA

Amy D. Amidon Naval Medical Center San Diego, San Diego, CA, USA

Rohul Amin Behavioral Health Directorate, Walter Reed National Military Medical Center, Bethesda, MD, USA

Paulette T. Cazares Naval Medical Center, San Diego, CA, USA

Jeffrey T. Cole Department of Neurology, Booz Allen Hamilton, McLean, VA, USA

Judith Cukor Department of Psychiatry, Weill Cornell Medical College, New York, NY, USA

Jonathan R. Dettmer 2d Marine Regiment Psychiatrist, Camp Lejeune, NC, USA

JoAnn Difede Department of Psychiatry, Weill Cornell Medical College, New York, NY, USA

Kerrie Earley Psychiatry Continuity Service, Walter Reed National Military Medical Center, Bethesda, MD, USA

Shannon C. Ford Department of Psychiatry, Walter Reed National Military Medical Center, Bethesda, MD, USA

Joshua N. Friedlander Behavioral Health Directorate, Walter Reed National Military Medical Center, Bethesda, MD, USA

Maryrose Gerardi Department of Psychiatry, Emory University, Atlanta, GA, USA

Geoffrey G. Grammer National Intrepid Center of Excellence, Walter Reed National Military Medical Center, Bethesda, MD, USA

Kyle J. Gray Department of Psychiatry, Walter Reed National Military Medical Center, Bethesda, MD, USA

Diego F. Hernandez College of Nursing, University of South Florida, Tampa, FL, USA

Anita H. Hickey Integrative and Interventional Pain Medicine, Department of Anesthesiology, USNH Okinawa, Okinawa, Japan

Charles W. Hoge Department of Psychiatry, Walter Reed Army Institute of Research, Bethesda, MD, USA

Erika M. Kappes National Capital Consortium Psychiatry Residency, Walter Reed National Military Medical Center, Bethesda, MD, USA

Marina Khusid Deployment Health Clinical Center, Defense Centers of Excellence for Psychological Health and Traumatic Brain Injury, Silver Spring, MD, USA

Kevin E. Kip College of Nursing, University of South Florida, Tampa, FL, USA

Robert Koffman Integrative Medicine and Behavioral Health, National Intrepid Center of Excellence, Walter Reed National Military Medical Center, Bethesda, MD, USA

Alexandra L. Laifer Veterans Medical Research Foundation, VA San Diego Healthcare System, San Diego, CA, USA

Ariel J. Lang VA San Diego Healthcare System, University of California San Diego, San Diego, CA, USA

Daniel J. Lee Department of Behavioral Health, Bayne-Jones Army Community Hospital, Fort Polk, LA, USA

Eugene Lipov Advanced Pain Centers, Hoffman Estates, Hoffman Estates, IL, USA

Brett T. Litz VA Boston Healthcare System, Boston University, Boston, MA, USA

Eric G. Meyer Department of Psychiatry, Uniformed Services University of the Health Sciences, Bethesda, MD, USA

Christopher S. Nelson Department of Psychiatry, United States Navy; Behavioral Health Directorate; Naval Hospital Camp LeJeune, Camp Lejeune, NC, USA

Remington Lee Nevin Department of Mental Health, Johns Hopkins Bloomberg School of Public Health, Baltimore, MD, USA

Michelle Nordstrom Occupational Therapy Mental Health Services, Walter Reed National Military Medical Center, Bethesda, MD, USA

Meg Daley Olmert Warrior Canine Connection, Brookeville, MD, USA

Marshall Peters Walter Reed National Military Medical Center, Bethesda, MD, USA

Cody J. Rall Department of Psychiatry, Walter Reed National Military Medical Center, Bethesda, MD, USA

Christopher Reist Department of Research, Long Beach VA Medical Center, Long Beach, CA, USA

Department of Psychiatry and Human Behavior, University of California, Irvine, CA, USA

Seema Reza Department of Rehabilitation, Walter Reed National Military Medical Center, Bethesda, MD, USA

Rita Richardson National Capital Consortium, Walter Reed National Military Medical Center Bethesda, Bethesda, MD, USA

Elspeth Cameron Ritchie Department of Psychiatry, Uniformed Services University of the Health Sciences, Bethesda, MD, USA

Albert Rizzo Medical Virtual Reality, Institute for Creative Technologies, Department of Psychiatry and School of Gerontology, University of Southern California, Playa Vista, CA, USA

Barbara O. Rothbaum Department of Psychiatry, Emory University, Atlanta, GA, USA

Michael Roy Division of Military Internal Medicine, Department of Medicine, Uniformed Services University of the Health Sciences, Bethesda, MD, USA

William D. Rumbaugh National Capital Consortium, Walter Reed National Military Medical Center Bethesda, Bethesda, MD, USA

Patcho N. Santiago National Capital Consortium Psychiatry Residency, Walter Reed National Military Medical Center, Bethesda, MD, USA

Paul Sargent LOGSU Medical Department, Naval Special Warfare Group ONE, San Diego, CA, USA

Caroline C. Scacca Department of Behavioral Health, Walter Reed National Military Medical Center, Bethesda, MD, USA

Matthew St Laurent Department of Rehabilitation, Walter Reed National Military Medical Center, Bethesda, MD, USA

Rachel Sullivan Child and Family Behavioral Health System, Department of Behavioral Health, Madigan Army Medical Center, Tacoma, WA, USA

Nicholas A. Tamoria Department of Psychiatry, Walter Reed National Military Medical Center, Bethesda, MD, USA

Connie L. Thomas Behavioral Health Directorate, Walter Reed National Military Medical Center, Bethesda, MD, USA

Wendi M. Waits Directorate of Behavioral Health, Fort Belvoir Community Hospital, Fort Belvoir, VA, USA

Christopher H. Warner Department of Psychiatry, Uniformed Services University of Health Sciences, Bethesda, MD, USA

Genelle Weits Behavioral Health Psychology Department, Navy Medical Center, San Diego, CA, USA

James C. West Department of Psychiatry, Uniformed Services University of the Health Sciences, Bethesda, MD, USA

Joseph E Wise Department of Psychiatry, Walter Reed Army Institute of Research, Walter Reed National Military Medical Center, Bethesda, MD, USA

Brian W Writer Department of Psychiatry, Adjunct Faculty, Audie L. Murphy VA Hospital, University of Texas Health Science Center San Antonio, San Antonio, TX, USA

Rick Yount Warrior Canine Connection, Brookeville, MD, USA

Hanna Zembrzuska National Capital Consortium, Walter Reed National Military Medical Center Bethesda, Bethesda, MD, USA

Part I
Introduction

Introduction and Overview: Posttraumatic Stress Disorder and Related Diseases in Combat Veterans

1

Elspeth Cameron Ritchie

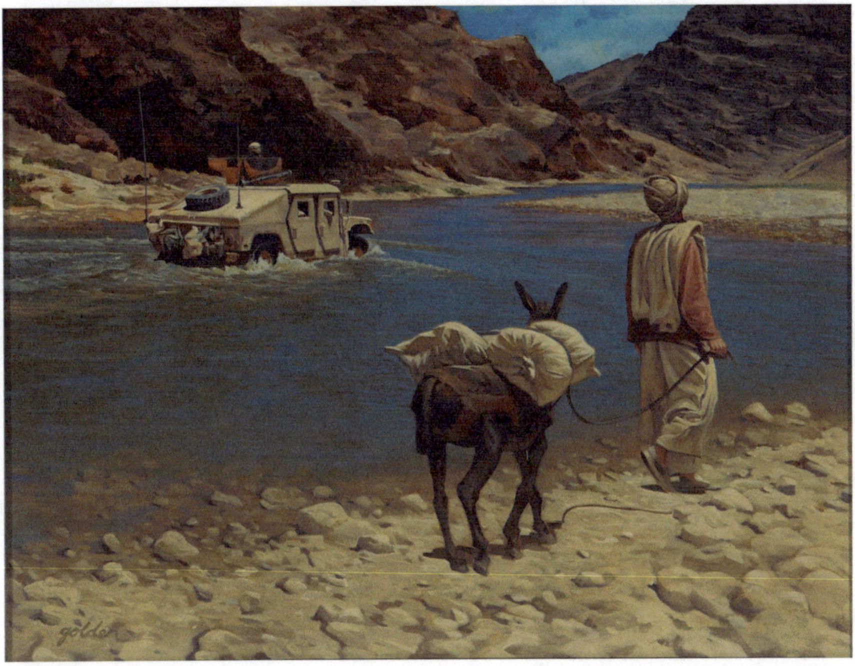

Tracking Bin Laden, by SFC Elzie Golden, courtesy of the Army Art Collection, US Army Center of Military History.

E. C. Ritchie (✉)
Department of Psychiatry, Uniformed Services University of the Health Sciences, 4301 Jones Bridge Road, Bethesda, MD 20314, USA
e-mail: elspethcameronritchie@gmail.com

E. C. Ritchie (ed.), *Posttraumatic Stress Disorder and Related Diseases in Combat Veterans*, DOI 10.1007/978-3-319-22985-0_1

Posttraumatic stress disorder (PTSD) is now a major topic in scientific literature and media, especially after the many years of the wars in Afghanistan and Iraq. This introductory chapter begins by covering some critical administrative and cultural competency issues. It briefly outlines the basics of prevalence, diagnostic criteria, evidence-based, and innovative therapy, in the context of the wars since 9/11. Later chapters delve into treatment with service members and veterans in far more detail. This introduction contains some caveats about the scientific basis of the therapies discussed.

Approximately 2.7 million service members have served in the conflicts since the planes dived into the Twin Towers and the Pentagon on 9/11/2001. Estimates of the numbers of service members who have deployed to Iraq and Afghanistan and have PTSD range from 15 to 25 % [1–3]. The number of diagnosed and treated PTSD cases is always lower than those who report symptoms on anonymous surveys, probably related to the concerns of active duty service members about their careers in the military [1, 2].

While about 50 % of recent veterans seek care in the Veterans Affairs (VA) health-care system, others do not, and/or get care in diverse settings. Some seek services in both the VA and through their job and educational (e.g., college and graduate school) clinic providers. Therefore, it is critically important that not just military and VA providers but also civilian mental health providers know how to recognize and treat PTSD.

PTSD does not occur just in combat veterans, of course. The symptoms of PTSD also follow sexual assault, crime, and disasters. However, this volume focuses on combat veterans. By combat veterans, we mean both active duty and those no longer on active duty (veterans), including those in the National Guard and reserves. The innovative therapies in this clinical casebook may also be useful in civilian populations, but that is not the focus of the volume.

1.1 Treatment Guidelines and "Refractory" Patients

There are well-established guidelines for the treatment of PTSD, developed by the American Psychiatric Association (APA) and the Department of Defense (DoD) and the Veterans Health Administration (VHA). These are often referred to as evidence-based treatments. These will be summarized later in this chapter and referred to in other chapters. However, there are many patients who are either unwilling or unable or do not respond to the evidence-based treatments.

While these patients may be called "treatment-resistant" or "refractory," it is the treatments themselves that are often not palatable to service members. That may be because of: (1) unacceptable side effects from medication; (2) difficulties with making frequent appointments, especially for the cognitive behavioral treatments; (3) the distaste of many service members to relive their trauma and/or talk about it; or (4) the stigma of seeking treatment from a mental health-care provider.

Thus this volume will focus on the more "refractory" patients, treated with newer and less conventional therapies, with a focus on how to engage reluctant veterans in treatment.

1.2 Administrative Issues and Medical Discharges

Service members need to be physically and mentally fit for duty, according to various regulations [4]. They need to be able to deploy to war zones and other austere environments. They may carry firearms, drive tanks, fly helicopters, and pilot ships.

Thus, if a service member has a severe mental illness, they usually will receive a medical evaluation board (MEB) to see if they are fit for duty. Severe mental illnesses include psychotic disorders, and may include mood disorders and PTSD. If found not fit for duty, they may be medically discharged. A medical discharge usually has some disability benefits attached.

They may also be "medically retired," depending on the severity of their condition. Retirement carries significant health-care and disability benefits (often at 50% of their base pay). A medical retirement is generally a lifelong benefit. The medical/physical evaluation board, now called the integrated disability evaluation system, is a complex process [5]. Many chapters within this volume refer to the MEB process, which is why it is discussed here.

PTSD does not necessarily lead to a medical discharge. If a service member responds to treatment, he or she may be found fit for duty. Alternatively, with actual practice varying according to the service, they may be administratively discharged, which comes without benefits. The financial discrepancy between a medical and administrative discharge is substantial.

Many of the complex cases described in this book have been referred by their physician to the MEB process. Service members may or may not want a medical discharge, which offers both benefits and potential shame.

There are in general two major drivers of not seeking or seeking treatment, in my experience. Service members who want to stay in the military do not want to go near a mental health provider, as they fear for their jobs. For example, Marines refer to a psychiatrist or psychologist as the "Wizard," as he or she makes Marines "disappear." This often leads to a medical or administrative discharge.

However, those who are nearing the end of their enlistment, or are planning to retire, have many pressures to endorse PTSD symptoms. The pressures include the financial benefits of medical retirement as well as priority for VA care.

1.3 Cultural Competency

A theme throughout the book is of cultural competency. Especially if you are a civilian provider, how do you understand the military culture?

As a start, one of the easy ways is to ask the patient about their military occupational specialty (MOS). Ask about basic and advanced training, and where they have been stationed. Ask when and where they have been deployed. Do not assume that the official DD 214 (official discharge paperwork) will list all their battle assignments.

Learn what their military rank is or was, and ask how they want to be addressed. Some will prefer to be addressed by rank, others by their first name. Patients who have been in the Special Forces, served at Guantanamo Bay, or have served in classified operations, may not be able to talk about the specifics of their experiences.

An important piece of cultural competency advice for providers: Today's combat veterans do not want to be seen as victims. Treat them as "battle-hardened" or maybe "battle-scarred." Respect their service [6].

1.4 Terminology and Health-Care Systems

The Military Health System (MHS) is separate and distinct from the VA health-care system, usually referred to as the VHA. The MHS mainly consists both of the direct health-care system, offered by hospitals and clinics on military posts, and also the purchased care system, commonly known as TRICARE. Technically, the direct health-care system and the purchased care system are all one in the MHS, but differences exist in eligibility. For example, retirees and dependents can go to the direct care system, but only if there is space available. Often they are referred to the purchased care system under TRICARE. (For more details on these health-care systems, see Ref. [7].)

"Service" refers to the branch of service, Army, Navy, Air Force, or Marines (although the Marines are actually part of the Department of the Navy). Correspondingly, the uniformed personnel are soldiers, sailors, airmen, or Marines. The term "service members" refers to all of the military personnel.

The term "veteran" has several uses. It usually means service members who are no longer on active duty. The term "combat veteran" is used for both service members and those no longer on active duty who have served in conflict zones.

Active duty service members wear the military uniform full time and receive care through the MHS. Reservists include many categories of reserve service members, as well as the National Guard. Reservists usually serve a weekend a month and 2 weeks a year, although there are many variations. Reservists may transition between active duty and veteran status. The National Guard belongs to their state, and may be mobilized in the event of state emergencies, or be called up to action for war.

All reserve components have seen deployments unprecedented since World War II. Their care is often complicated. They receive health care through the military health-care system while active, but are generally not eligible for care when on inactive status. However, they may be eligible for care within the VA system if they have served in combat, or met other eligibility criteria. Often reservists transition between the military health-care system, the VA, and civilian health-care organizations.

The cases discussed here are mainly of service members who have served in Iraq or Afghanistan. The Iraq War is usually called "OIF" for Operation Iraqi Freedom. Later, another term was Operation New Dawn. The conflict in Afghanistan was "OEF" for Operation Enduring Freedom.

But there have been many other conflicts in the last 20 years, including the first Gulf War (Desert Storm), Haiti, Somalia, and Bosnia. The latter three conflicts are often referred to as Operations Other than War (OOTW).

In addition, there have been many humanitarian missions that service members have been deployed to, such as the tsunami in 2004, and operations dealing with Ebola in West Africa in 2014 and 2015. They are not considered combat operations, but have their own share of trauma.

Again, overall, service members will not want to be seen as victims, or heroes, but as battle-hardened, or maybe battle-scarred.

1.5 Current Definition of PTSD

The *Diagnostic and Statistical Manual of Mental Disorders, Fifth Edition (DSM-5)* is the 2013 update to the APA classification and diagnostic tool which, in the USA, serves as a universal authority for psychiatric diagnosis [8]. PTSD used to be classified as an anxiety disorder (DSM-IV). The DSM-5 now includes PTSD with trauma- and stressor-related disorders. Although the new DSM-5 appeared in 2013, it is only beginning to be widely adopted. The MHS and VA were scheduled to adopt it on Oct 1, 2014. However, the implementation throughout the psychiatric world has been uneven.

These changes are summarized as follows: DSM-5 criteria now identify the trigger to PTSD as exposure to actual or threatened death, serious injury, or sexual violation. The diagnosis of PTSD is currently based on eight criteria from the DSM-5.

The first four criteria pertain to the "actual event" and must result from one or more of the following scenarios, in which the individual:

- directly experiences the traumatic event;
- witnesses the traumatic event in person;
- learns that the traumatic event occurred to a close family member or close friend;
- experiences first-hand repeated or extreme exposure to aversive details of the traumatic event.

Fear, helplessness and horror, as a result of the stressor, are no longer required. The disturbance, regardless of its trigger, causes clinically significant distress or impairment in the individual's social interactions, capacity to work, or other important areas of functioning. It is not the physiological result of another medical condition, medication, drugs, or alcohol.

Symptoms that accompany PTSD should be present for 1 month following the initial traumatic event and include the following: reexperiencing, avoidance, negative cognitions and mood, and arousal:

- *Reexperiencing* covers spontaneous memories of the traumatic event, recurrent dreams related to it, flashbacks, or other intense or prolonged psychological distress.
- *Avoidance* refers to distressing memories, thoughts, feelings, or external reminders of the event.

- *Negative cognitions and mood* represents myriad feelings, from a persistent and distorted sense of blame of self or others, to estrangement from others or markedly diminished interest in activities, to an inability to remember key aspects of the event.
- Finally, *arousal* is marked by aggressive, reckless or self-destructive behavior, sleep disturbances, hypervigilance, or related problems [8].

A study by Hoge in 2014 [9] compared diagnoses of soldiers under DSM-IV TR and DSM-5. In brief, about a third of the soldiers who met DSM-IV TR criteria for PTSD did not meet DSM-5 criteria. Almost a third were in the opposite camp, meeting DSM-5 but not the older criteria. The main discrepancy is related to the new Criterion C, which splits up avoidant symptoms from depressive symptoms [9].

1.6 A Brief Discussion of Comorbidities

While there are a few service members who have "pure" PTSD, in the experience of most clinicians that is the exception rather than the rule [2]. For example, insomnia may lead to drinking to try to sleep. Numbing and avoidance leads to relationship problems and, often, divorce.

Medications used to treat PTSD often have sexual side effects, including erectile dysfunction. The contribution of sexual side effects to divorce and suicide is only beginning to be evaluated. More details follow in various chapters which discuss medications.

PTSD, traumatic brain injury (TBI), and alcohol problems have long been associated with each other. As noted above, patients who "only" have PTSD are rare [2]. Many of the following chapters discuss the treatment of these common but still complex cases.

The physical stresses of military service, including wounds and injuries, contribute to musculoskeletal problems, with corresponding pain and disability. The musculoskeletal issues have led to service members being treated with opiates, which of course can cause dependence and addiction. In both military and civilian populations, many switch from legal opiates to illegal heroin. Many service members, especially after discharge from the military, thus start a sad slide into substance dependence, unemployment, and homelessness. Unfortunately, death by heroin overdose is increasingly common [6].

There is also the question of missed diagnoses. The antimalarial agent mefloquine (Lariam) has been associated with many neurological and psychiatric complaints, covered in detail in a later chapter. Thus, mefloquine toxicity may be confused with PTSD or TBI [10].

1.6.1 Evidence-Based Treatment

There are several forms of evidence-based treatment, covered in well-established guidelines for the treatment of PTSD, developed by the APA and the DoD and the VHA. The principal ones include: (1) pharmacotherapy or medication and (2) psychotherapy.

Pharmacotherapy includes two FDA-approved selective serotonin reuptake inhibitors (SSRIs), paroxetine (Paxil) and sertraline (Zoloft). However, most clinicians use a wide variety of SSRIs, with the choice depending on their side-effect profiles. Many other medications are also used, including second-generation antipsychotics and other standard medications for sleep. (More details will be covered further in later chapters.)

The evidence-based psychotherapies include: (1) cognitive processing therapy, a variant of cognitive behavioral therapy and (2) exposure therapy. The first one involves telling the combat-related trauma, and reframing the trauma. The second includes reexposure to the trauma in a gradual process. A variant of the latter includes "virtual therapy," a computer-aided reexposure process. Service members often like the virtual therapy techniques more than the face-to-face traditional approach.

Eye movement desensitizing processing (EMDR) is now also considered an evidence-based treatment. In the past it has been controversial. Many consider it another variant of exposure therapy. There is no separate chapter on it in this volume, because the senior editor could not find any military or VA authors who were practicing it. It is still used with some success in Israel. However, some consider accelerated resolution therapy (ART) an enhancement of EMDR. ART is covered later in the volume.

Acupuncture is now rising to the level of accepted therapies, but is not there yet. It is also covered in this volume. Another new and promising approach herein is stellate ganglion block (SGB). SGB has received considerable attention in recent years as an almost miraculous cure for some cases of refractory PTSD.

1.6.2 Select Populations: Female Service Members and Reservists

Approximately 15 % of the military are female. At present, 15 % of active military, 17 % of National Guard/Reserves, and 20 % of new recruits are women. The recent wars in Iraq and Afghanistan have engendered a growing population of female veterans seeking health care through the VA. Women are among the fastest growing segments of new users of VA health care; as many as 40 % of the women returning from Iraq and Afghanistan may elect to use the VA. However, in the available literature, female soldiers have about the same rate of PTSD as males [11].

Certain occupations may lead to an increased rate of PTSD. Some of these occupations are disproportionately drawn from reserve service members. For example, at the beginning of the war in Iraq, truck drivers had an elevated rate of PTSD symptoms, often feeling very vulnerable, "like sitting ducks", to improvised explosive devices and snipers [12].

Medical staff, another high-risk population, are exposed to both horrifically wounded service members and the injured local population. Severely wounded service members are usually evacuated quickly out of theater to Germany and beyond. However, the injured locals stay in the military facilities, sometimes for many months. Injured include children, third party nationals, and detainees.

Detainee missions have their own challenges. The detainees may try to hurt their caregivers, for example by grabbing their buttocks or trying to stab them while they are trying to deliver care. The mission is considered a "dirty one" [13].

Individual augmentees and other reservists are often "cross-leveled" to various units who they do not know. Reservists were assigned to the truck driving missions described above. They have made up a large share of those assigned detainee missions, such as at Guantanamo Bay, Camp Bucca, and Abu Ghraib [12, 13]. Reservists may not have the support of a cohesive unit when they return home.

1.6.3 Moral Injury

The concept of "moral injury" will be referred to in various chapters in this volume. Moral injury is related to but different from PTSD. In general, most authors conceptualize it as an insult caused by either the shame of killing or the guilt induced by having fellow service members die, while one has survived. It may also be caused by the belief that one's unit, or the military as a whole, has betrayed the service member. While not well studied by the medical community, most agree that it is a corrosive condition that contributes to relationship difficulties and suicide.

1.6.4 Suicide

Suicides among US Army personnel have been increasing since 2004, surpassing comparable civilian rates in 2008. Suicide rates peaked in active duty troops in the past few years, but are still rising in reservists. Suicides are consistently highest among young white males but have been rising in older ages and females as well.

Risk factors for suicide among active duty members are well known, since data are systemically collected. These include relationship difficulties, financial and occupational problems, pain and physical disability, and access to weapons [14, 15]. As alluded to above, we hypothesize a contribution of sexual impotence to suicidal thoughts, but there are no systematic data.

Suicides among veterans no longer on active duty are estimated at 22 a day. Less is known about risk factors among these post-services veterans. Anecdotally, suicides among recent veterans have the same risk factors as with active duty service members. For older veterans, they seem to be related to depression and substance dependence, risk factors more similar to the civilian population.

1.7 Case Examples and Clinical Pearls

Case examples are used in the following chapters extensively, and, by design, form the core of the teaching points. These are generally composite case examples, to both illustrate teaching points and to conceal identities. If actual case examples are used, the patient has given permission to use them.

Clinical pearls, also by design, are what clinicians have found useful in their practices. They are not usually borne out of practice guidelines, but rather what clinicians have found to have worked in their practice with combat veterans.

1.8 Conclusion

This casebook broadens the treatment options for PTSD and related comorbidities, by describing complex cases seen in clinical practice. These treatments include mindfulness, canine therapy, novel psychological and psychopharmacological interventions, psychoanalysis, virtual reality, and SGB. These are often received well by veterans, but we do not know which works for whom.

A related warning: Many of the treatments in this volume do not have the research background to affirmatively mandate their use. They are not yet FDA approved. It is imperative that the more promising ones receive more research scrutiny and funding.

References

1. Tanielian T, Jaycox LH. Invisible wounds of war. Rand Corporation. 2008. http://www.rand.org/content/dam/rand/pubs/monographs/2008/RAND_MG720.pdf. Accessed 3 Feb 2015.
2. Institute of Medicine. Treatment of posttraumatic stress disorder in military and veteran populations. Final assessment, June 20 2014. http://www.iom.edu/Reports/2014/Treatment-for-Posttraumatic-Stress-Disorder-in-Military-and-Veteran-Populations-Final-Assessment.aspx. Accessed 3 Feb 2015.
3. Joint Mental Health Advisory Team (J-MHAT). Report 7 2011. http://armylive.dodlive.mil/index.php/2011/05/joint-mental-health-advisory-team-vii-j-mhat-7-report/. Accessed 3 Feb 2015.
4. AR 40–501, Standards of Medical Fitness. 2011. http://www.apd.army.mil/pdffiles/r40_501.pdf. Accessed 3 Feb 2015.
5. The Army Integrated Disability Evaluation Process. 2015. http://www.wtc.army.mil/modules/soldier/s6-ides.html. Accessed 24 Aug 2015
6. Ritchie EC. Cultural competency and treatment of veteran and military patients with mental health disorders. Federal Practitioner, April 2015.
7. Ritchie EC. The DoD and VA health care system overview. In: Cozza S, Goldenberg M, Ursano RJ, editors. Care of military service members, veterans and their families. VA, USA: American Psychiatric Press Institute; 2014.
8. Diagnostic and Statistical Manual (DSM) 5. APA Press, 2013.
9. Hoge C. DSM-5 PTSD screening may miss previously diagnosed soldiers, August 28, 2014. http://www.healio.com/psychiatry/ptsd/news/online/%7B4e137bbf-4bc0-4c31-b6b2-77e83e9b09d9%7D/dsm-5-ptsd-screening-may-miss-previously-diagnosed-soldiers. Accessed 3 Feb 2015.

10. Ritchie EC, Nevin R, Block J. Psychiatric side-effects of mefloquine: relevance to forensic psychiatry. J Am Psychiatry Law. 2013;41(2):224–35.
11. Ritchie EC, Bell M, Milllikan A, Galloway M, Carino M, Bliese P, Thomas J. Psychological experiences of female soldiers during the long war. In: Ritchie EC, Naclerio A, editors. Women at war. Oxford: Oxford University Press; 2015.
12. MHAT II. 2005. https://timemilitary.files.wordpress.com/2012/07/2-oif-ii_report-105.pdf. Accessed 3 May 2015.
13. MHAT V. https://www.google.com/search?q=MHAT+V&oq=MHAT+V&gs_l=serp.3.0j0i22i30l4j0i22i10i30j0i22i30l2j0i22i10i30l2.3170.4745.0.6482.3.3.0.0.0.0.138.390.0j3.3.0.msedr...0...1c.1.64.serp.0.3.379.XMFiuSWVejw. Accessed 3 May 2015.
14. Ritchie EC. 2006. Suicides and the United States Army; Perspectives from the former Psychiatry Consultant to the Army Surgeon General. Cerebrum, Jan 2012.
15. Black S, Galloway S, Bell M, Ritchie EC. Prevalence and risk factors associated with suicides of army soldiers. Mil Psychol. 2011;23:433–51.

Posttraumatic Stress Disorder Screening in the US Military and VA Populations

2

Daniel J. Lee, Christopher H. Warner and Charles W. Hoge

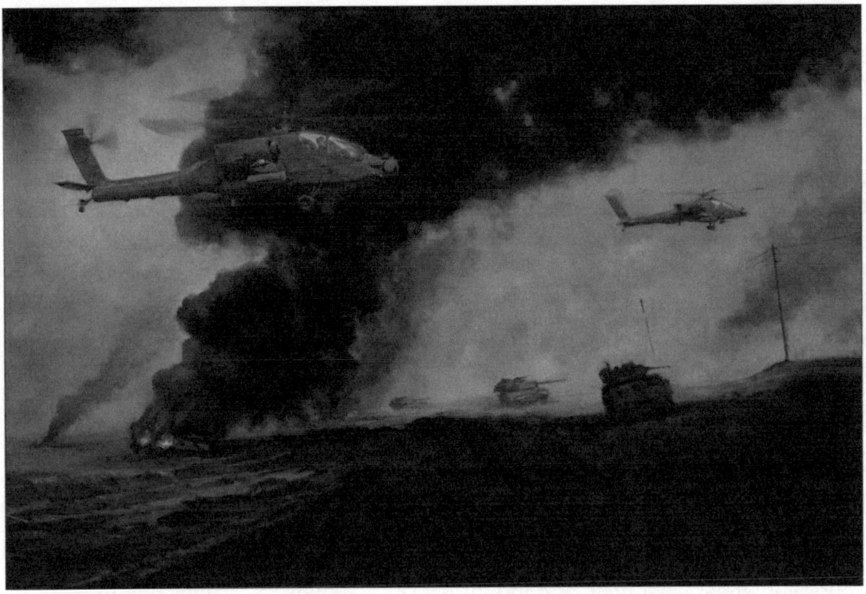

Satan's Sandbox, by SFC Elzie Golden, courtesy of the Army Art Collection, US Army Center of Military History.

C. H. Warner (✉)
Department of Psychiatry, Uniformed Services University of Health Sciences, Bethesda, MD, USA
e-mail: Christopher.h.warner.mil@mail.mil

D. J. Lee
Department of Behavioral Health, Bayne-Jones Army Community Hospital, Fort Polk, LA, USA
e-mail: Daniel.J.Lee82.mil@mail.mil

C. W. Hoge
Department of Psychiatry, Walter Reed Army Institute of Research, Bethesda, MD, USA

E. C. Ritchie (ed.), *Posttraumatic Stress Disorder and Related Diseases in Combat Veterans,* DOI 10.1007/978-3-319-22985-0_2

2.1 Case

Upon return from their second 12 month deployment to Iraq in early 2006, all members of the deployed unit completed a Department of Defense mandated Post-Deployment Health Assessment. Among them was a 24 year old, single, Caucasian male who endorsed having experiences which replayed as nightmares, feeling numb or detached from others, and constantly being on guard within the past month. As a result of his answers, he was asked to meet with a primary care provider. During this meeting, he cited three incidents in which he and his unit members were engaged by the enemy including two improvised explosive devices and one small arms ambush. During those engagements, two of his fellow unit members were wounded and one close friend was killed. The soldier was given a referral to speak with a behavioral health provider who conducted an evaluation the next day. He was found to meet DSM-IV-TR criteria for posttraumatic stress disorder (PTSD). The soldier was then enrolled into the installation medical facility's behavioral health service and underwent treatment with a course of trauma-focused psychotherapy. After 6 months of treatment, the soldier's symptoms were significantly improved and the soldier continued to successfully serve in the military.

Conversely, a second soldier from the same unit denied any difficulties or mental health symptoms during his post-deployment screening process. By 6 months following his return home, this previously even-tempered married soldier with no history of disciplinary problems had ongoing marital problems, was under investigation for domestic violence against his wife, and was cited by local police for driving under the influence of alcohol. Ultimately, he was administratively discharged from the military for patterns of misconduct, an outcome which could have likely been prevented.

2.2 Background

Maintenance of medical readiness is a top priority for all commanding officers in the military. Medical readiness is a shared responsibility of military commanders, military medical personnel, and individual service members. They should work in an integrated manner to ensure that our military personnel are ready to fight and win our nation's wars while taking all practical measures to minimize the risk of harm to indivdiuals and to the mission. Over the 14 year course of Operation Enduring Freedom (OEF) and Operation Iraqi Freedom (OIF), both commanders and the military health system (MHS) have primarily focused on treatment of symptoms and injuries following return from deployment, pre-deployment screening, and post-deployment screening. From a military mental health standpoint, common difficulties for service members have included PTSD, depression, traumatic brain injury, and substance misuse. OEF/OIF has involved unprecedented numbers of repeat deployments by service members and combat deployments by Guard and Reserve serve members; as these conflicts have continued, the impact on maintaining readiness has steadily increased [1–3]. The US Army alone has provided well over 1.5 million troop-years to OIF/OEF between 2001 and 2011, more than all other US services combined [3]. Since 2008, the cumulative amount of time an individual soldier has spent deployed increased by an average of 28 % [3]. The US Navy, Air Force, and Marine Corps have contributed 333,000, 309,000, and 280,000 troop-years to OIF/OEF from 2001 to 2011, respectively [3].

Epidemiologic studies estimate the current or 1-year prevalence of PTSD to be 3.5–5 % for the general population over 12 months, 4–31 % overall for military personnel returning from deployment, 13 % for infantry personnel returning from deployment, and upwards of 30 % for those seeking behavioral health care [4–9]. Rates of depression in similar populations have ranged from 3–25 % [10, 11] and traumatic brain injury has been identified in 19 % of the returning military personnel [12]. Service members with multiple combat deployments are at a higher risk of developing mental health problems than those deployed only once. Per the Office of the US Army Surgeon General, approximately 11.9 % of the individuals returning from their first deployment will have mental health problems [13]. This number climbs to 18.5 % with a second deployment, and 27.2 % with a third or fourth deployment [13]. National Guard and Reserve personnel also appear to be at higher risk of mental health problems when compared to active-duty peers. Longitudinal assessment by Miliken et al found that 35.5 % of the Guard and Reserve troops were at mental health risk 6 months after deployment compared with 27.1 % of the active-duty soldiers [14].

From these statistics, it appears the majority of service members exposed to trauma do not develop PTSD. Additionally, many service members who develop PTSD are able to pass screenings and deploy repeatedly, suggesting that the natural course of PTSD is to improve over time, even without treatment. Studies which have followed PTSD over time have come to similar conclusions [15]. Those that do not improve over time, even with treatment, have a poorer prognosis; a general trend among long-term PTSD trajectory and medication studies is that individuals with greater chronicity of symptoms demonstrate lower responses to treatment than those treated early following the index trauma [6, 16–28]. It is for this reason that screening is so vital; those treated earlier after onset of symptoms are much more likely to be returned to duty while those caught late are far more likely to require medical retirement or significant limitations in duty. Essentially, the primary purpose of screening service members for PTSD is to catch the small percentage of service members who are more likely to be treatment-refractory and get them help before symptoms become chronic.

Many veterans receive care from the Veterans Administration (VA) at some point in their careers. Relatively few of these individuals receive VA care due to retirement from active duty after serving 20 years or more or being medically retired due to one or more chronic medical conditions [29]. The majority of veterans seeks out care after serving one or two tours of duty [30, 31]. Of these, a substantial portion do not access, delay to access, or fail to complete an adequate course of treatment while on active duty [31, 32]. All Veterans of OIF/OEF have been entitled to 2 years of free health care through the VA since 2001, and this was raised to 5 years of free care in the 2008 National Defense Authorization Act (NDAA) [33]. As of 2008,

40 % of all the OIF/OEF veterans had enrolled with the VA [34] and 238,098 veterans received care through the VA [35]. Of these, 84,972 received new mental health diagnoses; 49,425 were new diagnoses of PTSD [35]. Given the impact of chronicity on treatment response for PTSD, it is clear that the VA faces a very difficult mission. VA treatment populations are comprised predominately of male veterans with chronic, treatment-refractory PTSD and a high percentage of comorbid conditions such as substance misuse [36]. Many experts feel that previously held distinctions between treatment response for men versus women and combat-trauma versus other traumas is better accounted for chronicity of symptoms in predominately male VA populations as opposed to anything unique about response to combat-trauma [36]. Unfortunately, no studies currently exist looking at these factors. Screening is less of a priority in this setting, though still important due to the proportion of service members who never seek out or receive treatment prior to enrolling with the VA.

2.3 History of Military/VA Screening

In 1991, nearly a quarter million US service members redeployed from Southwest Asia after participating in the Operation Desert Shield/Storm. At the time of their return they appeared healthy, but over the coming months to years reports emerged of illnesses and somatic complaints. This led to the development of large-scale epidemiological screening and special clinical programs to determine potential associated or causative factors; however, the lack of available deployment and post-deployment surveillance data served as a significant limitation to these efforts. In the wake of joint efforts by the Department of Defense, Department of Veteran's Affairs, and the Institute of Medicine, new guidelines were developed for post-deployment monitoring and management. In 1998, as part of the enactment of that protocol, the first Post-Deployment Health Assessment (PDHA) was introduced which included both a survey and a face-to-face interview and evaluation with a primary care provider [37].

Of note, the first PDHA contained a total of six questions of which only one focused on mental health (During this deployment have you sought, or intend to seek, counseling or care for your mental health?) [38]. Over the next 3 years, assessments conducted on personnel deploying to the Balkans allowed for refinement of the process and in 2001, the PDHA first included screening tools for depression (Patient Health Questionnaire-2) and PTSD (Primary Care-PTSD) [39, 40]. This process remained in place until 2006 when a second screening, called the Post-Deployment Health Re-assessment (PDHRA) was instituted.

The PDHRA, mandated as part of the 2005 National Defense Authorization Act, is required for all service members to complete 90–180 days after returning from a deployment [41]. This modification was based on initial studies in Afghanistan and Iraq veterans which showed that rates of service members with symptoms of PTSD increased after 90 days home [10, 14]. These studies also identified various barriers to care and stigmas about seeking mental health care which further influenced other mental health initiatives throughout the military and VA. During this time, multiple other initiatives and changes were considered to the process to include having all returning service members complete a face-to-face evaluation with a behavioral health provider or undergo a full behavioral health intake evaluation, but studies did not support the anticipated benefit of those initiatives and the general process of completing the initial questionnaire and reviewing with a primary care provider has remained intact [42]. The one augmentation that most post-deployment screening stations did add was the presence of on-site or tele-available mental health providers to allow for initial completion of mental health referrals if indicated, though this was not a Department of Defense requirement [43].

In conjunction with the post-deployment screening, the prolonged requirements in Iraq and Afghanistan placed a demand on the all volunteer military for service members to participate in repeated deployments to combat zones. This led to concerns over deploying service members with mental health conditions and led to the creation of minimum mental health standards for deployment. Specifically, these standards required at least 90 days of treatment (usually medication) stabilization before deployment and specified medications which precluded deployment regardless of duration of treatment (e.g., lithium, antipsychotics, and tricyclic antidepressants). When coupled with a coordination of care process, these standards were shown to be effective in reducing the incidence of mental health complications [44].

Even with the myriad of changes as well as the addition of questions on drug/alcohol abuse and family violence, many service members with PTSD were not identified prompting Congress to require additional screening. In the 2012 NDAA, lawmakers increased the frequency of screening to the current schedule of 120 days before deployment, upon return from deployment, 90–180 days after deployment, 180–365 days after deployment, and 18–30 months after deployment [45]. Additional screenings are also conducted on entry into the VA health-care system and prior to separation from the military.

In conjunction with the post-deployment screening process, the US Army also implemented a primary care PTSD and depression screening process called Re-engineering Systems of Primary Care for PTSD and depression in the military known as (RESPECT-Mil) [46, 47]. As part of this process, which is now being adopted by Department of Defense widely, service members were routinely screened for depression and PTSD at each of their primary care patient encounters. If the service member screened positive, then they were assigned a nurse case manager who helped both to establish and maintain consultative communication between primary care and mental health services, and also monitor the service member compliance and health status. More recently, this process now includes the presence of a licensed behavioral health provider working directly in the primary care clinic to provide supportive counseling needs and assist in the care coordination. Those receiving treatment through these programs or receiving treatment in a traditional behavioral health setting are screened periodically to gauge progress (see *Basic Epidemiology and Important Limitations of all Screening Instruments* for more about the problems associated with using screening instruments as outcome measures) [46, 47].

Most recently, the Department of Defense has introduced the Behavioral Health Data Portal (BHDP). This automated system contains multiple screening protocols which service members complete when attending their mental health appointments. The advantage of this system is that it is integrated throughout the military allowing for both a historical record of symptom scores and potential severity monitoring and it provides a standardized mechanism for assessment throughout the large, widespread military healthcare network. Through BHDP, patients complete screening questionnaires at each visit, which are immediately scored and saved. Data acquired through widespread use of this program may enable development of better instruments capable of being validated for repeated administration/gauging of symptoms over time [48].

2.4 Screening Tools

2.4.1 Basic Epidemiology and Important Limitations of All Screening Instruments

Effective screening requires appreciation of the general strengths and weaknesses of all screening instruments. An ideal screening instrument is simple to administer and grade, detects most of the cases of interest in a particular population (sensitivity), and does not cause the individual administering the test to be overwhelmed with false positives (specificity). While sensitivity and specificity are important in how an instrument functions, the most important consideration in screening is the predictive value which is driven largely by the prevalence of the condition in a given population. In most clinical situations, a lower cutoff score ensures the ability to detect most cases; however, since the prevalence of PTSD is generally low (<15%), most positive screening results will be false positives which may lead to a high number of unnecessary evaluations or referrals that could drain clinical resources away from higher priority needs. Determination of cutoff should take into consideration the purpose of the screening test, the estimated prevalence of PTSD in the population being screened, the predictive value and balance of false negatives and false positives, and the available clinical resources (4).

Another principal of psychometric testing that bears explanation is the difference between using an instrument for screening and using an instrument as an outcome measure. Many of the instruments for PTSD have been validated for screening purposes only, but are used as outcome measures by the military and VA. While these instruments appear to assess/quantify symptoms of a given disorder (face validity), scores obtained through repeated administrations become less reliable than those obtained on first administration [5, 49]. Screening instruments are validated in given populations for the ability to detect a condition when it is present. Detection involves an absolute cutoff score and answers the question "is the condition present?" Quantifying symptoms is inherently more labor intensive, requires more questions in order to more finely parse out symptoms, and involves clearly defined, symptom-based severity scales to grade severity to answer the question "to what degree is a condition present?" Adding a Likert scale to a patient-rated screening instrument questions does not turn a screening instrument into an outcome measurement. This limitation is immediately apparent when an individual attempts to explain his/her symptom scores on an instrument such as the PTSD Checklist (PCL); inevitably, explanations for self-reported severity scores are inconsistent. Differences between rating a symptom as a 2 or a 3 are variable from person-to-person and in how an individual rates his or her symptoms at the time. One person's 2 for nightmares may signify nightmares every single night that he can now fall asleep after. Another's may be two nights a week which are impacted by severe nightmares which prevent further sleep that night.

Another important caveat for screening interpretation is that all screening instruments provide snapshots of a particular point in time and are easily overwhelmed by an individual's distress at the time of instrument administration. For example, an individual who has been deemed well-treated can appear to have significantly worsened if the instrument is administered right after his/her spouse asks for a divorce or the bank forecloses on his/her home. Symptoms are worse in the moment, but will return to baseline after the individual has come to terms with the stressor. This is clearly demonstrated in a study by Bodkin et al.; his group found that 78% of the non-traumatized respondents screened positive for PTSD on the structured clinical interview for DSM-IV (SCID) if they were asked to complete that section using "something they had been worrying about" [50]. Given that the SCID, one of our single best assessments for PTSD, was fooled so easily, every PTSD screen should be correlated with an individual's life circumstances before the score is accepted as valid. It also underscores that no single instrument is sufficient for making a diagnosis of PTSD on its own.

Lastly, recent studies highlight two key limitations of the current US military PTSD screening program. The first is that all of the large-scale screening programs are non-anonymous, self-report screening tools which rely on the individual service member to honestly report their symptoms. Warner et.al., showed that in a population undergoing immediate post-deployment screening, the majority of those who had mental health symptoms did not endorse those symptoms on the self-report screening. While this assessment has not been repeated in other time intervals, it does highlight the ongoing concern for the impact of stigma towards seeking mental health assistance [51]. Additionally, all of the current screening tools in place were developed based on the DSM-IV-TR criteria for PTSD, not the recent DSM-5 changes. A recent study by Hoge et.al., indicates that the change in criteria may not represent a clinical improvement compared to the DSM-IV criteria that has been largely unchanged for 25 years. [40] A new PCL version, based on DSM-5 (PCL-5) was recently developed, but is not in wide use.

2.4.2 Different PTSD Assessments

Gold Standard instruments for diagnosis and/or grading of PTSD symptoms include the SCID (diagnosis only), Clinician Administered PTSD Score (CAPS), Short PTSD Rating Interview (SPRINT), and PTSD Symptom Scale-Interview (PSS-I).

These assessments are based on standardized interviews and are impractical for large-scale screening, necessitating the use of self-report instruments.

Current US military deployment screening is conducted before and after deployment and consists of a combination of self-administered questions and a face-to-face evaluation by a primary care provider trained to administer these screenings [10, 14, 51]. Questions cover deployment location, general health, physical symptoms, mental health symptoms, and trauma exposure [10, 14]. The mental health section consists of questions related to PTSD, depression, suicidal ideation, aggression, and interest in receiving mental health care [10, 14]. Questions regarding depression and PTSD are drawn from instruments commonly used in primary care, including the Patient Health Questionnaire-2 (PHQ-2) for depression and the Primary Care PTSD screen (PC-PTSD). Following completion of screening, the service member is interviewed by a credentialed physician, nurse practitioner, or physician assistant to determine if referral is required [10, 14]. Mental health personnel are often present as well to provide emergency care if the service member endorses suicidal or homicidal ideation and to assist high risk individuals with obtaining follow up if needed [10, 14, 44].

The majority of military PTSD screening is done using the PC-PTSD. The PC-PTSD contains four questions related to the major PTSD symptom clusters of re-experiencing, avoidance, hyper-vigilance, and emotional numbing [52]. Following a positive screen with the PC-PTSD, the PCL is often administered. Three very similar versions of the PCL, based on DSM-IV criteria, have been used, the military version (PCL-M), the civilian version (PCL-C), and the specific stressor version (PCL-S). A new PCL version, based on DSM-5 (PCL-5) was recently validated, but is not in wide use. The PCL consists of 17 questions related to DSM-IV criteria for PTSD as well as a Likert scale to assess symptoms severity, ranging from 1 (not at all) to 5 (extremely) [52]. Specific score cutoffs vary depending on the purpose of the test and population being tested.

The PC-PTSD and the PCL have been validated for screening in civilian populations, the US soldiers, and veterans in the VA system seen in primary and behavioral health care [4, 49, 52–54].The PCL has also been widely used by military services from other countries. Alternate versions of the PCL have been validated for multiple civilian trauma types [55] and subpopulations such as geriatric primary care patients [56], Brazilian first responders [57], and Sri Lankan military [58]. As alluded to above, evidence suggests that self-report instruments such as the PC-PTSD and PCL may not be as accurate over time. Neither of these were validated for repeated administration.

In a 9-month study with serial administration of the PCL, Forbes et al. found significant variations in accuracy of the PCL in determining presence and severity of individual symptom at each time point. As symptoms improved and approached minimum PTSD symptom criteria, the PCL demonstrated reductions in diagnostic accuracy [49]. Forbes et al. concluded that the PCL underrated improvement when compared against the clinician administered PTSD scale (CAPS). Although Monson et al. found that the PCL remains sensitive to symptom change over time [59], the potential for diminished accuracy is concerning as the PC-PTSD and PCL are built into most all of the current US military PTSD screening programs including the Behavioral Health Data Platform and all of the primary care centered programs.

Another presumptive weakness of the PC-PTSD and PCL is the overlap of PTSD symptoms with other mental health conditions. Studies of a similar instrument, the Davidson Trauma Scale (DTS), found a drop in sensitivity of 30–40 % when comorbid depression or another anxiety disorder was present [5]. In populations with large prevalence of comorbid disorders (e.g., military and VA populations), the PCL-S appears more optimal due to being anchored to a single traumatic experience, [60] and the PCL-S has been widely used in prevalence studies in military populations [7, 30, 61]. The new PCL-5 is also anchored in the same way as the PCL-S.

Other PTSD screening instruments widely used outside of the US military include the DTS, PTSD Symptom Scale—Self-Report (PSS-SR), and Harvard Trauma Questionnaire (HTQ). The DTS is similar to the PCL-M/PCL-C. Both share a 17-item structure tied to DSM-IV criteria with a 5-point Likert severity scale, demonstrate similar sensitivities and specificities, have been validated for use in US military and veteran populations, and are presumably equally nonspecific in differentiating between comorbid axis I disorders as the PCL [5, 62]. Like the PCL-S, the DTS is anchored to a single trauma [5]. It is widely used in PTSD medication research and appears in a few psychotherapy studies as well. The DTS was found to be sensitive to changes in selective serotonin reuptake inhibitor (SSRI) trials by its creator, Dr. Jonathan Davidson, when he analyzed his own medication trials [63]. However, due to the similarities with the PCL, the DTS likely demonstrates comparable performance overall.

The PSS-SR is a third 17-item questionnaire closely tied to DSM criteria with a 3-point Likert scale accompanying each symptom [64]. It is not widely used in the American or European studies and is not validated in the US military or veterans based on our literature search. The HTQ is a narrative-based assessment tool applied to an open-ended conversation. In a recent study of Iraq refugees, it took roughly 1 h to administer as well as time spent translating recorded responses [65]. Given its length and difficulty in administration, it is not widely used in research or clinical practice and is not validated for use in the US military or veterans.

2.4.3 Recommended CutOff Scores

Use of the PC-PTSD is fairly straightforward given its short length. It is generally agreed that a score of 2 or greater demonstrates sufficient sensitivity and specificity to be considered positive, though three or greater is sometimes used when greater specificity is sought [53]. This is a general screening tool and high rates of false positives are found when this tool is used for general population screening [4].

As referenced in our epidemiologic discussion, no single PCL cutoff is adequate for all purposes [4]. For research studies of PTSD prevalence in most general populations (where prevalence is expected to < 15 %), higher specificity cutoffs (e.g., 48 or higher), are necessary to ensure that estimates are not grossly inflated; for screening in a clinical setting where every individual will be receiving a clinical evaluation, a lower cutoff (33 -44) is preferred to reduce the number of false negatives [4]. This recommendation is contrary to guidelines from the National Center for PTSD which recommend the highest PCL cutoff scores be reserved for settings where prevalence is highest (e.g., >40 % prevalence in a VA mental health clinic). Terhakopian et al. provides an excellent illustration of the need for calibration in cutoff scores depending on the expected prevalence and clinical setting. In a population of returning veterans with a PTSD prevalence of 15 %, for example, a PCL cutoff of 30, which has been validated for use in clinical settings and estimated to have a sensitivity of 0.85 and specificity of 0.73, produces a prevalence estimate of 36 % (and a corresponding percent of the population needing clinical evaluation). This is more than double the actual prevalence, due to high numbers of false positives and low predictive value, [4] and can also potentially overwhelm mental health resources conducting clinical evaluations. If the cutoff is increased to 50, sensitivity decreases to 0.54 and specificity increases to 0.93 [4]. This results in nearly half of individuals with PTSD (46 %) being missed, but produces a prevalence estimate that is much more accurate (14 %). For the purpose of screening, clinical setting and clinical resources must be taken into consideration in when selecting appropriate cutoffs. Epidemiological studies of prevalence must utilize higher cutoffs, while screening in clinical settings must take into consideration an appropriate balance of identifying as high a number of individuals who have the disorder as possible while also not overwhelming clinic resources and the capacity to evaluate those who screen positive. One concern is that test performance may not be as reliable in the presence of comorbid conditions, and PCL results should be interpreted with caution in individuals with depression or other anxiety disorders. In terms of other instruments, the DTS appears to have no clear advantage over the PCL, though DTS validation studies are difficult to interpret because of subgroup analyses that limit accurate comparisons with PCL studies [5].

2.5 Future of PTSD Screening

The largest limitations of current screening programs is reliance on self-report data, which is impacted by concerns of a lack of anonymity due to stigma and appears to diminish in accuracy over time and as individuals improve [5, 49]. Use of standardized interview-based assessments such as the Clinician Administered PTSD Scale (CAPS), the Short PTSD Rating Interview (SPRINT), or the PTSD Symptom Scale—Interview (PSS-I) is impractical due to the time and special training required to administer each. To address this, a current research focus is the identification of potential biomarkers for PTSD, particularly early in its clinical course when it is most responsive to treatment [66–68]. Though still in its infancy, several potential markers such as p11 in peripheral blood cells and glucocorticoid receptor numbers have demonstrated potential utility in differentiating PTSD from other psychiatric conditions in humans, but not to the degree that they can be relied on clinically [67, 68]. Cortisol and inflammatory markers are also being studied, though their role in PTSD is very complex and variable [69, 70]. Should a viable biomarker for PTSD be identified, it would likely change the military's screening policies dramatically.

References

1. DoD. Deployment Health Policies. 2015 http://www.health.mil/Policies?&query=deployment. Accessed 25 Aug. 2015.
2. Kline A, Falca-Dodson M, Sussner B, Ciccone D, Chandler H, Callahan L, et al. Effects of repeated deployment to Iraq and Afghanistan on the health of New Jersey Army National Guard troops: implications for military readiness. AM J Public Health. 2010;100(2):276–83.
3. Baiocchi D. Measuring army deployments to Iraq and Afghanistan. Santa Monica: RAND corporation; 2013.
4. Terhakopian A, Sinaii N, Engel C, Schnurr P, Hoge C. Estimating population prevalence of posttraumatic stress disorder: an example using the PTSD checklist. J Trauma Stress. 2008;21(3):290–300.
5. McDonald S, Beckham J, Morey R, Calhoun P. The validity and diagnostic efficiency of the Davidson Trauma Scale in military veterans who have served since September 11th, 2001. J Anxiety Disord. 2009;23:247–55.
6. Martenyi F, Brown E, Zhang H, Koke S, Prakash A. Fluoxetine v. placebo in prevention of relapse in Posttraumatic stress disorder. Br J Psychiatry. 2002;181:315–20.
7. Kok B, Herrell R, Thomas J, Hoge C. Posttraumatic stress disorder associated with combat service in Iraq or Afghanistan: reconciling prevalence differences between studies. J Nerv Ment Dis. 2012;200(5):440–50.
8. Hotopf M, Hull L, Fear N, Browne T, Horn O, Iversen A, et al. The health of UK military personnel who deployed to the 2003 Iraq war: a cohort study. Lancet. 2006;367(9524):1731–41.
9. Lapierre C, Schwegler A, LaBauve B. Posttraumatic stress and depression symptoms in soldiers returning from combat operations in Iraq and Afghanistan. J Traum Stress. 2007;20(6):933–43.
10. Hoge C, Auchterlonie J, Milliken C. Mental health problems, use of mental health services, and attrition from military service after returning from deployment to Iraq or Afghanistan. JAMA. 2006;295:1023–32.
11. Vasterling J, Proctor S, Amoroso P, Kane R, Heeren T, White R. Neuropsychological outcomes of army personnel following deployment to the Iraq war. JAMA. 2006;296(5):519–29.
12. Tanielian T, Jaycox LH. Invisible wounds of war. Santa Monica: RAND Corporation; 2008.
13. US Army Medical Department. Mental Health Advisory Team (MHAT-V). Operation Iraqi Freedom06-08. 2008. http://armymedicine.mil/Pages/Mental-Health-Advisory-Team-V-Information-.aspx. Accessed 27 Aug 2015.
14. Miliken C, Auchterlonie J, Hoge C. Longitudinal assessment of mental health problems among active and reserve component soldiers returning from the Iraq war. JAMA. 2007;298(18):2141–8.
15. Santiago P, Ursano R, Gray C, Pynoos R, Spiegel D. A systemic review of PTSD prevalence and trajectories in DSM-5 defined trauma exposed populations: intentional and non-intentional traumatic events. PLoS ONE. 2013;8(4):e59236.
16. Brady K, Pearlstein T, Asnis G, Baker D, Rothbaum B, et al. Efficacy and safety of sertraline treatment of posttraumatic stress disorder. JAMA. 2000;283(14):1837–44.
17. Davidson J, Baldwin D, Stein D, Kuper E, Benattia I. Treatment of posttraumatic stress disorder with venlafaxine extended release: a 6-month randomized controlled trial. Arch Gen Psychiatry. 2006;63:1158–65.
18. Davidson J, Pearlstein T, Londborg P, Brady K, Rothbaum B, et al. Efficacy of sertraline in preventing relapse of posttraumatic stress disorder: results of a 28-week double-blind, placebo-controlled study. Am J Psychiatry. 2001;158:1974–81.
19. Davidson J, Rothbaum B, van der Kolk B, Sikes C, Farfel G. Multicenter, double-blind comparison of sertraline and placebo in the treatment of posttraumatic stress disorder. Arch Gen Psychiatry. 2001;58:485–92.

20. GlaxoSmithKline. A study of the maintained efficacy and safety of paroxetine versus placebo in the long-term treatment of posttraumatic stress disorder. Unpublished. 2001. http://www.gsk-clinicalstudyregister.com/study/29060/650#rs. Accessed 27 Aug 2015.
21. Martenyi F, Brown E, Zhang H, Prakash A, Koke S. Fluoxetine versus placebo in posttraumatic stress disorder. J Clin Psychiatry. 2002;63(3):199–206.
22. Martenyi F, Soldatenkova V. Fluoxetine in the acute treatment and relapse prevention of combat-related Posttraumatic stress disorder: analysis of the veteran group of a placebo-controlled, randomized clinical trial. Eur Neuropsychopharmacol. 2006;16:340–9.
23. Raskin M, Peskind E, Kanter E, Petrie E, Radant A. Reduction of nightmares and other PTSD symptoms in combat veterans by prazosin: a placebo-controlled study. Am J Psychiatry. 2003;160:371–3.
24. Raskin M, Peterson K, Williams T, Hoff D, Hart K. A Trial of prazosin for combat trauma PTSD with nightmares in active-duty soldiers returned from Iraq and Afghanistan. Am J Psychiatry. 2013;170:1003–10.
25. Schneier F, Neria Y, Pavlicova M, Hembree E, Jung Suh E, et al. Combined prolonged exposure therapy and paroxetine for PTSD related to the world trade center attack: a randomized controlled trial. Am J Psychiatry. 2012;169:80–8.
26. Shalev A, Freedman S, Peri T, Brandes D, Sahar T, Orr S. Prospective study of posttraumatic stress disorder and depression following trauma. Am J Psychiatry. 1998;155:630–7.
27. Shih R, Schell T, Hambarsoomian K, Marshall G, Belzberg H. Prevalence of PTSD and major depression following trauma-center hospitalization. J Trauma. 2010;69(6):1560–6.
28. van der Kolk B, Spinazzola J, Blaustein M, Hopper J, Hopper E, et al. A randomized clinical trial of eye movement desensitization and reprocessing (EMDR), fluoxetine, and pill placebo in the treatment of posttraumatic stress disorder: treatment effects and long-term maintenance. J Clin Psychiatry. 2007;68:37–46.
29. Goldberg M. Costs of military pay and benefits in the defense budget: Congressional Budget Office. 2012. https://www.cbo.gov/publication/43574. Accessed 26 Aug 2015.
30. Hoge C, Castro C, Messer S, McGurk D, Cotting D. Combat duty in Iraq and Afghanistan, mental health problems, and barriers to care. N Engl J. 2004;351:13–22.
31. Tanielian T, Jaycox L. Invisible wounds of war: Psychological and cognitive injuries, their consequences, and services to assist recovery. Santa Monica: RAND Corporation; 2008.
32. Hoge C, Castro C, Messer S, McGurk D, Cotting D, Koffman R. Combat duty in Iraq and Afghanistan, mental health problems, and barriers to care. N Engl J. 2004;351:13–22.
33. US Congress. National Defense Authorization Act (NDAA), F.Y. 2008, H.R. 1585, Section 1710. http://www.gpo.gov/fdsys/pkg/CRPT-110hrpt477/pdf/CRPT-110hrpt477.pdf. Accessed 28 Aug 2015.
34. Kang H. Analysis of VA health care utilization among US global war on terrorism veterans: operation Iraqi freedom and operation enduring freedom. Washington, DC: VHA Office of Public Health and Environmental Hazards; 2008.
35. Seal K, Maguen S, Cohen B, Gima K, Metzeler T, Ren L, et al. VA mental health services utilization in Iraq and Afganistan veterans in the first year of receiving new mental health diagnoses. J Traum Stress. 2010;23(1):5–16.
36. Friedman M, Marmar C, Baker D, Sikes C, Farfel G. Randomized, double-blind comparison of sertraline and placebo for posttraumatic stress disorder in a Department of Veterans Affairs setting. J Clin Psychiatry. 2007;68(5):711–20.
37. Hyams KC, Riddle J, Trump DH, Wallace MR. Protecting the health of United States military forces in Afghanistan: applying lessons learned since the Gulf War. Clin Infect Disease 2002;34(Suppl 5):S208–14.
38. Department of Defense. Post Deployment Health Assessment, DD Form 2796. May 1999. http://www.gulflink.osd.mil/medical/storyboard/dd2796.pdf. Accessed 25 Aug 2015.
39. Wright KM, Huffman AH, Adler AB, Castro CA. Psychological screening program overview. Mil Med. 2002;167:853–61.
40. Wright KM, Thomas JL, Adler AB, Ness JW, Hoge CW, Castro CA. Psychological screening procedures for deploying US forces. Mil Med 2005;170(7):555–62.

41. US Congress. Ronald W. Reagan National Defense Authorization Act (NDAA), F.Y. 2005, H.R. 4200, Section 723. http://www.gpo.gov/fdsys/pkg/PLAW-108publ375/html/PLAW-108publ375.htm. Accessed 25 Aug 2015.
42. Warner CH, Appenzeller GN, Mullen K, Warner CM, Grieger TS. Soldier attitudes towards mental health and seeking care upon return from combat. Mil Med 2008;173:563–69.
43. Warner CH, Breitbach J, Appenzeller GN, Yates VD, Grieger TS, Webster W. Division mental health: its role in the new Brigade Combat Team structure part II: re-deployment and post-deployment. Mil Med 2007;172:912–17.
44. Warner C, Appenzeller G, Parker J, Warner C, Hoge C. Effectiveness of mental health screening and coordination of in-theater care prior to deployment to Iraq: a cohort study. Am J Psychiatry. 2011;168:378–85.
45. US Congress. National Defense Authorization Act (NDAA), F.Y. 2012, H.R. 4310, Sections 582 & 1212. https://www.govtrack.us/congress/bills/112/hr4310/text. Accessed 25 Aug 2015.
46. Engel C, Oxman T, Yamamato C, Gould D, Barry S, et al. RESPECT-Mil: feasibility of a systems-level coliaborative care approach to depression and Posttraumatic stress disorder in military primary care. Milit Med. 2008;173(10):935–40.
47. Engel C, Oxman T, Yamamato C, Gould D, Barry S, et al. RESPECT-Mil: feasibility of a systems-level coliaborative care approach to depression and Posttraumatic stress disorder in military primary care. Mil Med. 2008;173(10):935–40.
48. http://digitalcommons.ohsu.edu/etd/929/
49. Forbes D, Creamer M, Biddle D. The validity of the PTSD checklist as a measure of symptomatic change in combat-related PTSD. Behav Res Ther. 2001;39:977–86.
50. Bodkin J. Is PTSD caused by traumatic stress? J Anxiety Disord. 2007;21:176–82.
51. Warner C, Appenzeller G, Grieger T, Belenkiy S, Breitbach J, et al. Importance of anonymity to encourage honest reporting in mental health screening after combat deployment. Arch Gen Psychiatry. 2011;68(10):1065–71.
52. Bliese P, Wrigh K, Adler A, Castro C, Hoge C, et al. Validating the primary care posttraumatic stress disorder screen and the posttraumatic stress disorder checklist with soldiers returning from combat. J Consult Clin Psychol. 2008;76(2):272–81.
53. Prins A, Ouimette P, Kimerling R, Cameron R, Hugelshofer D. The primary care PTSD screen (PC-PTSD): development and operating characteristics. Prim Care Psychiatry. 2004;9:9–14.
54. Dobie D, Kivlahan D, Maynard C, Bush K, McFall M. Screening for Posttraumatic stress disorder in female Veteran's Affairs patients: validation of the PTSD checklist. Gen Hosp Psychiatry. 2002;24:367–74.
55. Blanchard E, Jones-Alexander J, Buckley T, Forneris C. Psychometric properties of the PTSD checklist (PCL). Behav Res Ther. 1996;34(8):669–73.
56. Cook J, Elhai J, Arean P. Psychometric properties of the PTSD checklist with older primary care patients. J Traum Stress. 2005;18(4):371–6.
57. Passos R, Figueira I, Mendlowicz M, Moraes C, Coutinho E. Exploratory factor analysis of the Brazilian version of the Posttraumatic Stress Disorder Checklist—Civilian Version (PCL-C). Rev Bras Psiquiatr. 2012;34:155–61.
58. Semage S, Sivayogan S, Forbes D, O'Donnell M, Monaragala R, et al. Cross-cultural and factorial validity of PTSD check list—military version (PCL-M) in Sinhalese language. Eur J Psychotraumatol. 2013;4:19707.
59. Monson C, Gradus J, Young-Xu Y, Schnurr P, Price J. Change in posttraumatic stress disorder symptoms: do clinicians and patients agree? Psychol Assess. 2008;20(2):131–8.
60. Wilkins K, Lang A, Norman S. Synthesis of the psychometric properties of the PTSD checklist (PCL) military, civilian, and specific versions. Depress Anxiety. 2011;28:596–606.
61. Thomas J, Wilk J, Riviere L, McGurk D, Castro C. Prevalence of mental health problems and functional impairment among active component and National Guard soldiers 3 and 12 months following combat in Iraq. Arch Gen Psychiatry. 2010;67(6):614–23.
62. McDonald S, Thompson N, Stratton K, Calhoun P, MIRECC W. Diagnostic accuracy of three scoring methods for the davidson trauma scale among U.S. military Veterans. J Anxiety Disord. 2014;28(2):160–8.

63. Davidson J, Tharwani H, Connor K. Davidson Trauma Scale (DTS): normative scores in the general population and effect sizes in placebo-controlled SSRI trials. Depress Anxiety. 2002;15(2):75–8.
64. Foa E, Cashman L, Jaycox L, Perry K. The validation of a self-report measure of posttraumatic stress disorder: the posttraumatic diagnostic scale. Psychol Assess. 1997;9(4):445–51.
65. Shoeb M, Weinstein H, Mollica R. The Harvard trauma questionnaire: adapting a cross-cultural instrument for measuring torture, trauma, and posttraumatic stress disorder in Iraqi refugees. Int J Soc Psychiatry. 2007;53:447–63.
66. Zhang L, Li H, Benedek D, Li X, Ursano R. A strategy for the development of biomarker tests for PTSD. Med Hypotheses. 2009;73(3):404–9.
67. Su T, Zhang L, Chung M, Chen Y, Bi Y, Chou Y. Levels of the potential biomarker p11 in peripheral blood cells distinguish patients with PTSD from those with other major psychiatric disorders. J Psychiatric Res. 2009;43(13):1078–85.
68. van Zuiden M, Geuze E, Willemen H, Vermetten E, Maas M, Heijnen C, et al. Pre-existing high glucocorticoid receptor number predicting development of posttraumatic stress symptoms after military deployment. Am J Psychiatry. 2011;168(89–96):89.
69. von Känel R, Begré S, Abbas C, Saner H, Gander M, Schmid J. Inflammatory biomarkers in patients with posttraumatic stress disorder caused by myocardial infarction and the role of depressive symptoms. Neuroimmunomodulation. 2009;17(1):39–46.
70. Heim C, Ehlert U, Hellhammer D. The potential role of hypocortisolism in the pathophysiology of stress-related bodily disorders. Psychoneuroendocrinology. 2000;25(1):35.

3 Therapeutic Alliance in the Treatment of Combat PTSD

James C. West

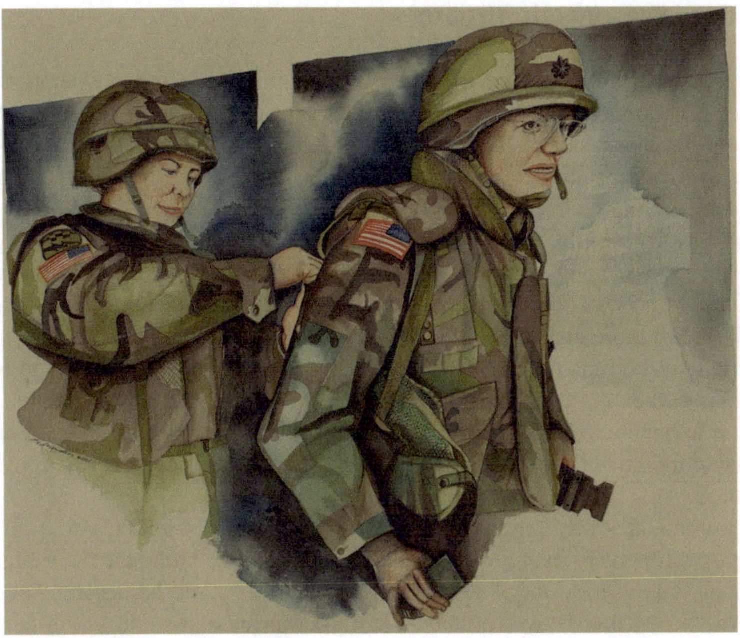

Buddy Assist, by Msg. Henrietta Snowden, courtesy of the Army Art Collection, US Army Center of Military History.

J. C. West (✉)
Department of Psychiatry, Uniformed Services University of the Health Sciences,
4301 Jones Bridge Rd., Bethesda, MD 20814, USA
e-mail: james.west@usuhs.edu

E. C. Ritchie (ed.), *Posttraumatic Stress Disorder and Related Diseases in Combat Veterans*, DOI 10.1007/978-3-319-22985-0_3

A common challenge in the treatment of veterans with combat trauma is getting them to engage in therapy. Whether due to the profound avoidance inherent in post-traumatic stress disorder (PTSD), distrust of authority, or overwhelming shame associated with either the trauma or resulting distress and impairment, veterans with psychological trauma have difficulty getting into and staying in treatment for PTSD. Studies examining the most effective treatments for PTSD identify dropout rates as high as 40% [1]. This leaves us to consider what can be done to improve retention and enable patients to recover from their trauma.

Therapeutic alliance may be just one such key to recovery. The following case illustrates the importance of therapeutic alliance in the care of a combat veteran. It can be a powerful tool in overcoming trauma, in this case the specific trauma of perpetration in combat.

3.1 Case Presentation/History

JP was a 23-year-old infantryman assigned as a military advisor in Operation Iraqi Freedom. He was deployed to Anbar Province during a time of high operational tempo for the Marines, and JP's small unit of advisors was no exception. Assigned to an Iraqi Army battalion, he and his fellow Marines were responsible for training and accompanying them on combat missions. He came to Operational Stress Control and Readiness (OSCAR) psychiatry voluntarily at the recommendation of his leadership for assistance with irritability and anger outbursts while on deployment.

JP thought he was doing fine, but not so well in the last 2 months since he deployed. He felt more distressed and edgy while performing combat patrols. He also started having nightmares related to his previous deployment to the same region 18 months earlier. As a result, he did not sleep very well. He also related his sleep problems to having to sleep alongside his Iraqi counterparts. While he knew he was assigned to train and support them, he had trouble trusting them and was constantly vigilant.

His commander was concerned because JP had recently gotten into a physical altercation with one of his fellow Marines. In the fight, JP broke the other Marine's collarbone, taking him out of operations for 3 weeks while he healed. The commander reported that JP was otherwise a good Marine and stood out in neither a positive nor negative light during the pre-deployment workup. He was not one he expected to be a disciplinary problem, and the commander seemed genuinely concerned that something was wrong.

During the initial interview, JP related a distressing incident from his first deployment. While on patrol in a convoy of Humvees, his squad came across a crowd of people gathered outside a mosque. The convoy had to stop because the crowd partially blocked the road. The vehicles stopped, and the crowd gathered around JP's vehicle. There was a lot of yelling and finger pointing as was typical when Americans were around. Since no one in the crowd appeared armed, the Marines tried to disperse the crowd peacefully. As they were getting out of their vehicles, a grenade rolled out of the crowd next to JP's Humvee, literally at his feet. He jumped back into the Humvee immediately and closed the door just as the grenade went off. The detonation did not significantly damage the vehicle or injure anyone.

JP exited the vehicle to see the crowd rapidly dispersing. He recalled seeing a young man staring him down in the crowd, and thought that this was the person who rolled the grenade.

JP's squad leader ordered the Marines to find and detain the person who dropped the grenade. JP saw the suspicious young man run down a side street and decided to pursue. He said it was hard to remember the specifics now, but he remembers several vivid moments he will never forget. He pursued for less than a minute and then realized he was separated from his squad. Realizing he did not have support and feeling vulnerable, he slowed. It was just then he saw the runner about to disappear. Without thought he raised his rifle to his shoulder, sighted in on the young man, and quickly fired several shots, dropping the fleeing individual to the ground. He remembers he did not take time to yell "stop" or "qef." He remembers seeing his shot hit the young man's head and blood and brains flying out.

The next thing he remembers is his squad catching up and walking up to identify the person. When he rolled over the body, he vividly recalls seeing the distorted face of an adolescent boy, somewhere between 12 and 16 years old. He recalls intense feelings of guilt and questioning whether he had done the right thing.

A distraught woman approached and began to cry over the body. He assumed she was the boy's mother. At that point the squad leader instructed the Marines to leave, and JP did not know what happened to the boy after that. He said this was the first time he had told anyone what happened, and he did not talk about it even with fellow Marines. The investigation found that he was justified in shooting, but he never felt as if it was.

He started having nightmares within days of the event. They continued on and off until about 2 months back home. He never sought any psychiatric treatment, and the nightmares resolved spontaneously. After that he did not think he had a problem. He did not have problems at home between deployments, and thought he would be fine on this one. The nightmares resumed within 2 weeks of returning to his old area of operations. He said he was operating in the same neighborhoods where the events had happened 2 years before. Whenever he went past that mosque he felt particularly uneasy, and did his best to choke it down and not tell anyone.

His nightmares were a vivid replay of running down the side street, feeling alone and vulnerable, shooting and seeing the boy's face, and the reaction of the woman. He would wake up with his heart pounding and feeling "amped up." He would go outside and smoke a cigarette and try to settle himself, but that usually took an hour or so to get back to sleep. He said he was worried that some of the Iraqis he worked with were giving information to insurgents and also worried that one of them might attack him or others on his team if they ever had an opportunity. He denied any dissociative episodes, and said he did not feel like he had problems getting distracted or confused, no matter how "amped up" he felt.

He felt intense guilt, still questioning himself whether he was justified in killing the boy. He viewed his actions as "messed up" and the entire mission that led to him shooting as "messed up" as well. These feelings spilled over into questions about his current mission. There was no way his actions could have a positive impact on the future of the country, so why was he putting himself in danger? He felt more and more disconnected from the rest of his team. They all seemed motivated, but they did not understand. Even though he felt this way most of the time, he acknowledged he still had a job to do whether he believed in it or not.

Further, psychiatric review of systems revealed that JP denied depressed mood, and he maintained his normal range of activities and interests prior to deployment. He drank alcohol on weekends with his peers, anywhere from two to ten beers on an occasion depending on whether he intended to get drunk or not. He denied any difficulty at work or in relationships as a result of his drinking. He smoked a pack of cigarettes every 3 days while at home, and that increased to one pack per day while deployed. He was not using any supplements and did not use caffeine. He never had any past episode consistent with mania, and he denied any psychotic symptoms now or in the past.

Describing the fight that got his commander's attention, JP said the other Marine was someone he never liked and he hated having to patrol with him. He thought the other Marine was overconfident, careless, and made the rest of the team vulnerable. JP got along fine with the other Marines in the unit, but generally kept to himself.

When asked about his reasons for becoming a Marine, he said he was in high school during 9/11, and from that day knew he wanted to serve. He chose the Marine Corps because he wanted to be part of a special group, and the Marines had that appeal for him. He was generally happy with his service to date, but was not sure if he would reenlist or not.

3.2 Diagnosis/Assessment

JP met criteria for PTSD with delayed expression. His trauma in this case was complex in that he was the person who did the killing. The resurgence of combat nightmares upon encountering the reminder of the same operating area fulfills the reexperiencing criterion. He avoided recalling or discussing his trauma, evidenced by not disclosing it for almost 2 years. His negative alterations in cognition and mood included distorted negative thoughts about himself and his exaggerated guilt, inability to recall details of that event, and his increasingly distorted and negative views about his current role. His disrupted sleep, irritability, and hypervigilance were all symptoms of increased arousal.

3.3 Treatment/Management

JP did not initially relate his current difficulty to his combat trauma. He came in looking for someone to vent to about his frustration over his current circumstances. He figured if he could "blow off some steam" he could get through the deployment, go home, and just forget about it. He was initially resistant to talking about his past combat experience. Initial approach required asking and allowing the patient to tell his story and allowing him to complete the narrative without commenting.

As the provider, I recall specifically using the words, "Tell me about the worst thing that happened to you on deployment, the thing that you least want to talk about with anyone." My intent was to allow him to open his suppressed narrative. He demonstrated significant physiologic arousal while telling the story. We engaged in a session of relaxation breathing, through which he was able to lower his physiologic arousal to a manageable level.

This relaxation served multiple purposes. First, it brought him down to a more tolerable state of arousal. On a therapeutic alliance level, it established my identity as someone who could guide him through a difficult story and offer him a means to contain the affect it generated. He returned for three further sessions over the next 2 weeks. Though this may seem like a very short course of treatment, it was limited by his need to remain connected to his unit, which continued daily patrols. In each session he repeated the narrative of the shooting, we discussed his perceptions of what happened, and he engaged in relaxation breathing before departing. After the fourth session, he indicated he felt better, was not having nightmares, and wanted to get on with his job.

3.4 Discussion

This case illustrates the importance of therapeutic alliance with the combat trauma patient. JP experienced unanticipated symptoms in an environment where he felt not only reminded of past acts but also exposed and vulnerable himself. His intense shame and guilt made establishment of a therapeutic alliance essential to successful treatment. This same shame and guilt also made him resistant to seeking treatment or acknowledging his problems.

A word that comes to mind in work with psychological trauma is *Paraclete*. It derives from the ancient Greek *parakletos*, which translates as advocate or intercessor [2]. It is a word frequently encountered in Christian writings as a description of the Holy Spirit. Within its Greek roots are the words "one called to the side." This is a helpful interpretation of the role of the therapist in early trauma work. A patient presents ambivalence about intentionally reexperiencing their trauma, often carrying intense shame or guilt. The therapist who begins by simply walking alongside the traumatized individual sets the stage for effective therapeutic alliance. This is a very passive and nonjudgmental approach, one of allowing the patient to relate and share affective states they normally avoid. The therapist as Paraclete walks with them and provides needed support initially.

Robert Stolorow describes trauma as the experience of unbearable affect associated with a poorly attuned response by those who would care for the traumatized individual [3]. The individual who experiences psychological trauma perceives themself as somehow detached from the world of others around them. Their shattering emotional experience leaves them unable to be understood by or relate to those around them. It was clear from the outset that JP experienced such detachment.

He viewed his act as one of unjustified killing. He was removed from the situation before achieving any closure or observing evidence that might have challenged his assumption that he killed a noncombatant. He continued to feel separate from those around him, even Marines with whom he had been in combat. There was no way for him to perceive others as capable of understanding what it was like to have his experience. Thus he reinforced his separateness and managed to suppress all thought of the shooting. This technique was effective until confronted with reminders of the trauma, at which point he became symptomatic. His response to increase symptoms was to further reinforce his separateness by being detached from his peers and finding fault with his unit and mission.

Ronnie Janoff-Bulman identifies three core assumptions that we carry prior to any traumatic exposure. These are: (i) the world is benevolent, (ii) the world is meaningful, and (iii) the self is worthy [4]. JP's experience effectively negated a benevolent world and challenged his view of a worthy self. Through his killing, he himself became the eliminator of benevolence in his world. Further, those whose orders put him in the ambiguous situation in which he chose to shoot and kill also presented a challenge to his assumption of a benevolent world.

This loss presents a challenge to the prospective therapist, particularly those in uniform or those that work for the government. Many veterans with psychological trauma tend to perceive authority figures, and therefore therapists with significant distrust. Authority figures put soldiers into the situations that traumatize them. As such the therapist may be subject to a negative transference with the expectation that we would be incompetent, uncaring, or unattuned to the needs of the patient. In this instance, efforts at developing alliance must focus on maintaining a nonjudgmental stance and empathic listening. We must also promptly demonstrate our capability to receive the patient in their intense affective state and demonstrate ways of managing such intense affects. Doing so is the first step in restoring previously destroyed assumptions about self and the world.

The uniformed provider in the deployed setting enjoys both advantages and handicaps in forging alliance with traumatized patients. On the one hand, sharing adversity alongside the individual seeking care promotes alliance. Many patients find it easy to relate to someone who they perceive as having an understanding of their experiences, even if not directly shared. On the other hand, deployed providers run the risk of patients perceiving them as out of touch with their traumatic experience, that they are either too attached to the comforts of large forward bases or too closely aligned with leadership.

Particularly relevant to JP's case is the presence of *moral injury*. Litz defines morally injurious experiences as, "Perpetrating, failing to prevent, bearing witness to, or learning about acts that transgress deeply held moral beliefs and expectations [5]." Such experiences generate enormous dissonance and conflict in affected individuals. This dissonance and conflict interacts with personal characteristics such as self-judging and difficulty managing internal conflicts leaving the individual in intense and unresolvable shame. This shame promotes withdrawal from attachments, and individuals continue to blame themselves or others they consider responsible for placing them in the morally ambiguous situation. Litz identifies development of a connection, a therapeutic alliance, as the first and most important step in attempting to treat morally injured individuals. It was clear that JP's anticipated response to disclosing his traumatic experience to the therapist was that he would be rejected or further shamed. He also feared that he might somehow be reported or disciplined as a result of disclosing his actions. Both of these would have reinforced his self-appraisal of intolerable shame. Therefore, the most constructive therapeutic stance in this case was one of nonjudgmental listening and reassurance of the privilege of the doctor–patient relationship. This created a safe space in which he could tell his story without fear of judgment or reprisal, and to experience the intense affects and begin the corrective experience.

There is evidence that suggests therapeutic alliance is a core component of effective therapy for trauma. In a study of therapist effects on evidence-based treatments for PTSD, Laska et al. identified therapeutic alliance as one of four significant effects [6]. They observed that a therapist's ability to meet the patient where they were exerted a significant positive effect on the outcome. Genuineness was a key trait related to alliance. What they hypothesized about genuineness was that it overcame a tendency on the part of traumatized veterans to be skeptical or resistant to authority figures based on past experience with "less-than-benign" authority while serving. Smith suggests that attending to the relationship in exposure-based therapies with individuals with perpetration trauma is an essential component of therapy [7].

Adaptive disclosure therapy has emerged in recent years as an effort to address the resistance to other evidence-based treatments [8, 9]. Adaptive disclosure entails three parts: reexperiencing, addressing traumatic loss, and addressing moral injury. It is a manualized six-session intervention tailored to fit the time limitations of young, employed, and active patients. The goal is to allow individuals to consider alternative interpretations of their traumatic experiences while also learning to manage intense affective states generated by those memories. Again, the value of therapeutic alliance with the nonjudgmental listener is core to the process.

3.5 Clinical Pearl

The therapist who begins the therapy by simply "walking alongside" the traumatized individual sets the stage for an effective therapeutic alliance, which has a significant positive effect on the outcome.

3.6 Outcomes/Resolution

JP completed four individual sessions of psychotherapy. In the first session, he fully disclosed his actions and feelings of shame and guilt over killing a noncombatant. He was unable to see any ambiguity in the circumstances, even though at the end of treatment his nightmares had resolved, and he expressed less anger toward his fellow Marines. In particular, he was able to tolerate the one that irritated him the most. He reported less guilt over his previous actions. He continued to express suspicion toward Iraqi soldiers, but this was not a focus of therapy. He continued to serve in his assigned role and completed the remaining 4 months of his deployment. He remained uncertain about whether or not he would reenlist.

This case demonstrates the importance of building, promoting, and maintaining therapeutic alliance in the treatment of veterans with combat trauma. Doing so requires recognition of the trauma patient's need to have another "walk alongside," their overwhelming sense of separation from others. This is particularly true when the patient's fundamental assumptions of safety and good in the world are shattered or when they struggle with moral injury. Therapeutic alliance is the foundation upon which successful therapy is built.

References

1. Jeffreys MD, Reinfeld C, Nair PV, Garcia HA, Mata-Galan E, Rentz TO. Evaluating treatment of posttraumatic stress disorder with cognitive processing therapy and prolonged exposure therapy in a VHA specialty clinic. J Anxiety Disord. 2014;28(1):108–14.
2. Merriam-Webster's Collegiate Dictionary. 10th ed. Springfield: Merriam-Webster Incorporated; 1993.
3. Stolorow R. Trauma and human existence: autobigraphical, psychoanalytic, and philosophical reflections. New York: Taylor & Francis Group; 2007.
4. Janoff-Bulman R. Shattered assumptions: towards a new psychology of trauma. New York: The Free Press; 1992.
5. Litz BT, Stein N, Delaney E, Lebowitz L, Nash WP, Silva C, et al. Moral injury and moral repair in war veterans: a preliminary model and intervention strategy. Clin Psychol Rev. 2009;29(8):695–706.
6. Laska K, Smith T, Wislocki A, Minami T, Wampold B. Uniformity of evidence-based treatments in practice? Therapist effects in the delivery of cognitive processing therapy for PTSD. J Couns Psychol. 2013;60(1):31–41.
7. Smith ER, Duax JM, Rauch SAM. Perceived perpetration during traumatic events: clinical suggestions from experts in prolonged exposure therapy. Cogn Behav Pract. 2013;20(4):461–70.
8. Steenkamp MM, Litz BT, Gray MJ, Lebowitz L, Nash W, Conoscenti L, et al. A brief exposure-based intervention for service members with PTSD. Cogn Behav Pract. 2011;18(1):98–107.
9. Gray MJ, Schorr Y, Nash W, Lebowitz L, Amidon A, Lansing A, et al. Adaptive disclosure: an open trial of a novel exposure-based intervention for service members with combat-related psychological stress injuries. Behav Ther. 2012;43(2):407–15.

Shame and Moral Injury in an Operation Iraqi Freedom Combat Veteran

4

Jonathan R. Dettmer, Erika M. Kappes and Patcho N. Santiago

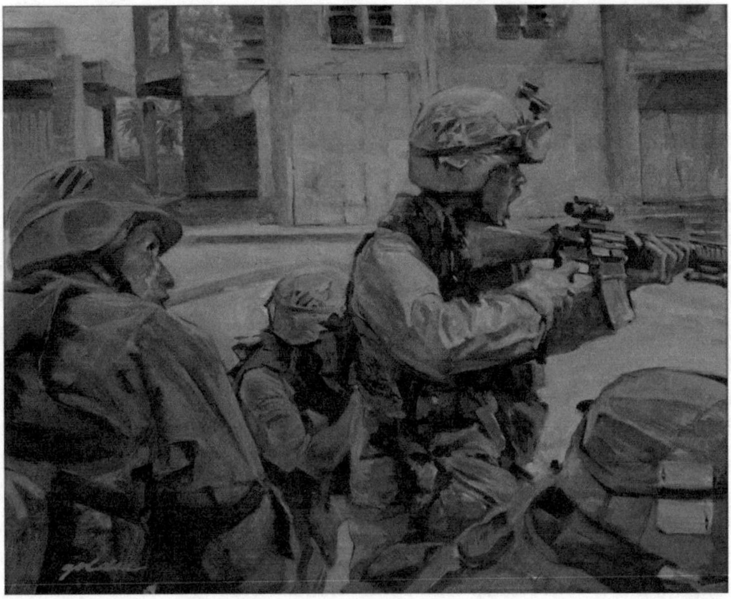

Street Fight, by SFC Elzie Golden, courtesy of the Army Art Collection, US Army Center of Military History.

J. R. Dettmer (✉)
2d Marine Regiment Psychiatrist, Camp Lejeune, NC, USA
e-mail: dr.jdettmer@gmail.com

E. M. Kappes · P. N. Santiago
National Capital Consortium Psychiatry Residency, Walter Reed National Military Medical Center, Bethesda, MD, USA

E. C. Ritchie (ed.), *Posttraumatic Stress Disorder and Related Diseases in Combat Veterans,* DOI 10.1007/978-3-319-22985-0_4

Posttraumatic stress disorder (PTSD) frequently develops in military combat veterans. Though symptoms broadly resemble PTSD that develops in civilian settings, the different index traumas and patient interpretations of those traumas have led to an increasingly recognized subset of this common disorder: moral injury. Gray and colleagues provided the following definition of moral injury: "a term used to describe a syndrome of shame, self-handicapping, anger, and demoralization that occurs when deeply held beliefs and expectations about moral and ethical conduct are transgressed [1]."

These beliefs and expectations, or "moral standards," can be defined as "an individual's knowledge and internalization of moral norms and conventions [2]." Conventions might be universal or culture specific. Generally, actions that cause adverse conscience experiences by other sentient beings get judged as "wrong," such as interpersonal violence and stealing [2]. Within the military, the rules of engagement typically vilify directing violence towards noncombatants and other vulnerable individuals [2, 3]. In this chapter, we discuss the experience of one soldier who developed moral injury secondary to violations of his moral standards.

4.1 Case Presentation/History

The pseudonym Sergeant (SGT) Smith will be used for a 27-year-old married male soldier with no prior psychiatric history who presented with symptoms of posttraumatic stress after his second combat tour in Iraq. The service member was in his usual state of good psychological health through the first half of a 6 month deployment. At that time the enemy began utilizing adolescents as young as 10 years old to load and fire mortars onto his base during night operations. Everyone in his unit recognized this practice and minimized return fire to limit injuries to these child soldiers. However, given mission interference and the vulnerability of their position, occasionally engagement became necessary to prevent American casualties.

The patient recalled one specific encounter when he fired the round that killed a teenage boy. Reflexively, he experienced a rush of excitement and euphoria that frequently accompanied engagement in firefights. After that event, his operational tempo did not allow him further reflection on this incident.

Upon return from deployment, SGT Smith remembered the cardinal event vividly whenever he attempted to spend time with his 9-year-old son. He developed multiple psychological symptoms over the course of the following months, including irritability, anhedonia, withdrawal from his nuclear family, exaggerated startle, depressed mood, poor sleep onset, frequent nightmares, self-loathing, suicidal thoughts, and paroxysmal physiologic anxious symptoms, namely flushed skin, muscle tension, and bounding heartbeat. Suicidal thoughts occurred in the context of his intense persistent dysphoria and belief that he did not deserve to live.

These symptoms interfered with his occupational functioning. He could not tolerate large congregations of people and he considered separating from his wife because of the arguments they were having, which he attributed primarily to his shortened temper. He presented voluntarily for mental health treatment at the urging of his unit medical provider.

SGT Smith suffered no other medical conditions and denied family history of psychiatric disorders. He took no medications and had no known drug allergies. He grew up in the Midwest to an intact union with three older siblings. Growing up, his favorite activity was participating in team athletics. He enjoyed the structure, traditions, and uniforms that were integral to sports culture. Additionally, contributing to something larger than the sum of its parts provided him a sense of purpose.

He enlisted in the Army immediately after high school, in part to cultivate these tendencies. He abstained from alcohol and illicit drugs, and his military performance until symptom development had been excellent.

Mental status exam revealed a well-groomed soldier of average build and no psychomotor abnormalities. He displayed a dysthymic and restricted affect, poor eye contact, and only surface-level rapport with the provider. He admitted to passive death wishes, but had no active suicidal or homicidal thoughts. Routine screening lab results were normal.

4.1.1 Pearls

1. Be patient while gathering history. Portions of this individual's history remained unrevealed even after several months of regular medication management appointments.
2. Become familiar with screening instruments available for moral injury. If suspected, consider administering the Moral Injury Events Scale or the Posttraumatic Cognitions Inventory [1, 4]. These instruments may help to characterize the contribution of moral injury to the service member's presentation.

4.1.2 Potential Pitfall

1. Being perceived as judgmental towards the actions of combat veterans. Be aware that military combat stories might not be savory, but the perception of negative appraisal by a provider could cause him or her to flee. SGT Smith's treatment course, detailed in following sections, illustrates this poignantly. Providing a sense of safety is one way to facilitate the therapeutic alliance, which seems to be particularly important treating individuals with PTSD [5].

4.2 Diagnosis/Assessment

4.2.1 Formal Diagnosis

The patient in this case exhibits all the classic PTSD symptom clusters, including avoidance, reliving experiences, and excessive physiologic hyperarousal. The fifth edition of the *Diagnostic and Statistical Manual of Mental Disorders (DSM-5)* reiterates these core areas but splits avoidance symptoms into two separate phenomena: avoidance and negative cognitions/mood. Currently, avoidance narrowly applies to internal ("memories, thoughts, or feelings") or external reminders of the traumatic event [6]. The category of "negative alterations in cognitions and mood" retains most avoidance symptoms that appeared in the text revision of DSM-IV, such as feelings of detachment and anhedonia [7]. However, critical features of this patient's presentation were not attributable to PTSD based on previous diagnostic symptom lists. New criteria added in DSM-5 include persistent and exaggerated negative beliefs and a persistent negative emotional state [6]. SGT Smith's self-loathing, negative mood, and negative self-perception grew out of shame for his actions and emotions experienced during combat, and can be accounted for without diagnosing another mental health disorder.

Despite the criteria modifications, available information and treatment recommendations for PTSD predominantly address symptoms as though they were caused from the intense fear associated with a life-threat incident. For instance, "fear situations" are systematically reevaluated using cognitive behavioral therapy (CBT) variants [1]. These variants include prolonged exposure (PE) and cognitive processing therapy (CPT), which are strongly recommended treatment protocols for PTSD [8]. Formulating cases with these cognitive models may be appropriate for most incidents resulting in PTSD in civilians.

Besides a perceived life threat, there are other recognized traumatic events that could precipitate symptoms, including significant loss of friends, bullying, chronic illnesses, killing, and exposure to malevolent environments [4]. Two things about SGT Smith's history differ from many other mental health patients by his inclusion in a military subculture and killing behavior, which he identified as his most significant combat experience. Although PTSD remained the coded diagnosis, moral injury more accurately captures the syndrome with which he presents.

4.2.2 Moral Injury

Specifically for this patient, killing a vulnerable youth represented the transgression that violated his view of how the world should operate. Moral transgressions that are stable, internal, and global lead to enduring emotional symptoms of shame and anxiety [3]. When asked, SGT Smith reported that taking the life of a teenager made him feel persistently bad about his character (stable), "less than human" (internal), and was not excused despite the operational context (global). He primarily exhibited shame as a result of this morally injurious event.

4.2.2.1 Shame

DSM-5 combines the experience of shame and guilt in a single criterion, yet a consequential distinction should be made [6]. Guilt involves believing that one committed an improper action or feeling. Usually, there is remorse for acting or experiencing events in a certain way. Those actions or emotions are judged harshly, and often there is a desire to "make amends" for them. In contrast, shame involves making implications about oneself, or one's own self-concept [9]. That is, the focus of negative assessment turns internally.

Shame and guilt are not mutually exclusive, though SGT Smith illustrates that they have the potential to exist independently. He did not regret his actions or feel a need to atone for them. If he had not returned fire his entire unit would have faced continuous and imminent lethal threat. However, the "pleasure" and "excitement" he reported during killing undermined his humanity. In his words, it "makes [him] no better than an animal." His pre-deployment self-concept became negatively altered because of how he felt after firing a round that ended the life of a youth.

Combat veterans can be differentially susceptible to shame development and the subsequent severity of PTSD symptoms. For example, Leskela, Dieperink, and Thuras administered the Test of Self-Conscious Affect (TOSCA) and the Military PTSD Checklist (PCL-M) to former prisoners of war [9]. The TOSCA has been utilized to measure proneness for feeling guilt or shame, with "proneness" defined by Tangney et al. as the "propensity to experience that emotion across a range of situations [2]." Results indicated that shame-proneness was positively correlated with PTSD symptom severity [9].

In contrast, the same study found that when isolated from other factors, guilt-proneness was negatively correlated with severity of PTSD symptoms. Although not conclusive, this implies that the ability to experience guilt for specific actions allows individuals to cope by atoning for their actions through alternative means available to them, such as volunteer work or mentoring. SGT Smith's shame has repercussions for his self-perception, and he did not feel that actions directed towards others might atone for his behaviors or earn forgiveness.

4.2.2.2 Killing

Military service members serving in combat missions bear the burden of participating in sanctioned killing. Killing is associated with multiple post-deployment problems. A study by Maguen and colleagues found that killing in combat is a predictor of relationship problems, alcohol abuse, and symptoms of PTSD [10]. Remarkably, when killing variables are controlled for, general combat experiences are not significantly related to PTSD severity in Vietnam vets [11]. This could imply that these behaviors mediate the severity of PTSD, not the sum of total combat exposure. Finally, in veterans with symptoms of PTSD or depression, a history of killing was associated with suicidal ideation [12]. These findings suggest a unique contribution of these behaviors to mental health problems.

While rare in civilian occupations, killing behaviors are common in veterans who have participated in war. Hoge et al. published survey-obtained statistics about those serving in the Iraq and Afghanistan conflicts. Service members believed they were responsible for the death of an enemy combatant at a rate of 32 %, while responsibility for the death of a noncombatant was reported at a frequency of almost 10 % [13].

In a study utilizing data from the National Vietnam Veterans Readjustment Study, 47 % of veterans killed or believed they killed someone during the war [11]. These data were obtained in nonclinical populations, but the association of killing with increased PTSD severity indicates that the percentage of veterans visiting mental health clinics who have engaged in killing behaviors may be higher than reported in those studies.

Although the reason for the link between these behaviors and mental health problems is not clear, empirical data suggests that a relationship exists between them. Whether it is rape, combat exposure, or childhood abuse, interpersonal traumas consistently lead to the development of PTSD at a rate of at least twice those of natural disasters or accidents [5]. Killing represents an extreme form of interpersonal violence, as participants typically have the intent to take another person's life. Humans ascribe meaning to events that occur to them, and not only does violence threaten physical health, it represents a "breakdown of social norms as well as the sense of safety associated with being a member of a rule-guided community [5]."

4.2.3 Understanding SGT Smith's Symptoms

As noted previously, the act of killing contributed to moral injury in SGT Smith. Prior to deployment he valued self-sacrifice while contributing to causes greater than himself. He identified with serving his country and appreciated the military culture. He valued the lives of vulnerable individuals, and saw himself as an enforcer of this principle.

Study data imply that combat experiences may selectively impact certain values. For instance, a cross-sectional study designed to identify the effect of personal values on the presence and severity of PTSD found those who highly regard the protection of others' welfare and respect cultural customs were more likely to suffer PTSD [14]. For SGT Smith, these values came into conflict after his index trauma. He no longer saw himself as a protector and was more ambivalent about being a member of the traditional and structured culture found within the military services. The violation of these moral standards contributed to alterations of his self-concept, which lay at the root of his moral injury.

No existing psychological theory singularly accounts for the symptoms manifested by SGT Smith secondary to his moral injury [3]. However, applying Ehlers and Clark's "cognitive model of PTSD" provides a partial understanding [15]. For example, the model posits that the patient sees himself as "a different person" and that "other people will respond negatively if they knew about" what he has done [15]. His low self-assessment makes him feel unworthy of his marriage or child, causing him to distance himself from them both.

Also, SGT Smith avoided all positive emotions that he felt during his identified trauma. This manifests as eliminating activities that can involuntarily induce excitement or thrill, which were the feelings he had while participating in the index event. This dysfunctional management strategy results in hiding from the memories and prevents him "from reorganizing [his] autobiographical memory knowledge base in a way that creates a continuous view of the self [15]." Therefore, the cognitive model seems to adequately explain the avoidance, dysphoria, and reliving symptoms that SGT Smith exhibits. Nevertheless, his excessive hyperarousal and interpersonal irritability beg an alternate view in cases of moral injury.

4.2.4 Pearls

1. Consider moral injury in diagnostic assessments of veterans. The index event might not be a classic life-threat incident involving firefights, but may include atrocities, heavy losses, the inability to help vulnerable populations, and feeling responsible for loss of life.
2. A history of killing behaviors might guide assessment and provide insight into prognosis. As noted previously, symptom severity, suicidality, and coping mechanisms could be impacted by these behaviors.
3. Appreciate the difference between shame and guilt. These emotions share similar characteristics, although they are not synonymous.

4.2.5 Potential Pitfall

1. Formulating patients with moral injury based on a single theoretical framework. Incorporating concepts from a variety of theoretical positions should increase conceptual understanding of patients suffering from this complex syndrome.

4.3 Treatment/Management

4.3.1 Psychopharmacologic Management

Medications do not address the underlying etiology of moral injury. Ultimately, SGT Smith's symptom severity required psychotropics. He reported excellent medication adherence since engaging with care. Medication regimens that have been sequentially trialed are listed in Table 4.1. All agents were titrated to maximum approved Food and Drug Administration (FDA) dose or as tolerated based upon side effects. Medications required changing for differing reasons.

For example, trazodone was ineffective for improving sleep onset or maintenance. Prazosin and clonidine helped with daytime hyperarousal but made no impact on nightmare frequency or intensity. Both alpha adrenergic agents were discontinued for unacceptable blood pressure variability and lack of positive impact on nightmares. Sertraline lacked efficacy for his low mood, hedonic drive, and isolationism. Venlafaxine improved his energy level and hedonic drive initially,

Table 4.1 SGT Smith's sequential medication regimens

1st	2nd	3rd	4th	Most recent
Sertraline (A)	Amitriptyline (B)	Venlafaxine (A)	Venlafaxine (A)	Paroxetine (A)
Trazodone (I)	Clonidine (I)	Zolpidem (I)	Quetiapine (I)	Olanzapine (I)
Prazosin (B)		Propranolol (I)	Propranolol (I)	Propranolol (I)

From the Veterans Administration/Department of Defense PTSD Pocket Guide [8]: (A) = "strong recommendation" with significant benefit; (B) = "fair evidence" of some benefit; (I) = insufficient evidence though this improvement was marginal. Also, at the upper level of the dosing range for venlafaxine, physiologic hyperarousal and agitation increased, which led to tapering of the medication. A beta-blocker was prescribed for daytime agitation and physiologic hyperarousal. The patient reported rapid and significant improvement in these symptoms. Zolpidem and quetiapine resulted in no improvement in sleep latency or maintenance. Finally, paroxetine and olanzapine were trialed with some initial response in mood, sleep onset, and nightmare frequency.

4.3.2 Psychotherapeutic Management

After intake, the patient was referred to a day program with components of group psychoeducation and supportive interventions. The service member walked out on day two of treatment because of physical symptoms associated with the group setting. He reported feeling embarrassed about how he would be accepted by the group for telling his combat stories. Individual cognitive therapy and exposure-based treatments began under a psychologist at the base clinic, though this was discontinued after three sessions. When discussed further, SGT Smith stated that he perceived the therapist as poorly receptive to discussions of suicidal thoughts and details of his killing in combat.

After these failures and the pressure his wife placed on him to receive help, he began marital therapy with a marriage and family life counselor off base. Despite having multiple failed individual therapists, he gained rapport with the marriage therapist during these sessions and started individual treatment with that provider as well. Both marital and individual therapy involved mostly supportive techniques including validation, nonjudgmental empathizing, and building cohesion with his spouse.

Evident in this patient's treatment summary is the attempt at using multiple standard psychotherapeutic treatments from the Department of Defense Clinical Practice Guidelines for PTSD [8]. According to the guidelines, patient education and group therapy garnered no general recommendation but have fair evidence for providing some benefit in treating PTSD. Individual cognitive and exposure therapies received strong recommendations. Trials of these interventions with SGT Smith proved largely unsuccessful. Exploration of his experience leading to termination of these treatments yielded much of the presenting history and reformulation of his case around the concept of shame. The evidence-based, indicated interventions including group, cognitive processing, and exposure techniques did not optimally address his symptoms in part because he did not establish a therapeutic alliance with the individuals administering therapy.

4.3.3 Pearls

1. Maintain flexibility during treatment. Standard PTSD treatment protocols did not seem to address the patient's most distressing symptoms. Supportive interventions that slowly built rapport and addressed his marital relationship proved to be the most beneficial.

4.3.4 Potential Pitfall

1. Relying primarily on medications to resolve symptoms. Even though medication contributed to management of SGT Smith's symptoms and possibly staved off crises, pharmacotherapy did not improve his self-concept or engagement with others.

4.4 Outcomes/Case Resolution

Progress was slow and incremental, but after eight biweekly sessions with the marriage therapist, he began to view his wife as an ally. SGT Smith shared with her his shame and negative self-perception, which was met with understanding and acceptance. This experience may support the notion set forth by Charavastra and Cloitre that improving social bonds facilitates emotional processing of trauma, which could relieve symptoms of PTSD even without exposure-based therapies [5].

More formal therapies to address moral injury have yet to attain convincing empirical support. However, adaptive disclosure and a modified CBT described by Litz and colleagues specifically address moral injury in their proposed treatment protocols [1, 3]. Both interventions de-emphasize challenging distorted thoughts relative to existing cognitive interventions. Instead, "emotion-focused disclosures" are utilized to ascribe meaning to the morally injurious events, which theoretically foster self-forgiveness, reparation, and reconnection with social supports [3].

Providers lacking familiarity with these models to conceptualize moral injury will usually still be familiar with sound principles that can aide in the management of this condition. Terms previously discussed, including "moral standard," "values," "self-concept," and "inner conflict" all relate to ideas espoused by other theoretical frameworks. These approaches, such as the biocognitive model, schema-focused CBT, and psychoanalytic intersubjectivity emphasize substantially similar concepts with variations in their respective underlying theories [16, 17, 18]. Each suggests that when individuals' self-perception is challenged by internal or external threats, symptoms develop. Resolution of these conflicts, à la adaptive disclosure discussed previously, should relieve manifested symptoms. Resolving these conflicts "through sustained empathic inquiry" should result in symptom reduction, regardless of theoretical orientation [18].

4.5 Conclusion

Identifying the particulars of combat that potentially lead to moral injury can inform further evaluation and treatment of this syndrome. Empathic exploration of killing behaviors could uncover unbearable shame and guilt in combat veterans. Moral injury can profoundly affect one's self-concept and participation in treatment. Management of PTSD symptoms in service members with moral injury may need modification to address associated shame and self-loathing. Ideally, more evidence will be generated that provide insight into optimal management techniques. Until such time, identifying the patient's values and how their experiences conflict with these values provides a viable starting point.

References

1. Gray MJ, Schorr Y, Nash W, Lebowitz L, Amidon A, Lansing A, Maglione M, Lang AJ, Litz BT. Adaptive disclosure: an open trial of a novel exposure-based intervention for service members with combat-related psychological stress injuries. Behav Ther. 2012;43:407–15.
2. Tangney JP, Stuewig J, Mashek DJ. Moral emotions and moral behavior. Ann Rev Psychol. 2007;58:345–72.
3. Litz BT, Stein N, Delaney E, Lebowitz L, Nash WP, Silva C, Maguen S. Moral injury and moral repair in war veterans: a preliminary model and intervention strategy. Clin Psychol Rev. 2009;29:695–706.
4. Nash WP, Marino Carper TL, Mills MA, Au T, Goldsmith A, Litz BT. Psychometric evaluation of the Moral Injury Events Scale. Military Med. 2013;178(6):646–52.
5. Charavastra A, Cloitre C. Social bonds and posttraumatic stress disorder. Ann Rev Psychol. 2008;59:301–28.
6. American Psychiatric Association. DSM-5 Task Force. Diagnostic and statistical manual of mental disorders: DSM-5. Arlington: American Psychiatric Association; 2013.
7. American Psychiatric Association. Diagnostic and statistical manual of mental disorders: DSM-IV-TR. 4th edn., text revision. Washington, DC: American Psychiatric Association; 2000.
8. Posttraumatic Stress Disorder Pocket Guide: To accompany the 2010 VA/DoD Clinical practice guideline for the management of PTSD. Veterans affairs Web site. http://www.healthquality.va.gov/guidelines/MH/ptsd/PTSDPocketGuide23May2013v1.pdf. Published May 23, 2013. Accessed 20 Aug 2014.
9. Leskala J, Dieperink M, Thuras P. Shame and posttraumatic stress disorder. J Trauma Stress. 2002;15(3):223–26.
10. Maguen S, Lucenko BA, Reger MA, Gahm GA, Litz BT, Seal KH, Knight SJ, Marmar CR. The impact of reported direct and indirect killing on mental health symptoms in Iraq war veterans. J Trauma Stress. 2010;23(1):86–90.
11. Maguen S, Metzler TJ, Litz BT, Seal KH, Knight SJ, Marmar CR. The impact of killing in war on mental health symptoms and related functioning. J Trauma Stress. 2009;22(5):435–43.
12. Maguen S, Luxton DD, Skopp NA, Gahm GA, Reger MA, Metzler TJ, Marmar CR. Killing in combat, mental health symptoms, and suicidal ideation in Iraq war veterans. J Anxiety Disord. 2011;25:563–67.
13. Hoge CW, Castro CA, Messer SC, McGurk D, Cotting DI, Koffman RL. Combat duty in Iraq and Afghanistan, mental health problems, and barriers to care. New Engl J Med. 2004;351(1):13–22.
14. Zimmermann P, Firnkes S, Kowalski JT, Backus J, Siegal S, Willmund G, Maercker A. Personal values in soldiers after military deployment: associations with mental health and resilience. Eur J Psychotraumatol. 2014;5:22939. doi:10.3402/ejpt.v5.22939
15. Ehlers A, Clark DM. A cognitive model of posttraumatic stress disorder. Behav Res Ther. 2000;38:319–45.
16. McLaren N. The mind-body problem explained: the biocognitive model for psychiatry. Ann Arbor: Future Psychiatry Press; 2012.
17. Westbrook D, Kennerley H, Kirk J. An introduction to cognitive behavioral therapy: skills and applications, 2nd Edn. London: Sage Publications; 2011.
18. Stolorow RD, Atwood, GE. The intersubjective perspective. Psychoanal Rev. 1996;83:181–94.

Part II
Established and Evidence-Based Treatments

Updates in Psychopharmacology for PTSD and Related Conditions: Focus on the Active Duty Service Member

5

Elspeth Cameron Ritchie and Christopher S. Nelson

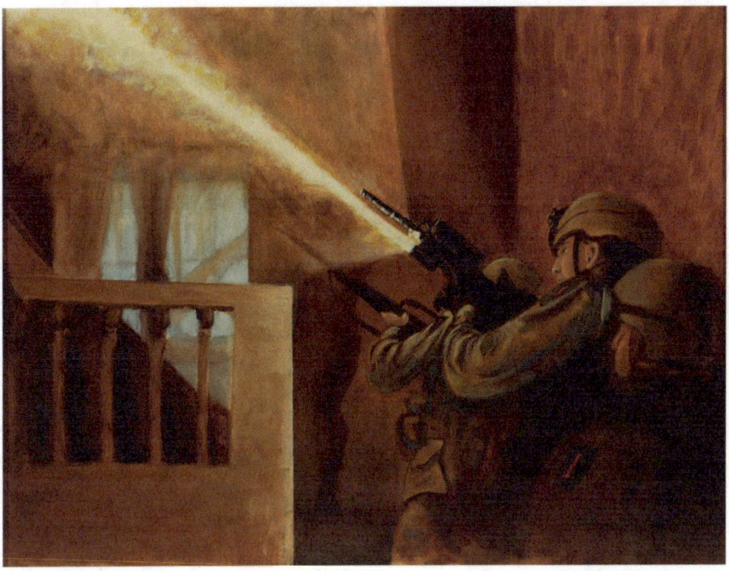

E. C. Ritchie (✉)
Department of Psychiatry, Uniformed Services University of the Health Sciences, 4301 Jones Bridge Road, 20314 Bethesda, MD, USA
e-mail: elspethcameronritchie@gmail.com

C. S. Nelson
Department of Psychiatry, United States Navy; Behavioral Health Directorate; Naval Hospital Camp LeJeune, Camp Lejeune, NC, USA
e-mail: ChrisSNelsonMD@aol.com

E. C. Ritchie (ed.), *Posttraumatic Stress Disorder and Related Diseases in Combat Veterans,* DOI 10.1007/978-3-319-22985-0_5

Another Day at the Office, by MSG Christopher Thiel, courtesy of the Army Art Collection, US Army Center of Military History.

This chapter focuses on psychopharmacology for posttraumatic stress disorder (PTSD) both in military service members and veterans. However, immediately one must realize that there are many military-specific issues involved in treating active duty military members with psychiatric medication. If a service member is no longer on active duty, then a wider variety of medications may be used without a negative impact on their career. The chapter will first cover these general issues and then get into some specifics of medications and their side effects.

The chapter is partly borne from personal experience, partly from clinical experiences, and partly from the scientific literature. The lead author served a career in the Army and was involved in many policy decisions about the use of psychiatric medications, especially in deployment. The second author went from civilian practice in New York to working as a civilian contractor at Camp Lejeune, a Marine base in North Carolina.

Themes of military cultural competency exist throughout this volume, specifically knowing the aspects of military life that intersect with psychiatric treatment. It is important for the clinician to know on which medications an active duty service member may deploy. While these restrictions vary somewhat depending on service (e.g., Army, Navy, Air Force, Marines) and military occupational specialty (MOS), in general the guidelines are covered under the Deployment Limiting Psychiatric Conditions policy [1].

5.1 Deployment-Limiting Psychiatric Conditions and Medications

Service members are not allowed to deploy on certain medications [1]. These include: (1) antipsychotics; (2) mood stabilizers that require therapeutic monitoring, such as lithium and valproic acid; and (3) medications like coumadin which could be dangerous if one were shot or injured. Thus, the clinician needs to realize that putting service members on these medications will limit their deployments, and could thereby end their careers, if they will need the medications for an extended period.

The restrictions on certain medications during deployment are borne out of the realities of the austere conditions of many operations, be they combat or humanitarian assistance missions. For example, one cannot get lithium or valproic acid levels at a field hospital, and it is easy to get dehydrated in a desert.

Another dimension is the public appearance of deploying service members on antipsychotic medications. However, many atypical psychotics are used "off-label," especially to augment antidepressants or to decrease trauma-induced nightmares. While clinicians and patients find them very useful, there are vocal anti-medication elements in society who highlight what they consider "overuse" of medication, especially antipsychotics. This is a very controversial area [2].

5.2 Psychiatric Medications and Military Service

There is a rich literature on evidence-based treatment of PTSD, developed by the American Psychiatric Association, the Department of Defense (DoD), the Department of Veterans Affairs (VA), and others [3–6]. These include: (1) pharmacotherapy or medication, and (2) psychotherapy. However, these guidelines do not take into account the deployment restrictions for active duty troops, discussed above. This chapter will highlight special considerations for active duty military troops.

Thirty years ago, chlorpromazine (Thorazine) and diazepam (Valium) were the only psychiatric medications in a deployed pharmacy. Beginning in the early 1990s, the services gradually increased the availability of medications allowed in the field environment.

Selective serotonin reuptake inhibitors (SSRIs) were developed for treatment of depression, with the first one, fluoxetine (Prozac), released in the early 1990s. Since then, many have been FDA approved for depression. Only two, paroxetine (Paxil) and sertraline (Zoloft), have been FDA approved for PTSD. Not surprisingly, clinicians use a wide range of SSRIs for PTSD. Usually the choice of SSRI is based on the side-effect profile.

Some SSRIs/serotonin–norepinephrine reuptake inhibitors (SNRIs) are equally effective, and may be helpful for other conditions. For example, Cymbalta (duloxetine) has been proven effective for some forms of concurrent neuropathic pain, and Effexor (venlafaxine) is established as useful for the prevention of migraine headache.

In general, service members may deploy on an SSRI, although certain military occupations, such as aviators, may not be allowed to take them. The clinically most important side effects in a military population are: (1) sedation, (2) weight gain, and (3) sexual side effects.

Other medications are also used for PTSD and related conditions, including second-generation antipsychotics, mood stabilizers, and medications for sleep. This chapter will cover the so-called "off-label" uses of other medications for PTSD. However, service members are not supposed to deploy on antipsychotics or mood stabilizers. Infrequent use of sleeping aids is permissible.

Sedation may either be useful or a problem, depending on whether the service member is suffering from insomnia, and what their job/life requirements are. Paroxetine is often considered the most sedating antidepressant, and fluoxetine the most activating. Sertraline (Zoloft) is usually considered neutral, although the side-effect profile varies based on the service member. Other middle-of-the-road choices include Celexa (citalopram) and Lexapro (escitalopram). However, sedating side effects vary in individuals.

Many service members and veterans with PTSD and/or traumatic brain injury (TBI) suffer from insomnia and PTSD-related nightmares. In that case, their insomnia should be treated. Standard sleeping aids may be used. Trazodone at low doses

(50–100 mg) is often used with good effect. The antidepressant effect of trazodone may also augment their other medications. Although rare, priapism can still occur even in this relatively young population, so the male service member being prescribed trazodone should be warned to seek help in the emergency department if he should develop a painful erection which does not subside.

Other sleeping aids should be used with caution. Diphenhydramine (Benadryl) is often used, but the anticholinergic properties may be problematic. Benadryl is very dangerous in overdose. Ambien (zolpidem) and Lunesta (eszopiclone) are useful if prescribed sparingly as they can be habit forming. There are new FDA warnings regarding the dosage of Ambien, recommending that dosages should be significantly reduced, especially in women, to avoid excessive morning sedation.

Most guidelines recommend against benzodiazepines, because of the dangers of tolerance and abuse. Furthermore, studies have shown that benzodiazepine worsens PTSD symptoms, making this class of medication generally contraindicated. While relatively safe by themselves in an overdose, they may be lethal if mixed with other medications, especially opiates. Finally, service members should not be operating heavy machinery or weapons on benzodiazepines.

Particularly useful for the military population is ramelteon (Rozerem), which by its action of affecting the natural production of melatonin can offer relief from insomnia without risk of dependence. To be most effective, the medication must be prescribed to be taken at least 1 h prior to bedtime rather than just as the service member plans to retire.

Mood stabilizers may be very useful, especially in service members with TBI-related symptoms, such as headaches or irritability and/or comorbid depression. Valproic acid (Depakote) use is common. Gabapentin is often helpful for pain syndromes. However, as mentioned above, neither lithium nor valproic acid levels can be obtained in a field environment. Both agents can cause weight gain. Topiramate (Topamax) is less likely to cause weight gain, but patients should always be warned about the possibility of acute glaucoma.

As mentioned above, atypical antipsychotics, such as quetiapine (Seroquel), are often used in a variety of psychiatric conditions, especially to augment antidepressants or to decrease trauma-induced nightmares. Quetiapine can be particularly helpful in those patients who are extremely hypervigilant at night, such that they are prone to "get up and clear the house" if they hear the slightest unfamiliar noise. With Seroquel (quetiapine), as with many second-generation atypical antipsychotics, longer-term use can cause increases in serum triglycerides. Weight gain is a major problem with this sedative as well, for which reason it should be used only if more traditional non-habituating sleep aids have failed.

For trauma-related nightmares, the "gold standard" for reduction or elimination of these ubiquitous symptoms is prazosin at bedtime. It is prudent to start dosing patients suffering from nightmares with 1 mg of prazosin at night, and increase by 1 mg every week to 2 weeks, as patients become accustomed slowly to the hypotensive effects of the medication. Although 1 or 2 mg is commonly the effective dose in most service members, patients with horrific recurring nightmares may require a dose as high as 10–12 mg, if their blood pressure will tolerate it. Reminding the patient to arise slowly from bed and drink water to avoid light-headedness can make the medication more easily tolerated and thereby encourage compliance.

5.3 Management of Other Side Effects, and Clinical Pearls

In all cases, caution should be used until any side effects are clear. In the military, consideration needs to be made that service members may be driving tanks, flying planes, and shooting artillery. Many of these medications cause aviators to be "dq'ed" (disqualified) from flight status.

As discussed above, many psychiatric medications cause weight gain. Service members are regularly weighed, and a determination made if they meet body fat standards. Weight gain above the standards is considered unacceptable by the military, and may lead to discharge from the service. Therefore, it is essential that the provider discuss these issues with the service members and develop strategies to avoid it.

Certain SSRIs, particularly sertraline (Zoloft), can cause or exacerbate preexisting dental bruxism. Some service members who take Zoloft, particularly in higher doses, may clench their teeth so vigorously at night with this medication that they awaken with a sore jaw. Since so many patients with PTSD also have TBI-related headaches from blast exposure, having chronic teeth-grinding at night can markedly worsen the frequency of their headaches. To reverse this side effect, low doses (10–15 mg) of BuSpar (buspirone) have been shown to be helpful to prevent dental bruxism in those patients.

Male service members may be bothered by sexual side effects of SSRIs, such as erectile dysfunction and ejaculatory delay. Female service members also can develop anorgasmia on these medications. These are extremely common with SSRIs, and patients should be warned to expect them. The most important principles for the clinicians are: (1) to ask about sexual health as part of the intake exam, (2) discuss potential side effects of medications with the patient, and (3) to continue to ask about sexual functioning during the course of therapy.

If a patient is having SSRI-related sexual side effects, bupropion (Wellbutrin) may be a helpful strategy, either as a primary treatment for PTSD or to assist with sexual functioning. It is especially useful if the service member is also addicted to nicotine, as it can reduce craving effectively. Although bupropion is not FDA approved for the treatment of PTSD, many clinicians have found it useful as a primary treatment. This is because it has generally no sexual side effects of its own, and its activating noradrenergic properties can often reverse the "numbing" or "dampening" of emotions which can sometimes be an unwanted side effect of SSRIs.

If Wellbutrin augmentation for the SSRIs does not reduce the sexual problems associated with Zoloft or Paxil, the next step is to offer the male service member Viagra (sildenafil), Cialis (tadakafuk), or Levitra (vardenafil), the three commercially available phosphodiesterase (PDE) inhibitors marketed for erectile dysfunction. These may be very helpful in maintaining intimacy with a spouse or partner.

Less commonly known is the utility of low-dose ciproheptadine (Periactin), which can be taken along with a PDE-inhibiting medication about 1 h prior to intercourse. This is helpful for male as well as female patients to reverse the anorgasmia associated with SSRIs. Whereas Viagra and its cousins will correct erectile problems, ciproheptadine can reverse the ejaculatory delay associated with SSRIs, a delay which many young male service members find particularly disturbing unless they are warned in advance that it is a common side effect. (It can be helpful to remind the male patients that premature ejaculation is often treated with an SSRI, such that a delay in achieving orgasm is common).

Some service members may find SSRIs ultimately intolerable due to the sexual side effects. For these patients, stand-alone Wellbutrin may be the first-line alternative, but mirtazapine (Remeron) is also an effective choice, since it is the only other commercially available antidepressant with no sexual side effects. Weight gain and sedation are expected with Remeron, however, due to its histaminic activity.

5.3.1 More Clinical Pearls

Very common among the military PTSD population is public hypervigilance, such that patients can develop severe anxiety bordering on panic when placed in crowds of strangers (such as at the shopping mall or movie theater). If SSRI and psychotherapy alone are not adequate to reduce this situationally induced or "triggered" anxiety, then small doses of beta-blocker, typically propranolol 10 mg, can be offered as a "p.r.n." Patients can be instructed to take this medication one half-hour prior to a situation wherein they know their anxiety will likely be triggered, and they will thereby more easily avoid the hypertension associated with near-panic. The medication has been used "off-label" in this way for years to assist performers in averting stage fright or performance anxiety.

Similarly, severe "flashes" of anger can occur in this population, such that their temper is typically described as "going from 0 to 100" even over minor irritations or provocations (e.g., while driving). Propranolol can be quite useful for this population as well. If used in the short-acting form on a t.i.d. basis, it may be helpful to switch the service member to the long-acting preparation, once it is clear he has tolerated the short-acting compound, in order to avoid having to take the medication as frequently.

Just as when starting prazosin for nightmares, patients who are beginning low-dose beta blocker must be counseled to arise slowly from a seated to a standing position (particularly for the first few doses), and to vigorously hydrate themselves in order to avoid feeling light-headed. Beta blockers cannot be prescribed for patients with bronchial asthma, who may require beta receptor agonists, such as albuterol to relieve their asthma attacks. It is therefore very important to first ask the patients if they have ever had asthma, and to document this in their chart.

In the asthmatic patient with anger problems, low-dose clonidine (0.05 mg b.i.d.) may be an effective alternative to propranolol, provided the patient is carefully warned about hypotensive side effects.

5.3.2 Case Example

This is a composite and does not represent a particular patient. SSgt Brown is a 27-year-old male Marine. He joined the military in 2005, and served two deployments, in Fallujah and otherwise in Anbar Province. During his deployments, he had a typical course: he shot and killed enemy soldiers; he engaged in firefights in which civilians were probably killed, and he lost four of his buddies to enemy fire, improvised explosive devices, and training accidents. He also suffered at least two documented TBIs, and may have suffered more from IEDs.

He was first diagnosed and treated for probable PTSD and TBI by his battalion surgeon, but shortly afterwards referred for psychiatric care at the local military hospital. Symptoms included nightmares, insomnia, avoidance, irritability, and marital problems. He was placed on sertraline for his PTSD symptoms and prazosin for nightmares. Depakote was added for headaches related to his repeated TBI. He did not do well, with complaints about work performance and continued marital problems, as well as a driving under the influence (DUI) charge. He was referred for a medical board, to assess fitness for duty. He was subsequently referred to the Deployment Wellness Clinic, a specialty clinic.

There he complained of weight gain and sexual dysfunction, specifically problems of getting and maintaining an erection. The valproic acid was tapered off. Bupropion was added to the Zoloft and the sexual problems abated. Prazosin successfully and significantly reduced his trauma-related nightmares. Taking occasional Viagra and Periactin for sexual problems also improved his intimate life with his wife, and reassured him regarding his libido.

After 3 months, his symptoms had resolved, and the decision was made to return him to duty. He was promoted 3 months later.

5.4 Conclusion

This chapter focuses on medications. However, it is increasingly clear that a broad array or approaches are warranted, to include psychotherapy and other integrative treatments discussed elsewhere in this volume. Medications can be extremely effective for the treatment of PTSD and other war-related symptoms. Nonetheless, it is essential for the clinician to be aware of, and warn the patient about, related side effects. For active duty patients, there may be consequences of being placed on medication. It can either save or end a career.

References

1. Policy Guidance on Deployment Limiting Psychiatric Conditions and Medications. Nov 7, 2006. http://www.health.mil/~/media/MHS/Policy%20Files/Import/Guidance_20061107_deplo_limiting_psyc_cond.ashx. Accessed 2 Feb 2015.
2. Chekedel L, Kauffman M. Policies on mentally troubled troops questioned. Hartford Courant, May 16, 2006. http://articles.baltimoresun.com/2006-05-16/news/0605160124_1_depression-mental-health-iraq. Accessed 2 Feb 2015.
3. Guidelines VA-DoDP. 2006. http://www.healthquality.va.gov/guidelines/MH/ptsd/. Accessed 2 Feb 2015.
4. American Psychiatric Association Practice Guideline for the Treatment of Patients with Acute Stress Disorder and Posttraumatic Stress Disorder. 2004. http://psychiatryonline.org/pb/assets/raw/sitewide/practice_guidelines/guidelines/acutestressdisorderptsd.pdf. Accessed 2 Feb 2015.
5. Ritchie EC. Psychiatric medications for deployment. Mil Med. 1994;159(10):647–9.
6. Thompson, M. America's medicated army. June 5, 2008. http://content.time.com/time/magazine/article/0,9171,1812055,00.html. Accessed 2 Feb.

Prolonged Exposure for Combat Veterans with PTSD

6

Connie L. Thomas, Rohul Amin and Joshua N. Friedlander

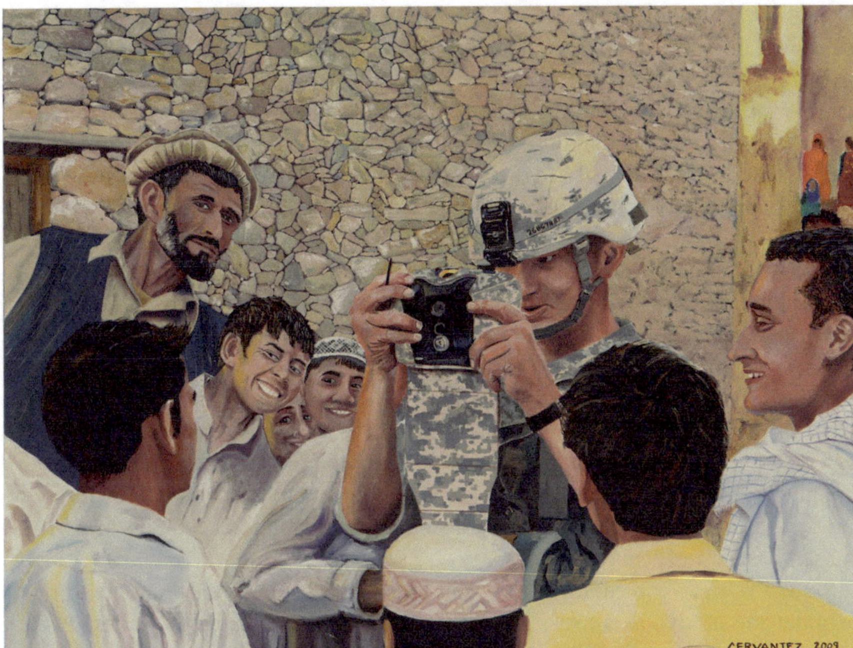

Picture Day in the Village, by MSG Martin J. Cervantez, courtesy of the Army Art Collection, US Army Center of Military History.

C. L. Thomas (✉) · R. Amin · J. N. Friedlander
Behavioral Health Directorate, Walter Reed National Military Medical Center, Bethesda, MD, USA
e-mail: connie.l.thomas29.mil@mail.mil

E. C. Ritchie (ed.), *Posttraumatic Stress Disorder and Related Diseases in Combat Veterans,* DOI 10.1007/978-3-319-22985-0_6

6.1 Clinical Case

The patient is a 25-year-old service member who sustained a gunshot wound in combat without any immediate psychological sequelae. He underwent approximately 8 months of surgical and rehabilitative care. Around that time frame, he presented with his military commander to the behavior health clinic due to public alcohol intoxication and suicidal ideation. He was diagnosed with alcohol abuse and posttraumatic stress disorder (PTSD) with delayed onset per the *Diagnostic and Statistical Manual of Mental Disorders (DSM) IV-TR* [1].

His predominant symptoms were reexperiencing his trauma through nightmares and flashbacks; avoidance of crowds, driving, and traffic; persistent negative beliefs about the world; persistent negative emotional state; and hyperarousal with insomnia, profuse hyperhidrosis at night, hypervigilance, and panic attacks. This presentation resulted in depressed mood and suicidal ideations secondary to feelings about guilt of being a burden on his family with perceived loss of independence. He reported that drinking alcohol would help him cope with his emotional pain.

Basic laboratory evaluation including thyroid panel, urine drug screens, and markers for heavy alcohol use was assessed and found to be normal, which helped narrow the differential diagnosis. Based on his presentation, several treatments were initiated: psychosocial interventions for alcohol abuse, somatic treatments of sertraline for anxiety and prazosin for nightmares, and prolonged exposure (PE) for PTSD.

Due to his history of index trauma with subsequent symptom development 8 months later, he was diagnosed with delayed-onset PTSD. The most disabling feature of his presentation was noted to be his avoidance behaviors. Premorbidly, the patient was a highly independent and socially engaged individual. After the trauma, he had to rely on others to accomplish his activities of daily living and instrumental activities of daily living. For example, he had to be escorted and chauffeured everywhere due to his fear of driving and inability to go to crowded places like the shopping market. These resulted in overwhelming social isolation. His inability to perform basic activities of daily living also had significant impact on his self-image and sense of self-efficacy.

Since PE gives considerable attention to treating avoidance symptoms through imaginal and in vivo exercises, PE was initiated using standardized techniques per the manual by Foa and colleagues [2]. In vivo exercises are based on PEs theory that the conditioned response (fear and avoidance) to the feared stimulus (avoidance of daily activities, such as driving) will reduce or extinguish through prolonged and repeated habituation-based exercises. It is conceptualized that the reduction or extinction of the fear and avoidance response would result in an increased sense of mastery.

Given the practical limits of a clinic setting and the patient's preference, the recommended 90 min sessions from the manual were reduced to standard 60 min sessions. Safety assessments were routinely conducted since the patient initially presented with suicidal ideation. Although PE does not directly treat suicidality, it may reduce the psychiatric distress of the patient's PTSD symptoms, which were conceptualized to be contributory to his suicidality. The clinician was prepared to shift the therapy focus as appropriate to address his suicidality more directly. The PTSD Checklist-Military (PCL-M) was administered at every visit as part of standard practice. In the early sessions of PE, he was educated on the basic concepts and rationale for PE therapy. Relaxation breathing techniques were reviewed.

Despite encouragement from the clinician, the patient declined to use breathing techniques. It was unclear at the time why he was reluctant to use these, but the therapist elected to not emphasize the relaxation skills to avoid endangering or fracturing the therapeutic alliance. It was later revealed that a relaxed state was threatening to the patient. He reported a belief that he may be caught unprepared for potential emergencies if he became too relaxed using such techniques. Since those relaxation skills are a critical component of PE treatment, it was noted as a possible contributor to the slow progression of treatment.

During the next several sessions, he was educated on the subjective units of distress scale (SUDS) and aided in creating an in vivo SUDS hierarchy using standard PE forms. The patient selected activities corresponding to SUDS levels of 40 and 50 as part of his in vivo exposure. The sessions were recorded on his smartphone. The initial in vivo exposure homework exercise was to watch a war-related video that was similar to the patient's reported trauma memory of gunshot wound sustained during combat.

He successfully accomplished this task, but had more difficulty completing assignments related to imaginal exposure via listening to the recorded session of his index trauma due to significant fear and anxiety. He described that the anticipation of hearing his voice and traumatic experience caused him to feel shortness of breath, chest tightness, racing heart, and fear of losing control. He reported a belief that his hypervigilance was protective because it was what kept him safe. During the third session, he was introduced to in-session imaginal exposure. While initially hesitant, he was able to progress with significant encouragements. He provided data on his SUDS during the detailed description of his trauma, which lessened with repeated exposure (Fig. 6.1).

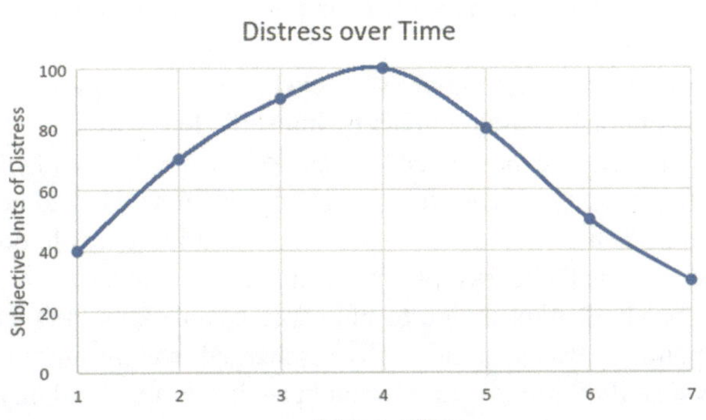

Fig. 6.1 SUDS scores during imaginal exposure over time demonstrating the gradual initial increase with increasing details in trauma narrative, eventually reaching a peak and then dropping over time

Despite much support from the clinician, he continued to avoid listening to his trauma from the session. Modifications were attempted, such as listening to just the initial 5 min of the tape. However, he reported becoming extremely anxious when attempting to open the recordings on his smartphone. Since imaginal exposure is a critical component of PE, the clinician and patient decided to use a less overwhelming method of exposure. Rather than listening to his trauma, he was asked to write a narrative.

While this seemed like a reasonable alternative to the patient, he still avoided doing this until the ninth session. He did well with in vivo exposure assignments such as going to the mall or watching certain anxiety-provoking videos, although continued to avoid driving. Exploring his avoidance revealed his beliefs that the world is a dangerous place, something bad would happen, and he would die. Over the course of several sessions, he was able to advance to higher level stimuli on his in vivo and imaginal exposure SUDS hierarchy peaking to 100 and demonstrated expected drops during the session.

The PE therapy continued for 12 sessions and then care was terminated due to the anticipated transfer of the clinician. The patient's goals were discussed, with the dyad agreeing that the patient continued to show much disability and should continue with PE. While the patient demonstrated some success with in vivo exposure, he maintained his fear and avoidance of driving and dependency on family members. However, his mood symptoms had significantly improved. He no longer had thoughts or desire to kill himself. He also maintained his sobriety following brief psychoeducational interventions.

Given his persisting symptoms, he was transferred to another therapist. They continued modified PE with imaginal exposure without in vivo exposure for an additional 20 sessions. Some modifications that were made to help the patient better engage in imaginal exposure included using the past tense, keeping his eyes open, writing the trauma instead of speaking it, and not using audio recordings. Since the patient was hesitant to complete the PE exercises due to these maladaptive beliefs, the clinician modified his approach to include a greater emphasis on cognitive therapy in order to address those beliefs. As the patient was able to increase the intensity of imaginal exposure over time, he progressed to having better tolerance for in vivo exposure.

Initially, he performed these homework exercises with family supervision, but over time, he accomplished assignments by himself. He reported an increased ability to tolerate anxiety, and possessed a sense of accomplishment. At the end of therapy, the patient had significant functional improvement. He had begun to drive, was engaged to be married, and was reporting euthymia. It was hypothesized that the improvement of his PTSD symptoms, particularly avoidance and emotional estrangement from others, contributed to improved socialization and led to his marriage. At that point, he was also medically discharged from military service due to significant physical limitations from his combat-related injury and inability to carry on his duties as an active duty service member.

6.2 Diagnosis and Assessment

When assessing a patient such as in the clinical case example, standardized diagnostic criteria should be used. With the recent update of the *Diagnostic Statistical Manual* [3], it is important to consider the significant differences between the DSM IV-TR and DSM-5 in the diagnostic criteria of PTSD and how this may impact patient selection for treatment. In DSM-5, PTSD is no longer classified as an anxiety disorder, but as a separate category, trauma-stressor-related disorders. One impetus for this classification was growing research supporting that PTSD is characterized by a range of emotional and behavioral reactions, which are not exclusive to anxiety. Changes in definition and diagnostic criteria, even if minor, do create dilemmas for clinicians with regard to external validity of preceding evidence and its application to the new criteria.

The clinical case described in this chapter illustrates the diagnostic uncertainty that often accompanies diagnosing mental disorders. The differential diagnosis of PTSD can be especially challenging. First of all, the temporal relationship between traumatic event and the development of symptoms can vary. In this case, the patient did not present with immediate psychological sequelae after his trauma. After approximately 8 months of surgical and rehabilitative care, he was evaluated by behavioral health due to alcohol intoxication and suicidal ideation. His presentation was delayed in onset and calls into question whether that patient's symptoms are attributable to a different disorder.

Delayed-onset PTSD is defined in the DSM-5 as the onset of the symptoms occurring at least 6 months after the traumatic event. It is theorized that many soldiers do not develop symptoms immediately because stress reactions are adaptive in combat [4]. Additionally, one study of soldiers evacuated from combat in Iraq and Afghanistan found some evidence that severe injuries tend to postpone the development of PTSD by several months [5]. Other literature suggests that patients may display milder symptoms initially that are not immediately detected, which become more functionally impairing over time [6]. For example, in the clinical case described, the patient may have been so occupied with surgery and rehabilitation that his symptoms were not readily apparent in such a protective environment.

Another reason that the differential diagnosis can be so challenging is that there is a high comorbidity between PTSD and other psychiatric diagnoses [7]. In this case, the patient's presentation was also complicated by alcohol use disorder, which can present as anxiety during periods of withdrawal and mimics other mental health disorders. Literature indicates that PTSD often occurs with at least one or more psychiatric diagnoses [8, 9]. Some of the more common comorbid diagnoses are mood, anxiety, and substance use disorders. The co-occurrence of PTSD with traumatic brain injury is also problematic because there is a significant overlap of symptoms to include problems with memory, concentration, irritability, and insomnia [10].

Similarly, PTSD-related symptoms can be shared with or misinterpreted to be secondary to other mental disorders. For example, specific phobia, agoraphobia, and PTSD share a psychological and physiological response to exposure to cues resulting in avoidance behaviors. Anhedonia, social isolation, restricted emotional range, insomnia, difficulty concentrating, and excessive guilt are common symptoms of both PTSD and depression, making it difficult to distinguish the two disorders. PTSD flashbacks may also mimic hallucinations secondary to a psychotic process. Given shared phenotypical presentations and overlap between PTSD and other disorders, it becomes important for the provider to understand the context and motivation for why symptoms emerge. For example, specific phobia and PTSD share an irrational fear of specific objects or situations. Asking patients to explain the reason for their fear helps determine the diagnosis. In PTSD, individuals avoid certain objects or situations because they signify the traumatic event.

6.3 Treatment and Management

6.3.1 Selection Criteria

When selecting patients for PE therapy, specific selection criteria can be applied. Individuals should be chosen who have a diagnosis of PTSD, ideally with a major index trauma as the designated target of imaginal exposure. PE focuses on one event, the index event, even though the patient may have several traumatic events. This criterion appears to serve both cases of rape victims who suffer index sexual trauma and military combat trauma with a singular major violent event.

There are several exclusion criteria for patients who are not ideal candidates for PE therapy. Patients with safety concerns—suicidal or homicidal ideations and behaviors or self-injurious behavior within 3 months prior to treatment—are typically excluded from PE [2, 11]. Presentations characterized by unstabilized risk for harm to self or others may be better served by interventions targeting risk stabilization [12, 13]. Some literature suggests that patients with psychotic disorders are not ideal candidates for PE since there is an absence of intact reality testing and treatment could lead to negative outcomes [11].

There are also some criteria that are not exclusionary, but should be evaluated on a case-by-case basis. For example, patients with substance abuse and dependence could be receiving concurrent treatment with PE, as demonstrated in the case example [2, 14]. Ongoing alcohol use through its sedating properties can chemically inhibit the treatment of anxiety by preventing habituation, which is required to benefit from PE. Depending on the severity of symptoms, dissociation can also be a limiting factor in this form of therapy due to elevated levels of anxiety triggering dissociative symptoms.

6.3.2 Structure of Therapy

The structure of PE therapy averages 10 sessions that are 90 min in duration. The number and length can be modified based on the provider's or patient's needs and goals. In our case vignette, the patient participated in 60 min sessions due to practical clinical necessity and patient preference. More sessions were added since the patient's symptoms did not show a satisfactory response to treatment. However, before adding sessions, it is important to conceptualize the reasons for an unsatisfactory response, and to determine if extending the therapy will address those reasons. In this case, the patient's nonadherence to imaginal and in vivo assignments due to overarousal and the patient's lack of adherence to prescribed relaxation strategies may have contributed to the lack of satisfactory response. Given these reasons, modifications were made, such as writing the trauma memory instead of speaking it and revising the in vivo exercises by initially allowing the patient to be in the company of his fiancé. These modifications seemingly promoted greater treatment adherence and a satisfactory treatment response.

The first PE session is focused on understanding the trauma [2]. A detailed history is obtained in which the diagnosis of PTSD is confirmed. It also includes identifying the index trauma, a single distressing event to serve as the basis of symptom inquiry and focal point for PE. A rationale for treatment procedures is introduced, describing the overview of therapy, the time-limited nature of the sessions, and its ultimate long-term goal. The patient is also educated on relaxation techniques to include how the pathophysiology of hyperventilating produces bodily reactions that resemble fear. The patient is instructed that slow breathing, focused on exhalation, can reduce tension and stress. Deep breathing should be performed outside of treatment sessions at least three times a day for 10 min. Finally, a therapeutic alliance is established in the first encounter in order to serve as a basis of trust for future sessions.

In the clinical case, the patient chose not to perform relaxation breathing due to his belief that a relaxed state was threatening and he may be caught unprepared for potential emergencies if he became too relaxed using such techniques. The provider chose not to pressure him to adhere to the techniques in order to maintain the therapeutic alliance. Ultimately, this decision likely contributed to the initial lack of an adequate treatment response. In retrospect, the therapist could have spent more time addressing the patient's beliefs about the threatening nature of relaxation exercises. With more practice, he may have become comfortable with them and learned to challenge those beliefs, which in turn may have strengthened the therapeutic alliance.

In session 2, psychoeducation about common responses to trauma is provided. This discussion involves both eliciting the patient's reactions to trauma while normalizing and validating his or her experiences. Finally, instilling hope that these symptoms can improve other time can help further reinforce the therapeutic alliance and patient compliance with treatment. In vivo exposure is also introduced in session 2. The provider educates the patient about the role of avoidance in the maintenance of PTSD symptoms. In order to decrease anxiety, the patient has learned to avoid certain situations or activities.

There are generally three real-life types of situations that patients avoid: situations viewed as dangerous because the world is viewed as a dangerous place, situations that are reminders of the trauma, and situations and activities that the patient has lost interest in doing. The goal of therapy is to help the patient realize that when he or she confronts avoided situations that nothing bad or dangerous actually occurs. This acknowledgment helps the patient learn that the situation no longer needs to be avoided.

One misconception among many patients is that they believe if they remain in a situation, the provoked anxiety will continue at the same level. In actuality, the anxiety should decrease over time—called habituation—which should be explained to the patient. Ultimately, confronting these fears will help patients feel competent and enhances self-esteem. For example, in the clinical case described, the patient was able to drive himself again and go to public places like the mall, which decreased his feelings of guilt and thoughts that he was a burden to his family and increased his feelings of self-sufficiency.

To conceptualize how much anxiety the patient is experiencing, the subjective units of distress scale (SUDS) is used. The scale ranges from 0 to 100, with the latter representing severely debilitating anxiety that often manifests in physical symptoms. The patient may want to select "anchor points" of 25 and 75 to serve as benchmarks. These activities can then be compared with symptoms produced in each session and during homework assignments in order for patients to more accurately report perceived distress.

The therapist can then help the patient establish an avoidance hierarchy by asking him or her to create a rank order list of avoided activities and situations and describe their SUDS for each. Ultimately, the patient's initial score can be compared over time and at the final session of therapy to measure symptom improvement. The provider will give in vivo exposure homework to be performed outside sessions, in which the patient will attempt to complete these activities and log their SUDS score. Usually, homework assignments last approximately 30 min.

The therapist will help the patient select two or more activities within this avoidance hierarchy that the patient will have a high likelihood of being successful completing outside of the session. Activities that are initially selected are usually in the 40–50 SUDS range. In the case example, the patient selected to watch a war-related video and instructed to record his SUDS. At the beginning of subsequent meetings, homework is first reviewed and the therapist helps the patient process the outcome and meaning of these experiences. Avoidance of homework is usually addressed in a nonthreatening way.

In the third session, the theory behind imaginal exposure is introduced: to relive the memory repeatedly during and outside therapy sessions in order to enhance the patient's ability to process the traumatic memory and tolerate distress. Imaginal exposure is based on the principle of habituation. Through imaginal exposure, the anxiety to the traumatic memory reduces, there by decreasing avoidance of it as well. General benefits of imaginal exposure include processing and organizing the memory, emphasizing the difference between remembering and being retraumatized by a memory, habituation, emphasizing the difference between the traumatic event and similar events, and increasing mastery and sense of control. Imaginal exposure can be an area of significant avoidance, as displayed by the case example, due to its ability to significantly heighten anxiety.

For example, the clinical case had an index trauma of a gunshot wound obtained in combat. He developed the belief from this experience that the world is a dangerous place and something bad would happen if he allowed himself to go out in crowded public places or situations in which he felt vulnerable to attack, like shopping markets and in the car. Due to the heightened anxiety associated with these beliefs, the patient did not perform homework assignments and even had difficulty engaging in therapy in session as displayed by arriving late or preferring to talk about current life stressors rather than on PE exercises. Additional components of cognitive therapy could be considered in this type of presentation to address significantly exaggerated thought patterns post-trauma.

The provider should first describe the process of imaginal exposure before allowing the patient to attempt the technique during the session. The therapist instructs the patient to close his or her eyes in order to recall memories of the index trauma. These sessions are recorded with audiotape for patients to listen to after the session. Smartphones can be useful tools to record sessions since the patient can easily take the device home and listen to the recordings at any time. While retelling the traumatic experience, the therapist periodically assesses the patient's distress using the SUDS scale. The purpose of the exercise is for the patient's retelling to be repeated and prolonged, as much as the patient can tolerate. Each narrative should last 30–60 min. The therapist can inform the patient before starting the narrative that he or she may be asked to start over again after they are finished based on how much time remains in the session. The purpose of this exercise is to demonstrate to the patient that remembering the trauma does not lead to a catastrophic outcome and is not dangerous.

It is important to remember to provide supportive comments to help decrease the patient's distress during imaginal exposure. It can also be helpful for providers to comment on the habituation you observe during the session and compared to previous sessions. For homework, the patient is instructed to listen to the recording every day at home for 30–60 min.

In sessions 4–10, the therapist will continue to review in vivo and imaginal exposure homework from previous meetings and help the patient process the experiences outside of these sessions. Each session, the therapist will spend 15–20 min processing these experiences. The patient will also continue to perform imaginal exposure during the session with subsequent recordings of the narrative being viewed for homework.

6.4 Outcomes, Clinical Pearls, and Pitfalls

6.4.1 Literature

The premise of PE is based on learning theory. Through classical conditioning, a preliminary phase of fear acquisition results in neutral stimuli procuring the ability to arouse fear by their association with the unconditioned stimulus, or those aspects of the traumatic event that produce fear [15]. Peripheral stimuli could then acquire fear-eliciting properties through stimulus generalization and higher order conditioning [16, 17]. Normally, repeated exposure to memories and cues of the traumatic event extinguish these associations.

PE, based on learning theory, targets avoidance of trauma-associated stimuli through in vivo and imaginal exposure (conditioned stimuli) in a manualized manner. The recurrent exposure without the occurrence of feared outcome (unconditioned stimuli) is theorized to result in extinction and reduction in anxiety symptoms and disconfirms any erroneous beliefs which may have developed [2, 16]. While there is substantially less emphasis on cognitive interventions in PE as contrasted with cognitive processing therapy (CPT), PE posits that eventual cognitive restructuring likely results secondarily to the behavioral interventions [18].

Currently, the empirically validated therapies for PTSD. CPT , eye movement desensitization and reprocessing (EMDR), PE , and stress inoculation therapy (SIT) have been shown to effectively decrease PTSD-related symptoms [19]. The Department of Veterans Affairs/Department of Defense (VA/DOD) guidelines for PTSD strongly recommend that patients who are diagnosed with PTSD should be offered one of the evidence-based trauma-focused psychotherapeutic interventions that include components of exposure and/or cognitive restructuring or SIT [12].

Since there are several evidence-based psychotherapy options, it raises the question of how to match the best treatment for each patient. There is no compelling evidence yet to inform this decision. The VA/DOD guidelines (2010) recommend that treatment selection should be driven by clinician expertise and patient preference. Other authors have posited that treatment selection should be guided by individually tailored case formulation [20].

With regard to the idea for treatment matching, there is some preliminary data from a head-to-head study, which show that guilt, an associated symptom in DSM IV-TR and DSM-5, responds better to CPT than to PE therapy [21]. In this study, the overall results, however, were largely equivalent. CPT may prove to be a better match for those specific symptoms, given that CPT more explicitly targets changes in cognition. Alternatively, the head-to-head trial also demonstrated that PE led to reductions in negative alterations in cognition, despite CPT's relatively greater focus on changing negative alterations in cognition. At this point, there is not yet an empirical consensus to guide treatment selection.

In medical and social sciences, interpretation of differences in outcomes is challenging, particularly in small studies. One way to overcome this is by pooling data from multiple studies in systematic reviews and meta-analysis with corrections for design differences. A common statistical tool used to communicate in a quantitative way whether results are meaningful is effect size (ES). There are numerous recommended cutoffs for "clinical meaningfulness" for either a difference or an association between two groups. A good rule of thumb for data showing a group difference in social sciences is using the minimal ES estimate cutoff of $d=0.41$, with $d=1.15$ suggesting moderate effect and $d=2.70$ suggesting a very strong effect [22]. Hence, a study reporting ES of less than 0.41 would be less likely to demonstrate a clinically relevant difference. Another important tool for appraising the internal validity of primary literature is the use of intention to treat (ITT) analysis in therapeutic studies. ITT is a preferred design because all data including from those subjects who prematurely leave the study, or the control arm, are analyzed in order to reduce bias.

PE has been studied extensively in civilian sexual trauma and is noted to have a robust ES in that population with ITT analysis yielding an ES of 1.46 and those who completed all the sessions had improved ES of 1.92 [23]. The efficacy of PE in combat-related PTSD was unclear until more recently. One meta-analysis of PTSD treatment in veterans only included three studies, two of which were unpublished, using PE with a total of 53 subjects that showed a combined ES of 1.79 [24]. The same meta-analysis looked at several studies, including some controlled trials, and showed exposure-based therapies overall yielded an ES of 1.1 in veterans with PTSD.

The best evidence for PE in combat PTSD comes from a recent trial [25]. It was conducted among combat veterans with a heterogeneous population including females, and veterans from different conflicts including Vietnam, Iraq, Afghanistan, and the Persian Gulf with a total of 1888 subjects showing an ITT ES of 0.87 and among completers (N=1354) of 1.21.

Despite the robust results seen in these studies, implementation of PE in clinical practice continues to face barriers. One study reports only 6.3 % of veterans in the Veterans Affairs medical system receive evidence-based, trauma-focused therapy [26]. It is unclear what barriers prevent more clinicians from utilizing PE, but one hypothesis is that using a manualized therapy may be too resource intensive and appears unapproachable to clinicians.

In spite of the good effect size of PE in PTSD, the external validity in manualized therapies is unclear. Findings in efficacy studies may not be generalizable to diverse patient samples across different clinical settings, as evidenced by the need for numerous modifications in real-world clinical settings. Some efforts have been made to overcome this barrier by the implementation of smartphone applications and computer-based therapy programs that may be a more convenient and approachable option for clinicians since patients can use them independently. While there is some support for its use in depressive and anxiety disorders, there is still insufficient evidence for the use of computer-based therapy programs among patients with PTSD and may be an area of future research [27].

6.4.2 Clinical Pearls

When performing PE, there are several clinical pearls that are important for providers to remember. Although PE is a manualized treatment, it often requires flexibility and willingness to modify it in order to meet the patient's needs. For example, in this clinical vignette, the patient's encounters were reduced from 90 to 60 min. This was done due to practical demands of the clinic. His total number of sessions also exceeded the 10 recommended due to the severity of his symptoms and the patient's avoidance of some aspects of treatment.

At the same time, PE is a time-limited therapy with a central focus. Due to the severity and complexity of symptoms, the patient may need to access other resources in the future if he or she continues to require help. In patients with chronic multiple-incident traumas, it may be helpful to focus on one distressing memory, which is typically the worst memory, or index trauma. It is often found that the benefit of improvement on one memory typically generalizes to other traumatic memories.

When utilizing PE, even though it is not explicitly a cognitive therapy, it is certainly within the model to address any maladaptive beliefs using cognitive therapy strategies. Elements of cognitive therapy may be used to address the maladaptive beliefs underlying a patient's avoidance, particularly if these thoughts interfere with optimal treatment engagement and response [2]. In the case described, the patient avoided performing in vivo exposure assignments for several sessions because of the underlying belief that the world is a dangerous place and something bad would happen. Incorporating cognitive strategies with the patient in the clinical case helped the patient complete homework assignments and be more readily engaged during PE sessions.

Additionally, the patient's symptoms of panic proved to be a barrier for participating in in vivo exposure. The provider could have considered adding components of treatment for panic disorder [28], or considered a more systematized integration of treatment of panic attacks in the context of PTSD, such as in multiple channel exposure therapy [29].

There are some emotional states that may limit the effectiveness of PE [30]. For example, anger is often secondary to a sense of injustice resulting from the context of the trauma and is a common symptom of PTSD. It is hypothesized that severe and constant anger impedes activation of fear associated with the trauma. In such cases, it may be helpful to implement cognitive restructuring initially, such as identifying automatic negative thoughts and underlying negative schema, labeling cognitive distortions, and challenging maladaptive thinking, so that the patient can be able to elicit fear and anxiety while reliving traumatic experiences in exposure therapy.

Similarly, high levels of anxiety can decrease the effectiveness of PE by interfering with information processing. To benefit from PE, anxiety should be titrated to a tolerable level, which may necessitate a modification to standard treatment recommendations. In the clinical case, allowing the patient to keep eyes open or the use of short breaks helped control the patient's anxiety to encourage optimal engagement in therapy.

Commonly, the patient may be reluctant to attend and participate in sessions that focus on confrontation of distressing cues associated with their trauma. To help mitigate this difficulty, providers must be active and directive in encouraging the patient to attend the sessions, do homework, adhere to therapeutic instructions, and apply new skills. Alternatively, providers often do not encourage patients to go far enough due to the therapist's fear that such interventions may exacerbate symptoms and lead to patient dropout. For example, patients with anxiety disorders typically generate concerns that are unrealistic and irrational. Providers must carefully determine the extent to which the participant's fears are realistic and rational when the avoidance hierarchy is constructed and in vivo exposure homework is assigned. Using supportive therapy and reassurance can help enable patients to confront trauma-related material. Therefore, the therapeutic alliance becomes an essential part of treatment.

6.5 Conclusion

The goal of this chapter is to introduce PE therapy by using this clinical vignette involving combat-related PTSD. It provides an example of how PE can be applied in the behavioral health setting and highlights challenges when applying controlled research protocols to real-world cases and barriers to external validation of therapeutic research protocols. Despite these challenges, this chapter aimed to provide some direction for how to adapt such protocols to real-world cases. Ultimately, it will give therapists more treatment options, which will increase the chances of patient's access to the most efficacious treatments. Although PE is a manualized form of a therapy, It can be adapted on a case-by-case basis to meet patient and provider needs.

References

1. American Psychiatric Association. Diagnostic and statistical manual of mental disorders: DSM-IV-TR. 4th ed., text revision. Washington: American Psychiatric Association; 2000.
2. Foa EB, Hembree EA, Rothbaum BO. Prolonged exposure therapy for PTSD: emotional processing of traumatic experiences: therapist guide. New York: Oxford University Press; 2007.
3. American Psychiatric Association. American Psychiatric Association, DSM-5 Task Force. Diagnostic and statistical manual of mental disorders: DSM-5. Arlington: American Psychiatric Association; 2013.
4. Andreasen NC. Acute and delayed posttraumatic stress disorders: a history and some issues. Am J Psychiatry. 2004;161:1321–3.
5. Grieger TA, Cozza SJ, Ursano RJ, Hoge C, Martinez PE, Engel CC, Wain HJ. Posttraumatic stress disorder and depression in battle-injured soldiers. Am J Psychiatry. 2006;163:1777–83.
6. Andrews B, Brewin CR, Philpott R, Stewart L. Delayed-onset posttraumatic stress disorder: a systemic review of the evidence. Am J Psychiatry. 2007;164(9):1319–26.
7. Bradley KT, Killeen TK, Brewerton T, Lucerini S. Comorbidity of psychiatric disorders and posttraumatic stress disorder. J Clin Psychiatry. 2000;61 Suppl 7:22–32.
8. Scherrer JF, Xian H, Lyons MJ, Goldberg J, Eisen SA, True W, et al. Posttraumatic stress disorder, combat exposure and nicotine dependence, alcohol dependence, and major depression in male twins. Compr Psychiatry. 2008;49(3):297–304. doi:10.1016/j.comppsych.2007.11.001.
9. Stander VA, Thomsen CJ, Highfill-McRoy RM. Etiology of depression comorbidity in combat-related PTSD: a review of the literature. Clin Psychol Rev. 2014;34:87–98. doi:10.1016/j.cpr.2013.12.002.
10. Hoge CW, McGurk D, Thomas JL, Cox AL, Engel CC, Castro CA. Mild traumatic brain injury in U.S. soldiers returning from Iraq. N Engl J Med. 2008;358(5):453–63. doi:10.1056/NEJMoa072972.
11. Van Minnen A, Harned MS, Zoellner L, Mills K. Examining potential contraindications for prolonged exposure therapy for PTSD. Eur J Psychotraumatol. 2012;3. doi:10.3402/ejpt.v3i0.18805.
12. Department of Veterans Affairs. VA/DoD clinical practice guideline for the management of posttraumatic stress. Washington: Veterans Health Administration, Department of Defense 2010; 149–66.
13. Foa EB, Keane TM, Friedman MJ, Cohen JA. Effective treatments for PTSD: practice guidelines from the International Society for Traumatic Stress Studies. 2nd ed. New York: Guilford; 2009.

14. Back SE, Dansky BS, Carroll KM, Foa EB, Brady KT. Exposure therapy in the treatment of PTSD among cocaine-dependent individuals: description of procedures. J Subst Abuse Treat. 2001;21(1):47–54.
15. Mowrer OH. Learning theory and behavior. Huntington: R.E. Krieger Pub. Co; 1973.
16. Keane TM, Zimering RT, Caddell JM. A behavioral formulation of posttraumatic stress disorder in Vietnam veterans. Behav Ther. 1985;8:9–12.
17. Brewin CR, Holmes EA. Psychological theories of posttraumatic stress disorder. Clin Psychol Rev. 2003;23:339–76. doi:10.1016/S0272-7358(03)00033-3.
18. Resick PA, Monson CM, Chard KM. Cognitive processing therapy: veteran/military version. Washington: Department of Veteran's Affairs; 2007.
19. International Society for Traumatic Stress Studies. Effective treatments for PTSD: practice guidelines from the International Society for Traumatic Stress Studies. New York: Guilford; 2000.
20. Zayfert C, Becker CB. Cognitive-behavioral therapy for posttraumatic stress disorder: a case formulation approach. New York: Guilford; 2007.
21. Resick PA, Nishith P, Weaver TL, Astin MC, Feuer CA. A comparison of cognitive-processing therapy with prolonged exposure and a waiting condition for the treatment of chronic posttraumatic stress disorder in female rape victims. J Consult Clin Psychol. 2002;70:867–79.
22. Ferguson CJ. An effect size primer: a guide for clinicians and researchers. Prof Psych Res Prac. 2009;40(5):532–8. doi:10.1037/a0015808.
23. Foa EB, Dancu CV, Hembree EA, Jaycox LH, Meadows EA, Street GP. A comparison of exposure therapy, stress inoculation training, and their combination for reducing posttraumatic stress disorder in female assault victims. J Consult Clin Psychol. 1999;67:194–200.
24. Goodson J, Helstrom A, Halpern JM, Ferenschak MP, Gillihan SJ, Powers MB. Treatment of posttraumatic stress disorder in U.S. combat veterans: a meta-analytic review. Psychol Rep. 2011;109:573–99. doi:10.2466/02.09.15.16.PR0.109.5.573-599.
25. Eftekhari A, Ruzek JI, Crowley JJ, Rosen CS, Greenbaum MA, Karlin BE. Effectiveness of national implementation of prolonged exposure therapy in Veterans Affairs care. JAMA Psychiatry. 2013;70:949–55. doi:10.1001/jamapsychiatry.2013.36.
26. Shiner B, D'Avolio LW, Nguyen TM, Zayed MH, Young-Xu Y, Desai RA, Schnurr PP, Fiore LD, Watts BV. Measuring use of evidence based psychotherapy for posttraumatic stress disorder. Adm Policy Ment Health. 2013;40:311–8. doi:10.1007/s10488-012-0421-0.
27. Dedert E, McDuffie JR, Swinkels C, Shaw R, Fulton J, Allen KD, et al. Computerized cognitive behavioral therapy for adults with depressive or anxiety disorders. Washington: Department of Veterans Affairs (US). http://www.ncbi.nlm.nih.gov/books/NBK269001/. Accessed Oct 2013
28. Craske M, Barlow DB. Panic disorder and agoraphobia. In: Barlow D, editor. Clinical handbook of psychological disorders: a step-by-step treatment manual. 5th ed. New York: Guilford; 2014.
29. Falsetti SA, Resnick HS, Davis J. Multiple channel exposure therapy: combining cognitive-behavioral therapies for the treatment of posttraumatic stress disorder with panic attacks. Cogn Behav Ther. 2008;37(2):117–30. doi:10.1080/16506070801969088.
30. Jaycox LH, Foa EB. Obstacles in implementing exposure therapy for PTSD: case discussions and practical solutions. Clin Psychol Psychother. 1996;3:176–84. doi:10.1002/(SICI)1099087 9(199609)3:3<176::AID-CPP100>3.0.CO;2-1.

Virtual Reality Exposure Therapy for Combat-Related PTSD

7

Judith Cukor, Maryrose Gerardi, Stephanie Alley, Christopher Reist, Michael Roy, Barbara O. Rothbaum, JoAnn Difede and Albert Rizzo

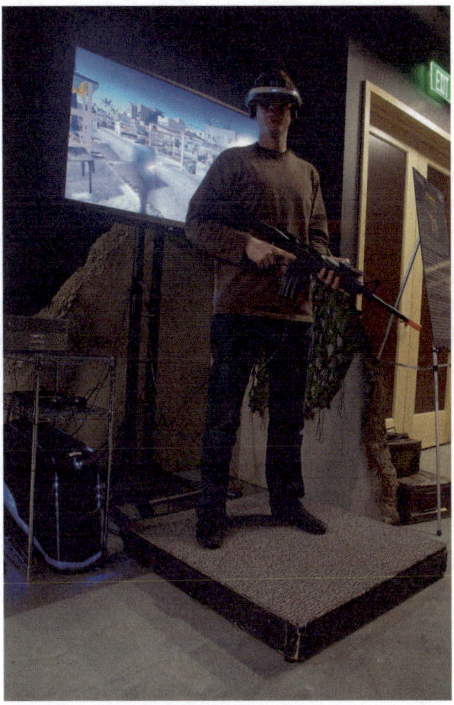

Courtesy of Albert Rizzo, PhD.

A. Rizzo (✉)
Medical Virtual Reality, Institute for Creative Technologies, Department of Psychiatry and School of Gerontology, University of Southern California, Playa Vista, CA, USA
e-mail: rizzo@ict.usc.edu

J. Cukor · J. Difede
Department of Psychiatry, Weill Cornell Medical College, New York, NY, USA

E. C. Ritchie (ed.), *Posttraumatic Stress Disorder and Related Diseases in Combat Veterans,* DOI 10.1007/978-3-319-22985-0_7

A virtual revolution is ongoing in the use of simulation technology for clinical purposes. When discussion of the potential use of virtual reality (VR) applications for human research and clinical intervention first emerged in the early 1990s, the technology needed to deliver on this "vision" was not in place. Consequently, during these early years, VR suffered from a somewhat imbalanced "expectation-to-delivery" ratio, as most users trying systems during that time will attest. Yet it was during the "computer revolution" in the 1990s that emerging technologically driven innovations in behavioral healthcare had begun to be considered and prototyped.

Primordial efforts from this period can be seen in early research and development that aimed to use computer technology to enhance productivity in patient documentation and record-keeping, to deliver cognitive training and rehabilitation, to improve access to clinical care via Internet-based teletherapy, and in the use of VR simulations to deliver exposure therapy for treating specific phobias. Over the past 20 years, the technology required to deliver behavioral health applications has significantly matured.

This has been especially so for the core technologies needed to create VR systems where advances in the underlying enabling technologies (e.g., computational speed, 3D graphics rendering, audio/visual/haptic displays, user interfaces/tracking, voice recognition, intelligent agents, and authoring software) have supported the creation of low-cost, yet sophisticated, immersive VR systems capable of running on commodity-level personal computers. Partly driven by digital gaming and entertainment sectors, and a near-insatiable global demand for mobile and networked consumer products, such advances in technological "prowess" and accessibility have provided the hardware and software platforms needed to produce more usable and high-fidelity VR scenarios for the conduct of human research and clinical intervention. Thus, evolving behavioral health applications can now usefully leverage the interactive and immersive assets that VR affords as the technology continues to get faster, better, and cheaper moving into the twenty-first century.

During the same time frame, dramatic geopolitical events in the form of terrorist attacks and war put a high-profile public spotlight on the effects of trauma on its human victims. For example, following the September 11 terrorist attacks on the World Trade Center (WTC), a significant number of persons were seen to be in

M. Gerardi · B. Rothbaum
Department of Psychiatry, Emory University, Atlanta, GA, USA
e-mail: brothba@emory.edu

S. Alley
Southern California Institute for Research and Education, Long Beach VA Medical Center, Long Beach, CA, USA

C. Reist
Department of Research, Long Beach VA Medical Center, Long Beach, CA, USA

Department of Psychiatry and Human Behavior, University of California, Irvine, CA, USA

M. Roy
Division of Military Internal Medicine, Department of Medicine, Uniformed Services University of the Health Sciences, Bethesda, MD, USA
e-mail: rizzo@ict.usc.edu

need of treatment for posttraumatic stress disorder (PTSD). This event provided an impetus for clinical researchers to develop and evaluate the use of VR simulations of the 9/11 attacks as tools for delivering trauma-focused exposure therapy to treat PTSD [1].

However, it was the onset of Operation Enduring Freedom/Operation Iraqi Freedom (OEF/OIF) and the subsequent need to provide treatment for the significant numbers of US service members (SMs) returning from the battlefront with traumatic injuries that drove an intensive focus on how computer technology could be marshaled to enhance, expand, and extend the reach of clinical care. The urgency of war led to substantial US government funding that served to foster innovative efforts in behavioral health technology. This increased US Department of Defense (DoD) and the Department of Veteran Affairs (VA) focus and funding support was dramatically seen in research efforts to study how VR technology could enhance the understanding and treatment of PTSD and comorbid health conditions. It is within this historical context that this chapter will discuss the approach to using VR as a method to deliver prolonged exposure for the treatment of PTSD.

7.1 PTSD Due to Combat Exposure

War is perhaps one of the most challenging situations that a human being can experience. The physical, emotional, cognitive, and psychological demands of a combat environment place enormous stress on even the best-prepared military personnel. Thus, it is no surprise that the stressful experiences that have been characteristic of the OEF/OIF combat theatres have produced significant numbers of SMs and veterans at risk for developing PTSD and other psychosocial/behavioral health conditions.

For example, as of December 2012, the Defense Medical Surveillance System reported that 131,341 active duty SMs have been diagnosed with PTSD [2]. In a meta-analysis across studies since 2001, 13.2% of OEF/OIF operational infantry units met criteria for PTSD with the PTSD incidence rising dramatically (ranging from 25 to 30%) in infantry units with the highest levels of direct combat [3]. During this same time period, the prevalence of PTSD among discharged veterans receiving treatment at VA clinics has been reported to be 29% [2]. These findings make a compelling case for a continued focus on developing and enhancing the availability of diverse evidence-based treatment options to address this military behavioral healthcare challenge.

7.2 The Rationale for Virtual Reality Exposure (VRE) Therapy

7.2.1 Prolonged Exposure

Prolonged Exposure (PE) is a form of individual psychotherapy based on the Foa and Kozak emotional processing theory [4], which posits that phobic disorders and PTSD involve pathological fear structures that are activated when information represented in the structures is encountered. Emotional processing theory purports that fear memories include information about stimuli, responses, and meaning and fear structures are composed of harmless stimuli that have been associated with danger and are reflected in the belief that the world is a dangerous place. This belief then manifests itself in cognitive and behavioral avoidance strategies that limit exposure to potentially corrective information that could be incorporated into and alter the fear structure. As escape and avoidance from feared situations are intrinsically (albeit, temporarily) rewarding, phobic disorders can perpetuate without treatment.

Consequently, several theorists have proposed that conditioning processes are involved in the etiology and maintenance of anxiety disorders. These theorists invoke Mowrer's two-factor theory [5], which posits that both Pavlovian and instrumental conditioning are involved in the acquisition of fear and avoidance behavior. Successful treatment requires emotional processing of the fear structures in order to modify their pathological elements so that the stimuli no longer invoke fear, and any method capable of activating the fear structure and modifying it would be predicted to improve symptoms of anxiety. Imaginal PE entails engaging mentally with the fear structure through repeatedly revisiting the feared or traumatic event in a safe environment. The proposed mechanisms for symptom reduction involve activation and emotional processing, extinction/habituation of the anxiety, cognitive reprocessing of pathogenic meanings, the learning of new responses to previously feared stimuli, and ultimately an integration of corrective non-pathological information into the fear structure [6, 7].

When PE is used for PTSD, the approach typically involves the graded and repeated imaginal reliving and narrative recounting of the traumatic event by the patient within the therapeutic setting. Although PE relies primarily on sensory memory and imagination, the exposure process is not passive. Patients are asked to verbally recount their trauma experience in the first person with their eyes closed, as if it were happening again with as much attention to sensory detail as they can. Using clinical judgment, the therapist might prompt the patient with questions about their experience or provide encouraging remarks as deemed necessary to facilitate the recounting of the trauma narrative. This approach is believed to provide a low-threat context where the patient can begin to confront and therapeutically process trauma-relevant memories and emotions as well as decondition the learning cycle of the disorder via a habituation/extinction process.

7.2.2 Virtual Reality Exposure for Anxiety Disorders and PTSD

VR can be seen as an advanced form of human–computer interaction [8] that allows the user to "interact" with computers and digital content in a more natural or sophisticated fashion relative to what is afforded by standard mouse and keyboard input devices. Immersive VR can be produced by combining computers, head-mounted displays (HMDs), body-tracking sensors, specialized interface devices, and real-time graphics to immerse a participant in a computer-generated simulated world that changes in a natural/intuitive way with head and body motion.

One common configuration employs a combination of an HMD and head tracking system that allows delivery of real-time images and sounds of a simulated virtual scene rendered in relation to user movements that corresponds to what the individual would see and hear if the scene were real. Thus, an engaged virtual experience creates the illusion of being immersed "in" a virtual space within which the user can interact.

The use of VR to address psychological disorders began in the mid-1990s with its use as a tool to deliver exposure therapy targeting anxiety disorders, primarily for specific phobias (e.g., heights, flying, spiders, and enclosed spaces). At the time, VR was seen to be capable of immersing an individual in a digital 3D graphic rendering of a feared environment, within which activation and modification of the fear structure was possible. Exposure was the first psychological treatment to use VR in part due to the intuitive match between what the technology could deliver and the theoretical requirement of gradual exposure to systematically expose users to progressively more challenging stimuli as needed to activate the fear structure. Moreover, even during the early days of VR, this was not so technically challenging to achieve. Virtual environments (VEs) could be created that required only simple navigation within a simulation where users were presented with scenarios that resembled key elements of the targeted fear structure that could be made progressively more provocative (views from tall buildings, aircraft interiors, spiders in kitchens, etc.). And even with the limited graphic realism available at the time, phobic patients were observed to be "primed" to suspend disbelief and react emotionally to virtual content that represented what they feared.

In general, the phenomenon that users of VR could become immersed in VEs provided a potentially powerful tool for activating relevant fears in the treatment of specific phobias in the service of therapeutic exposure. A growing body of controlled studies targeting specific phobias has emerged since 1995; two meta-analyses of the early literature concurred with the finding that VRE is an efficacious therapeutic approach [9, 10], and a more recent meta-analysis and a systematic review of this literature have expanded on the findings in this area [11, 12]. These initial reviews support the notion that VR is an effective tool for fostering therapeutic exposure within an evidence-based cognitive behavioral therapy (CBT) protocol to treat these types of anxiety disorders.

7.2.3 Virtual Reality Exposure for PTSD

In the late 1990s, researchers began to test the use of VRE for the treatment of PTSD by systematically immersing users in simulations of trauma-relevant environments. While the efficacy of imaginal PE for PTSD has been established in multiple studies with diverse trauma populations [13–15], it is reported that some patients are unwilling or unable to effectively visualize the traumatic event [1]. This is a crucial concern since avoidance of cues and reminders of the trauma is one of the cardinal symptoms of the DSM 5 diagnosis of PTSD [16]. In fact, research on this aspect of PTSD treatment suggests that the inability to emotionally engage (*in imagination*) is a predictor for negative treatment outcomes [17].

Similar to its use in treating specific phobias, the rationale for using VR as a tool to deliver PE for PTSD is clear and compelling. Clients can be immersed in simulations of trauma-relevant environments in which the emotional intensity of the scenes can be precisely controlled by the clinician to customize the pace and relevance of the exposure for the individual patient. In this fashion, VRE offers a way to circumvent the natural avoidance tendency by directly delivering multisensory and context-relevant scenes and cues that aid in the retrieval, confrontation, and processing of traumatic experiences. Within a VR environment, the hidden world of the patient's imagination is not exclusively relied upon.

The first effort to apply VRE for PTSD began in 1997 when researchers at Georgia Tech and Emory University began testing the *Virtual Vietnam* VR scenario with Vietnam veterans diagnosed with PTSD [18]. This occurred over 20 years after the end of the Vietnam War. During those intervening years, in spite of valiant efforts to develop and apply traditional psychotherapeutic and pharmacological treatment approaches to PTSD, the progression of the disorder in some veterans significantly impacted their psychological well-being, functional abilities, and quality of life, as well as that of their families and friends. This initial effort yielded encouraging results in a case study of a 50-year-old, male Vietnam veteran meeting DSM IV-R criteria for PTSD [19]. Results indicated posttreatment improvement on all measures of PTSD and maintenance of these gains at a 6-month follow-up, with a 34 % decrease in clinician-rated symptoms of PTSD and a 45 % decrease in self-reported symptoms of PTSD.

This case study was followed by an open clinical trial with Vietnam veterans [18]. In this study, 16 male veterans with PTSD were exposed to two HMD-delivered virtual environments, a virtual clearing surrounded by jungle scenery and a virtual Huey helicopter, in which the therapist controlled various visual and auditory effects (e.g., rockets, explosions, day/night, and shouting). After an average of 13 exposure therapy sessions over 5–7 weeks, there was a significant reduction in PTSD and related symptoms. *For more information, see the 9-minute Virtual Vietnam Documentary video at*: http://www.youtube.com/watch?v=C_2ZkvAMih8.

Initial positive results were reported in a case study by Difede et al. [1] for PTSD related to the terrorist attack on the WTC using VRE with a patient who had failed to improve with traditional imaginal exposure therapy. The authors reported a 90 % reduction in PTSD symptoms as measured by the "gold standard" clinician-administered PTSD scale (CAPS), and an 83 % reduction in depressive symptomatology as measured by the Beck Depression Inventory [20]. This research group later reported positive results from a wait-list-controlled study using the same WTC VR application [21]. The VR group demonstrated statistically and clinically significant decreases on the CAPS relative to both pretreatment and to the wait-list control group with a between-groups posttreatment effect size of 1.54. Seven of the ten people in the VR group no longer carried the diagnosis of PTSD, while all of the wait-list controls retained the diagnosis following the waiting period and treatment gains were maintained at 6-month follow-up. Also noteworthy was the finding that five of the ten VR patients had previously participated in imaginal PE with no clinical benefit, and showed a 25–50 % improvement following VRET. Such initial results were encouraging and suggested that VR may be a useful component within a comprehensive treatment approach for persons with terrorist attack-related PTSD. *For more information, see the Virtual World Trade Center video at*: http://www.youtube.com/watch?v=XAR9QDwBILc.

Initial clinical tests of the Virtual Iraq/Afghanistan PTSD VRE system have also produced promising results. Three early case studies reported positive results using this system [22–24]. In the first open clinical trial [25], analyses of 20 active duty treatment completers (19 male, 1 female, mean age=28, age range: 21–51) produced positive clinical outcomes with statistically and clinically meaningful reductions in PTSD, anxiety, and depression symptoms resulting in 16 clients no longer meeting PTSD criteria on the PCL-M [26]. These improvements were also maintained at 3-month posttreatment follow-up. Another open clinical trial with active duty soldiers ($n=24$) produced significant pre-/postreductions in PCL-M scores and a large treatment effect size (Cohen's $d=1.17$) [27]. After an average of 7 sessions, 45 % of those treated no longer screened positive for PTSD and 62 % had reliably improved. In a small preliminary quasi-randomized controlled trial [28], 7 of 10 participants with PTSD showed a 30 % or greater improvement with VR, while only 1 of 9 participants in a "treatment as usual" group showed similar improvement. The results are limited by small size, lack of blinding, a single therapist, and comparison to a set relatively uncontrolled usual care condition, but it did add to the incremental evidence suggesting VR to be a safe and effective treatment for combat-related PTSD.

Positive results from uncontrolled open trials are difficult to generalize and caution is necessary such that excessive claims are not made on the basis of these early results. However, the overall trend of these positive findings (in the absence of any reports of negative findings) is encouraging for the view that VRE is safe and may be an effective approach for delivering an evidence-based treatment (PE) for PTSD. Three randomized controlled trials (RCTs) are currently ongoing using the Virtual Iraq/Afghanistan system with SMs and veteran populations. One RCT is focusing on comparisons of treatment efficacy between VRET and imaginal PE [29], and another is testing VRET compared with VRET + a supplemental care approach [30]. One other RCT is investigating the additive value of supplementing VRET and PE with a cognitive enhancer called D-cycloserine (DCS) [31, 32].

DCS, an N-methyl-d-aspartate partial agonist, has been shown to facilitate extinction learning in laboratory animals when infused bilaterally within the amygdala ("fight or flight" conditioning center in the brain) prior to extinction training. Recent evidence of both VRET and DCS effectiveness has been reported by Difede et al. [33] in a clinical trial with WTC PTSD patients. In a double-blinded controlled comparison between VRET + DCS and VRET + Placebo, both groups had clinically meaningful and statistically significant positive outcomes, with the DCS group achieving statistically greater gains at 6-month follow-up. Significant funding support for these RCTs underscore the interest that the DOD/VA has in exploring this innovative approach for delivering PE using VR.

7.3 The Implementation of VRE Therapy for PTSD: Technical Development

In anticipation of the impending military behavioral health needs, the USC Institute for Creative Technologies developed an initial prototype Virtual Iraq VRE system in 2004 for running initial user tests to determine feasibility. This was followed by the creation of a full Virtual Iraq/Afghanistan VRE system developed during 2005–2007, funded by the US Office of Naval Research. This early version system was the product of both theory-driven design and iterative user-centered feedback cycles with OEF/OIF service members to maximize its ultimate relevance for clinical users. Preclinical user-testing was conducted at Ft. Lewis, Washington, and within an Army Combat Stress Control Team in Iraq [34]. This feedback from nondiagnosed SMs (and later by clinical users) has provided essential input for an iterative design process that has served to continuously evolve the content and usability of the clinical VRE system to the current day.

The 2007 system consisted of four customizable scenarios designed to represent relevant contexts for VRE: three Humvee driving scenarios within Iraq, Afghanistan, and USA-themed settings and a 24-block middle-eastern city that was navigable in a dismounted patrol format. General navigation for driving used a standard game pad and when interacting in the dismounted foot patrol, a thumb mouse affixed to a user-held mock M4 gun supported travel. The visual stimuli presented within an orientation-tracked *Emagin Z-800* HMD. Directional 3D audio, vibrotactile, and olfactory stimuli of relevance could also be delivered to users. Such stimuli could be controlled and modified in real time by the clinician via a separate "Wizard of Oz"-type clinician interface.

This interface is a key feature that allows clinicians to customize the therapy experience to the individual needs of the client. Using the interface, clinicians can place users in various VR scenario locations that resemble the settings in which the client's trauma-relevant events had occurred. Ambient lighting and sound conditions can be modified to match the client's description of their experience and the clinician can then gradually introduce and control real-time trigger stimuli (e.g., gunfire, explosions, and insurgent attacks). This level of clinician control is required to foster the anxiety modulation needed for therapeutic exposure and emotional processing in a fashion customized to the client's past experience and treatment progress. The use of a VR HMD to immerse the user within these controlled stimulus environments is believed to help support user engagement with typically avoided trauma-relevant experiences as required to activate the emotions needed for therapeutic exposure to occur. This system was disseminated to over 60 early-adopter clinical sites (e.g., VA Medical Centers, military, university, and private clinics) for use as a tool to deliver PE and to collect outcome data as to its effectiveness.

In 2011, the US Army funded the development of an updated and expanded version of the Virtual Iraq/Afghanistan system. Now referred to as *BRAVEMIND*, one of the primary goals for this effort was to increase the diversity of the VR scenario content and improve the customizability of stimulus delivery to better address the needs of clinical users who have had a diverse range of trauma experiences. This effort was supported by drawing on the vast amount of user feedback generated from both clients' and clinicians' feedback from use of the previous 2007 VRE system. The system was rebuilt from the ground up using the state-of-the-art current software. The 4 original 2007 environments have been completely rebuilt and 10 additional scenarios have been added for a total of 14, including separate Iraq and Afghanistan cities, a rural Afghan village, an industrial zone, a roadway checkpoint, slum and high-end residential areas, a mountainous forward operating base, and a Bagram Air Force Base setting. New features include selectable Humvee/MRAP/Helicopter vehicles, vehicle-to-foot patrol transitioning, expanded weather and time of day controls, customizable sound trigger profiles, and an updated clinical interface designed with clinician feedback to enhance usability. The system was also designed to use off-the-shelf components with the aim to reduce equipment costs to under $5000 and a detailed equipment/software manual is available from the last author. *For more information, see the Virtual Iraq/Afghanistan BRAVEMIND video at*: https://www.youtube.com/watch?v=nrgUPVFY44o.

7.4 The Implementation of VRE Therapy for PTSD: Clinical Delivery

7.4.1 General VRE Treatment Procedures

The VRE treatment procedure follows the standard evidence-based protocol for "imagination-only" PE therapy [35] and consists of weekly, 90–120 min individualized and patient-driven sessions over approximately 10 weeks. During the first session, the clinician generally aims to develop a working therapeutic alliance with the patient as is standard for most clinical approaches. The clinician may attempt to identify and discuss some of the patient's trauma experiences, provide psychoeducation on trauma and PTSD, and present instruction on a deep breathing technique for general stress management purposes. Session 2 follows up on topics from session 1 as needed and then focuses on providing the patient with a clear explanation and rationale for PE. In some cases, the patient is engaged in light practice with imaginal exposure that focuses on less provocative elements of their trauma experience.

In session 3, the rationale for VRET is introduced and the patient engages in a personally relevant area of the simulation environment, usually while recounting the trauma narrative for approximately 30 min, with no provocative trigger stimuli introduced. The purpose of this is to allow the participant to learn how to navigate the system, and to function as a "bridge session" from imaginal alone to imaginal exposure combined with VRET. Sessions 4–10 are when the VRET proper is conducted with the participant engaging in the VR while verbally recounting the trauma narrative. The goal of this active exposure approach is for the patient to experience a moderate, yet manageable level of anxiety as they are encouraged to activate, confront, and process difficult trauma memories and emotions that they have typically avoided (and in some cases never discussed with anyone). When conducted in the safe and supportive clinical setting, at a pace that the patient can handle, anxiety typically habituates by way of a learning process referred to as "extinction." As this occurs, the patient is encouraged to further confront more provocative elements in the VR scenarios that the clinician can introduce in real time via the clinician control panel. The treatment also includes homework, such as requesting the participant to listen to an audiotape of their exposure narrative from the most recent session as a form of continual exposure for processing the trauma outside of the treatment setting. Assessment of PTSD status is typically done with a combination of self-report symptom questionnaires, structured interview methods, and sometimes active psychophysiological reactivity tests. A more detailed description of this system, PTSD assessment procedures, and the methodology for a standard VRET clinical protocol can be found in [36].

7.4.2 Virtual Iraq/Afghanistan Case Study

John was a 30-year-old army veteran of the war in Iraq. He deployed twice during his military service, and had been home for 3 years at the time of treatment. John was married with a young child, and attending school to learn a trade. He reported experiencing intrusive thoughts, especially at night when trying to fall asleep, nightmares, very strong startle reaction to any loud or unpredictable noise, irritable mood, impatience with a "short fuse," and tension and distance in his marriage. He also had some difficulty with concentration in school, and described being easily angered by the comments of fellow students who he saw as "clueless," sometimes resulting in him having to leave class. John was very avoidant of any situation he perceived as dangerous, such as being in crowds, and only attended mandatory events such as classes. He also kept a weapon at home, and was extremely vigilant when night fell. He acknowledged drinking too much, as he reported that it was the only thing that helped him stop thinking about events in Iraq and allowed him to eventually fall asleep. He reported being tired of hearing family and friends tell him that they are worried about him and that he is not the guy he was before he deployed. He came to treatment with the understanding that he needed to do something to keep his marriage intact, although he was ambivalent about the relationship, stating, "I just don't seem to care." He reported that he does not engage much with his daughter, and that he felt bad about that.

During the first session, John's symptoms of PTSD and their impact on his life were discussed, and the rationale for exposure therapy was explained, along with a description of the immersive nature of virtual reality exposure therapy. John was also taught a breathing/relaxation technique to use between sessions. He was asked to identify and describe his index (most distressing) trauma in detail in order to prepare for the VR therapy to follow. John had not spoken about the event previously, and was wary of doing so, but managed to follow through. The identified event occurred while John was driving the lead Humvee vehicle in a convoy going through a city area of Iraq, late in the afternoon on a sunny day. John described noticing the people on the street starting to thin out as he drove, and then an insurgent holding an AK-47 suddenly coming around a corner up ahead, holding a young woman in front of him as a shield. John kept driving, yelled out to alert others in the vehicle, hesitated briefly, and then shot the insurgent, also killing the woman. He recalled looking in his side view mirror as he drove, and seeing her lying on the street, receding in his view. The therapist later matched the most appropriate VR scenario and available cues to John's reported traumatic event.

John began the VR therapy seated in the Humvee driver position, feeling the vibration under his feet and using the controller to drive ahead down a Baghdad-like city street. Humvee radio sounds were introduced, and John described his thoughts and feelings in the first person as he moved down the street (e.g., beginning to suspect something was wrong as the crowd thinned out, feeling a sense of apprehension, and feeling his heart start to pound). He then described the sudden appearance of the insurgent, and this image was introduced. John continued to describe his experience of disbelief and then his training "kicking in" as he took action, simultaneously making a split-second decision around saving the hostage and taking the chance that the insurgent (and possible accomplices) would then take out the following trucks in the convoy, versus eliminating the threat. The sound of John's weapon was also introduced into the VR scenario. John's subjective units of distress (SUDS) ratings were monitored via a self-reported 1–100 level scale throughout his repeated recounting of the event. After going through the event multiple times, John then processed the experience, expressing exhaustion, surprise at all of the details he remembered as he went through the repetitions, and commenting on the realistic nature of the virtual environment leading him to feel as if he was "there, but safe here."

Subsequent sessions focusing on the "hot spots" of the memory allowed John to put the event in context, identify emotional reactions which were put aside out of necessity at the time, and realizing the complexity of the "no-win" situation he was placed in. He was able to both express and feel sorrow over the loss of an innocent life, and to acknowledge all of the factors that came together at that moment which were not in his control, especially the decision of the insurgent to place the woman's life in such grave danger. As he progressed in treatment, John was able to acknowledge the fact that his decision likely resulted in the saving of lives, and that he had done the best that he could in that moment. He began to talk with his wife about what was happening in treatment, and reported that she was feeling more included and more able to understand some of what he had been through. John also noticed a softening of feelings toward his daughter, which pleased him. Additionally, John reported improvement in his ability to sleep without nightmares waking him, and began challenging some of his fears around going to restaurants, movies, etc. At follow-up, John's symptoms continued to decrease in frequency and intensity, and he reported improved ability to be comfortable in public situations.

7.5 Conclusions

Interest in using VR technology to deliver exposure therapy for PTSD has grown in recent years as positive outcomes have been reported with its initial implementation. When clinicians were surveyed as to interventions predicted to increase in the next decade, VR ranked 4th out of 45 options with other computer-supported methods occupying 4 out of the top 5 positions [37]. VR for exposure-based treatment may have particular appeal to clinicians in that it uses the latest advances in human–computer interaction to deliver consistent, controllable, and immersive trauma-relevant stimulus environments that do not rely exclusively on the variable nature and ultimately hidden world of a client's imagination.

VR also provides an objective and consistent format for documenting the sensory stimuli that the client is exposed to that can be precisely linked to physiological and self-reported reactions for treatment documentation and research. In addition to these functional stimulus/response quantification assets, the use of VR as a PE delivery system may also be found to break down barriers to care by improving treatment appeal, acceptability, and adherence by those in need of care. The current generation of young military SMs and veterans, many having grown up with digital gaming technology, may be more attracted to and comfortable with participation in a VR therapy approach [38] and this could lead to increased accessing of care by those in need. Thus, more research is needed to determine if VRE is perceived with less stigma by "digital generation" SMs and veterans relative to what they perceive as traditional talk therapies.

While it can be said that VR simply provides a novel and engaging mechanism for delivering an already endorsed, evidence-based approach (CBT with exposure), more research is needed to provide scientific support for that claim. Although the current state of the literature is promising (especially with the solid evidence for VRE effectiveness in the treatment of specific phobias), the existing research for VRE therapy with PTSD provides only preliminary evidence for its efficacy. Positive results from three published case reports, two open trials, two wait-list-controlled studies, and one small RCT have formed the initial basis for support thus far, but RCTs with larger sample sizes are still needed to provide confirmatory evidence for the efficacy of VRE with PTSD.

It will be important to conduct dismantling studies to better specify what elements of VRE are crucial for differentiating VRE from standard CBT exposure approaches, for improving the treatment, and for providing a better understanding of the mechanisms that may predict who this treatment may appeal to and who will benefit from it. Subject variables including gender, age, video game experience, number of deployments, and past trauma history may provide useful covariates to support better prediction as to who might benefit from what form of exposure. As well, research on variations from the standard protocol delivery of VRE in terms of the frequency and duration of sessions, the additive value of multisensory stimuli—i.e., olfaction—and the addition of pharmacological agents (D-Cycloserine) or CNS focused procedures (vagal nerve stimulation) could also be usefully studied for their impact on treatment outcomes within the controlled stimulus environment that a VR simulation provides.

Such clinical research efforts are now more feasible, with the rapid advances in the technology that have driven the recent availability of off-the-shelf VR equipment that is cheaper, less complex, and of higher quality than what was available just 2 years ago. Thus, it is likely that VRE interventions for PTSD will continue to drive novel research and address the significant clinical and social welfare challenges that exist with those who suffer from the experience of trauma.

Moreover, if one reviews the history of the impact of war on advances in clinical care, it could be suggested that VR is an idea whose time has come. For example, during WW I, the Army Alpha/Beta test emerged from the need for better cognitive ability assessment and that development later set the stage for the civilian intelligence testing movement during the mid-twentieth century. As well, the birth of clinical psychology as a treatment-oriented profession was borne out of the need to provide care to the many veterans returning from WW II with "shellshock." The Vietnam War then drove the recognition of PTSD as a definable and treatable clinical disorder. In similar fashion, one of the clinical "game changing" outcomes of the OIF/OEF conflicts could derive from the military's support for research and development to advance clinical systems that leverage new interactive and immersive technologies such as VR. As we have seen throughout history, innovations that emerge in military healthcare, driven by the urgency of war, typically have a lasting influence on civilian healthcare long after the last shot is fired.

Based on these examples, one of the outcomes of the OEF/OIF conflicts could be the military's support for research and development in the area of clinical VR that could potentially drive increased recognition and use in the civilian sector. However, this will only occur if positive cost-effective outcomes are produced with military VRET applications. It should also be noted that any rush to adopt VRET should not disregard principles of evidence-based and ethical clinical practice. While novel VR systems can extend the skills of a well-trained clinician, they are not intended to be automated treatment protocols that are administered in a "self-help" format. The presentation of such emotionally evocative VR combat-related scenarios, while providing treatment options not possible until recently, will most likely produce therapeutic benefits when administered within the context of appropriate care via a thoughtful professional appreciation of the complexity and impact of this behavioral health challenge.

For an extensive collection of videos on this project (simulation videos, patient interviews, media reports, etc.), the reader is directed to: http://www.youtube.com/watch?v=2wmM2aCZ3JAandlist=PLMuMO5eoYy_BDmAfZrFSLBLlniAtvAdad.

References

1. Difede J, Hoffman HG. Virtual reality exposure therapy for World Trade Center posttraumatic stress disorder: a case report. Cyberpsychol Behav. 2002;5(6):529–35.
2. Fischer H. United States military casualty statistics: operation New Dawn, Operation Iraqi Freedom, and Operation Enduring Freedom. Congressional Research Service Report. December 2012;7-5700:RS22452. http://www.fas.org/sgp/crs/natsec/RS22452.pdf. Accessed 5 Feb 2013.
3. Kok BC, Herrell RK, Thomas JL, Hoge CW. Posttraumatic stress disorder associated with combat service in Iraq or Afghanistan: reconciling prevalence difference between studies. J Nerv Ment Dis. 2012;200(5):444–50.
4. Foa EB, Kozak MJ. Emotional processing of fear: exposure to corrective information. Psychol Bull. 1986;99(1):20–35.

5. Mowrer OA. Learn behaviour. New York: Wiley; 1960.
6. Bryant RA, Moulds ML, Guthrie RM, Dang ST, Nixon RDV. Imaginal exposure alone and imaginal exposure with cognitive restructuring in treatment of posttraumatic stress disorder. J Consult Clin Psychol. 2003;71:706–12.
7. Foa EB, Franklin ME, Perry KJ, Herbert JD. Cognitive biases in generalized social phobia. J Abnorm Psychol. 1996;105(3):433–9.
8. Rizzo AA, Buckwalter JG, Neumann U. Virtual reality and cognitive rehabilitation: a brief review of the future. J Head Trauma Rehabil. 1997;12(6):1–15.
9. Parsons T, Rizzo AA. Affective outcomes of virtual reality exposure therapy for anxiety and specific phobias: a meta-analysis. J Behav Ther Exp Psychiatry. 2008;39:250–61.
10. Powers M, Emmelkamp PMG. Virtual reality exposure therapy for anxiety disorders: a meta-analysis. J Anxiety Disord. 2008;22:561–9.
11. Opris D, Pintea S, Garcia-Palacios A, Botella C, Szamoskozi S, David D. Virtual reality exposure therapy in anxiety disorders: a quantitative meta-analysis. Depress Anxiety 2012;29(2):85–93.
12. Scozzari S, Gamberini L. Virtual reality as a tool for cognitive behavioral therapy: a review. In: Brahnam S, Jain LC, editors. Advanced computational intelligence paradigms in healthcare, 6, SCI 337. Berlin: Springer; 2011. pp. 63–108.
13. Bryant RA. Psychosocial approaches of acute stress reactions. CNS Spectr. 2005;10(2):116–22.
14. Rothbaum BO, Schwartz A. Exposure therapy for posttraumatic stress disorder. Am J Psychother. 2002;56:59–75.
15. Van Etten ML, Taylor S. Comparative efficacy of treatments of posttraumatic stress disorder: an empirical review. JAMA. 1998;268:633–8.
16. American Psychiatric Association, editor. Diagnostic and statistical manual of mental disorders (Revised 5th editor). Washington, DC: American Psychiatric Association; 2012.
17. Jaycox LH, Foa EB, Morral AR. Influence of emotional engagement and habituation on exposure therapy for PTSD. J Consult Clin Psychol. 1998;66:186–92.
18. Rothbaum BO, Hodges L, Ready D, Graap K, Alarcon R. Virtual reality exposure therapy for Vietnam veterans with posttraumatic stress disorder. J Clin Psychiatry. 2001;62:617–22.
19. Rothbaum BO, Hodges LF. The use of virtual reality exposure in the treatment of anxiety disorders. Behav Modif. 1999;23:507–25.
20. Beck AT, Steer RA, Brown GK. Manual for the beck depression inventory-II. San Antonio: Psychological Corporation; 1996.
21. Difede J, Cukor J, Jayasinghe N, et al. Virtual reality exposure therapy for the treatment of posttraumatic stress disorder following September 11, 2001. J Clin Psychiatry. 2007;68(11):1639–47.
22. Gerardi M, Rothbaum BO, Ressler K, Heekin M, Rizzo AA. Virtual reality exposure therapy using a virtual Iraq: case report. J Trauma Stress. 2008;21(2):209–13.
23. Reger G, Gahm G. Virtual reality exposure therapy for active duty soldiers. J Clin Psychol. 2008;64:940–6.
24. Rizzo AA, Graap K, Mclay RN, et al. Initial case reports from a VR exposure therapy application for combat-related post traumatic stress disorder. IEEE XPlore Virtual Rehabilitation International Conference; 2007. pp. 124–30.
25. Rizzo A, Difede J, Rothbaum BO, Reger G. Virtual Iraq/Afghanistan: development and early evaluation of a virtual reality exposure therapy system for combat-related PTSD. Ann N Y Acad Sci. 2010;1208:114–25.
26. Blanchard EB, Jones-Alexander J, Buckley TC, Forneris CA. Psychometric properties of the PTSD Checklist (PCL). Behav Res Ther. 1996;34(8):669–73.
27. Reger GM, Holloway KM, Rothbaum BO, Difede J, Rizzo AA, Gahm GA. Effectiveness of virtual reality exposure therapy for active duty soldiers in a military mental health clinic. J Trauma Stress. 2011;24(1):93–6.

28. McLay RN, Wood DP, Webb-Murphy JA, et al. A randomized, controlled trial of virtual reality exposure therapy for Posttraumatic stress disorder in active duty service members with combat-related Posttraumatic stress disorder. Cyberpsychol Behav Soc Netw. 2011;14:223–9.
29. Reger G, Gahm G. Comparing virtual reality exposure therapy to prolonged exposure. Randomized Controlled Trial: 2010. http://www.bmedreport.com/archives/25530. Accessed 19 Aug 2015.
30. Beidel DC, Frueh BC, Uhde TW. Trauma management therapy for OIF/OEF Veterans. Department of Defense United States Army Military Operational Medical Research Program: 2010. http://www.psych.ucf.edu/faculty_beidel.php. Accessed 19 Aug 2015.
31. Difede J, Rothbaum BO, Rizzo A. Enhancing exposure therapy for PTSD: virtual reality and imaginal exposure with a cognitive enhancer. Randomized Controlled Trial: 2010–2015. http://clinicaltrials.gov/ct2/show/NCT01352637. Accessed 19 Aug 2015.
32. Rothbaum BO, Ressler KJ. D-cycloserine and virtual reality exposure to treat Iraq war Veterans with TSD: 2008. http://clinicaltrials.gov/ct2/show/NCT00356278?term=Barbara+Rothbaum&rank=4.
33. Difede J, Cukor J, Wyka K, et al. D-cycloserine augmentation of exposure therapy for post-traumatic stress disorder: a pilot randomized clinical trial. Neuropsychopharmacology 2013;39:1052–8.
34. Reger GM, Gahm GA, Rizzo AA, Swanson RA, Duma S. Soldier evaluation of the virtual reality Iraq. Telemed J E Health. 2009;15:100–3.
35. Foa EB, Hembree E, Rothbaum BO. Prolonged exposure therapy for PTSD: emotional processing of traumatic experiences, therapist guide. New York: Oxford University Press; 2007.
36. Rothbaum B, Difede J, Rizzo A. Therapist treatment manual for virtual reality exposure therapy: posttraumatic stress disorder in Iraq combat veterans. Atlanta: Virtually Better Inc; 2008.
37. Norcross JC, Pfund RA, Prochaska JO. Psychotherapy in 2022. A Delphi poll on its future. Prof Psychol: Res Pr. 2013;44(5):363–70.
38. Wilson J, Onorati K, Mishkind M, Reger M, Gahm GA. Soldier attitudes about technology-based approaches to mental healthcare. Cyberpsychol Behav. 2008;11:767–9.

8 Psychoanalytic Approaches to Treatment-Resistant Combat PTSD

Joseph E Wise

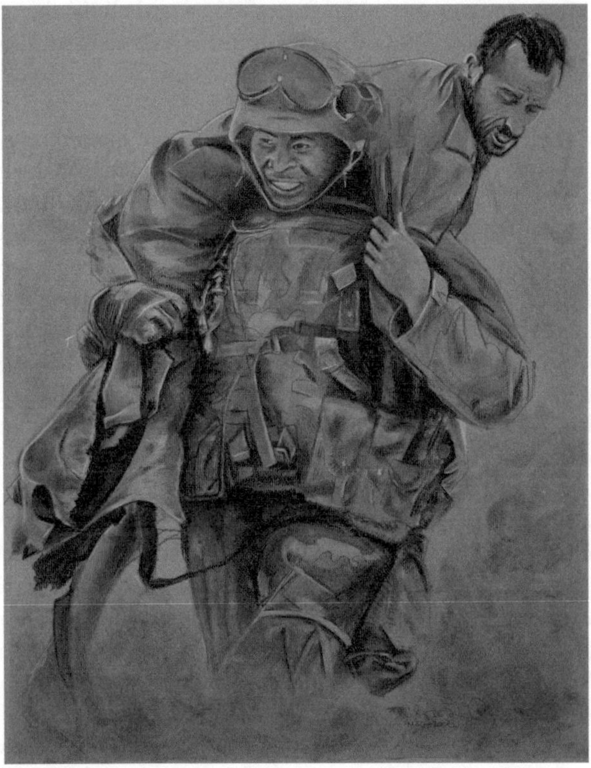

Brothers in Arms, by MSG Christopher Thiel, courtesy of the Army Art Collection, US Army Center of Military History.

J. E. Wise (✉)
Department of Psychiatry, Walter Reed Army Institute of Research, Walter Reed National Military Medical Center, 8901 Wisconsin Ave, Bethesda, MD, USA
e-mail: joseph.e.wise.mil@mail.mil

E. C. Ritchie (ed.), *Posttraumatic Stress Disorder and Related Diseases in Combat Veterans,* DOI 10.1007/978-3-319-22985-0_8

Since September 11, 2001 to the beginning of 2015, approximately 2.5 million service members have deployed in support of the wars in Iraq, Afghanistan, and related activities [1]. Early on in the current wars, surveys determined that an average of 15% of deployed soldiers had symptoms of posttraumatic stress disorder (PTSD) [2]. Additionally, many of those who screened positive for behavioral health (BH) symptoms were hesitant about getting care [2]. Moreover, those who were identified as having symptoms did not seek care in traditional ways or as a result of a positive screen [3, 4]. More recently, in active duty soldiers with PTSD, about half dropped out of care prematurely or got an inadequate number of sessions [5].

The historical connection between military and psychoanalysis runs deep. Notably, many of the early psychoanalysts were conscripted in World War I [6]. Freud experienced World War I personally, living in the capital Vienna and having his children drafted. It was partly due to these experiences that Freud elaborated on his theories. For Freud, trauma was when excitation overwhelmed the protective ego shield of the psyche [7, 8]. Moreover, the early analysts such as Sandor Ferenczi described cases of what would be considered PTSD, in modern psychiatric nosology [9, 10].

In World War II, many psychiatrists came back from the military expecting to apply psychodynamic concepts [11]. Across the Atlantic, the British psychoanalytic experiences in World War II were monumental. For example, Wilfred Bion and collaborators at Northfield Military Hospital developed what was to evolve as group psychotherapy and an understanding of unconscious forces in groups [12]. Fairbairn, as early as 1943, posited a "military neurosis" whereby a patient may project his internal object relations in the military organization [13].

For PTSD, the Department of Defense/Veterans Affairs (DoD/VA) Practice Guidelines identify psychotherapy with cognitive restructuring and/or exposure and selective serotonin reuptake inhibitor (SSRI) medications, as first-line treatment [14]. The American Psychiatric Association (APA) Guidelines, including updates, have similar recommendations but do recognize the need for psychoanalytic approaches as well [15]. Recognized manualized evidenced-based psychotherapies for PTSD include prolonged exposure (PE) [16], cognitive processing therapy (CPT) [17], and eye movement desensitization and reprocessing (EMDR) [18]. Core principles from these treatments include narration, cognitive restructuring, in vivo exposure, stress inoculation/relaxation skills, and psychoeducation [19].

Limitations of the manualized treatments include concerns that many of these were tested in civilian, not active duty military populations. Moreover, although generally efficacious for those patients who complete the protocol, there are a significant proportion of patients who drop out of the treatment. Many DoD providers self-identify as using evidence-based psychotherapies, but likely less than half report fidelity to the researched manualized protocol [20]. For those who cannot tolerate medications or do not respond to initial trials of psychotherapy (i.e., treatment-resistant), additional interventions are needed. As mentioned in the APA Guidelines, a psychodynamic/psychoanalytic approach may be helpful for these patients (here, the terms psychoanalytic and psychodynamic are used synonymously).

There is increasing evidence of efficacy of psychoanalytic psychotherapy in randomized controlled trials for a variety of psychiatric disorders. Milrod has demonstrated efficacy in panic disorder, where there was 73% response rate compared to 39% for a type of relaxation training [21]. Bateman, Fonagy, and collaborators, using mentalization-based therapy in the UK, have demonstrated good effect in borderline personality disorder (BPD), including in long-term follow-up [22–25]. Kernberg and collaborators with transference-focused psychotherapy (TFT) have shown efficacy, even compared to the well-known dialectical behavioral therapy (DBT) in BPD [26]. Gunderson, who developed "good psychiatric management" for character disorders, has shown efficacy with this approach, which is easily adaptable to routine psychiatric practice in many clinics, rather than specialized BPD units [27]. A meta-analysis for long-term psychodynamic psychotherapy (LTPP) showed superior efficacy, especially in patients with complex mental disorders [28]. Gerber and colleagues reviewed trials from 1974 to 2010 and found psychodynamic psychotherapy to having "promising" results and "mostly show superiority of psychodynamic psychotherapy to an inactive comparator" [29]. Finally, in a recent widely disseminated article, Shedler reviews the efficacy of psychodynamic psychotherapy, and he finds these psychotherapies to have effect sizes as large as those reported for other psychotherapies [30].

Psychoanalytic psychotherapies also seem to have a particular niche in treatment-resistant cases. The Austen Riggs psychoanalytic hospital has written extensively on this approach with patients who have not responded to traditional community interventions [31]. The present chapter focuses on psychoanalytic approaches in the situation of treatment resistance in combat PTSD. If symptoms can significantly mitigate by 12 sessions/6–12 weeks, with/without a medication trial of 6 months, then there is little reason to engage in more rigorous time- and resource-intensive therapy. As noted above, many patients do not respond to initial attempts of treatment or have complex comorbidities, and it is for this population that psychoanalytic approaches can be considered for the treatment of PTSD.

There is limited writing on psychoanalysis as an approach to PTSD from modern military operations. There is only one published psychoanalytic case, which was an approximately 3-year analysis of a Vietnam veteran, during which developmental trauma was linked with combat trauma [32]. Within the post-9-11 Global War on Terror (GWOT), Carr has published a few cases using psychoanalytic psychotherapy, especially highlighting the relational and intersubjective aspects [33–35].

The following account will (1) present a case, (2) describe the course of treatment, including outcome measures of complex treatment-resistant PTSD, (3) give two transcripts of actual sessions of psychoanalysis for combat PTSD, and (4) present a psychodynamic formulation with unique considerations for military patients. The conclusion summarizes the case and identifies areas for future research to further clarify the contribution of psychodynamic psychotherapies to treatment of PTSD.

8.1 Case Presentation/History

This case describes a 30-year-old male lower enlisted soldier in the combat arms with one GWOT deployment (material is used with his consent and identifying details/dates are disguised). The patient had no premorbid (pre-combat) treatment or identified BH conditions. He did have a comorbid gastrointestinal condition, which was diagnosed early in his military career, and this condition is often considered psychosomatic or at least significantly influenced by emotional stress. The patient, a married man, in his early 30s, is a self-described "country person" from a long line of "poor country people." He grew up in the rural South. He joined the army in his mid-twenties because he always wanted to be in the army and be a policeman, and the army afforded him the opportunity to do both. He said he would have joined the army earlier, but he had to take care of his family first. In so doing, owning a home at age 21, prior to enlisting, was one of the accomplishments for which he was most proud, and something that no one else in his family was able to do.

He was raised by his biological parents, who were married. His father was often unemployed due to the unpredictability of construction work. His mother worked as a secretary and provided stable income and "held the family together." He had a close family member of approximately the same age who had "some sort of emotional problems." The patient described frequent angry outbursts from this relative and emotional lability/affective instability, with which the parents were apparently frequently engaged.

After graduating from high school, he went to work at a warehouse. Soon after graduating from high school, his mother was diagnosed with colon cancer and died after battling the cancer with surgery and radiation/chemotherapy. He described how, growing up, he learned to tell the truth, keep his word, work hard, take care of the family, and respect others.

He had been in the army for 5 years when I saw him. His first duty station was outside of the continental US, where he worked in the military corrections facility for a year. He was then stationed for 2 years at a large army base in the Midwest. He reenlisted to be stationed at a post in the southern USA so that he could be closer to his roots. It was from there that he was deployed to the Middle East for a year.

Consistent with most complex treatment-resistant patients in the military, his course had several stages, including initial treatment from primary care manager (PCM), then walk-in BH, then being followed by a psychiatric nurse practitioner, a series of consults from a neurologist, my initial assessment, my initial psychotherapy, then psychoanalysis. The patient presented in early September 2012 to primary care with complaints of pervasive anxiety, hypervigilance in crowds, nightmares, sleep problems, and an upper arm tremor. Consistent with military programs to emphasize primary care screening and management of BH conditions (Respect.mil), his PCM consulted (via electronic communication) with the Respect.mil psychiatrist. The consultation was essential to start SSRIs and refer for specialist care. After 2 days of his PCM appointment and with his PCM's guidance, the patient walked in to "sick call." The "sick call" psychiatrist continued him on paroxetine (a medication FDA approved for the treatment of PTSD), and propranolol was added. Additionally, the provider referred the patient to neurology for his tremor, a definitive management in the BH clinic, and told the patient to continue follow-up in "sick call" while this was being arranged.

Due to demand for BH services and neurology, the patient was not able to be scheduled for another 2 months. My colleague, the walk-in psychiatrist, had three visits in the "sick call" clinic, during which supportive psychotherapy and attempts at adding adjunctive buspirone, prazosin, and buproprion were attempted.

By December 2012, 3 months after presentation, the patient had his first appointment with his assigned provider, a psychiatric nurse practitioner, who switched him to venlafaxine and continued supportive psychotherapy. These visits continued for the next few months. It was during the December-through-March time period that I learned of the case since I had the responsibility of reviewing the cases managed by the nurse practitioner. I worked with the neurologist to ensure completion of the brain magnetic resonance imaging (MRI), electroencephalogram (EEG), neurological exams, all of which were normal and showed no neurologic cause for the tremor. In an attempt at symptomatic treatment, propranolol was continued and primidone was added but were discontinued after a few months due to lack of effect on the tremor.

It was in early April that I, on behalf of the entire treatment team, contacted the unit commander since there had been some questions about duty limitations. He was essentially given a non-deployable profile, and his other duty limitations were formalized (the unit had—months ago—limited his work to administrative duties due to his "shakes"). At the patient's request, I also met him with his wife for a session, and she confirmed the various anxiety and PTSD symptoms and confirmed the time line of the symptoms, as being a change from baseline and starting during deployment.

8.2 Treatment/Management

Since I was already significantly involved, the psychiatric nurse practitioner and I agreed that he would terminate and that I would manage the patient, whose symptoms had remained basically unchanged since presentation. It was in early May 2013 that the patient and I had our first formal appointment (this was approximately 8 months after he had initially presented to our clinic). Since he had already experienced initial evidence-based psychopharmacology (SSRI) and supportive psychotherapy, I consider this as the point that he transitioned to a treatment-resistant category. Moreover, the neurologist had also shared the normal MRI, EEG, and exam findings with the patient and was ending care with a "non-physiologic" diagnosis. When I met with the patient in early May, I shared my discussion with the neurologist and that "anxiety might be contributing or causing this." The patient seemed to take this without much reaction. He was tacitly agreeable and accepting, but my impression was that the patient still held out that there may be a physical etiology for his tremor. The patient and I also noted that coming in seemed to be helpful for him as well as the venlafaxine, by now, 225 mg/d. So, I recommended that we embark on a more formal course of psychotherapy, and I would continue to monitor his prescription. I suggested that we meet twice a week for the next 6 weeks in a 12-session brief treatment and then make some decisions about the longer term at the end. Our scheduled 12 sessions ran throughout May and June.

Regarding the content of our twice weekly psychotherapy, it presaged the themes of the psychoanalysis. Psychotherapy themes included: coming from a family where not expressing emotions was valued; beliefs that angry emotions were necessarily linked with destructive actions; anger was adjudged as a "bad" emotion; significant resistance to combat discussion with anxious tearful affect and worsening tremor when discussing combat; he did connect his "stress" with his psychiatric and tremor symptoms; beliefs that he needed to comply with authority and sorting through interpersonal experiences to figure out what was wanted by authority, especially military authorities; controlling emotions was very important to him, and when he was not in complete control he feared becoming overwhelmed. The details of traumatic events from deployment were probed directly, but the patient was unable to elaborate much since the process of telling his story in detail generated overwhelming levels of anxiety (the transcribed sessions below do include some narration of traumatic events which occurred while he was deployed). Consistent with many combat veterans, the trauma often involves several demarcated events, but it also seems to be a cumulative experience of the deployment being traumatic in total. At the very least, this veteran had been on several patrols during which he perceived his life to be in imminent danger.

At the end of our scheduled sessions, with no remission, I felt like I could offer a proper military retention decision. I opined that he needed a medical discharge since he remained symptomatic despite full evaluation and treatment trials and due to the possibility of decompensation if he would to deploy again. With regard to the initial psychotherapy, manualized treatments, such as CPT or PE or EMDR, were not tried. Consistent with the treatment guidelines, our work did involve cognitive restructuring and elements of exposure in addition to narration, relaxation skills, and psychoeducation.

Since he got benefit from the psychotherapy (though clearly not curative), I recommended that we continue to meet starting the next month in psychoanalysis. This next phase is what I want to specifically highlight in a treatment approach for a treatment-resistant PTSD patient. I told him we would continue in ways similar to our recent meetings but that he would come in four times per week, lie on the couch, and speak aloud what was coming to mind. I also told him that I would be sitting behind him and probably ask less than he was used to in the therapy sessions. Regarding the technique, I saw it as my role, as an analyst, to set the psychological frame to allow the possibility of having his mental experiences symbolized with words, in the context of appropriate containment and psychological holding.

In order to demonstrate the process, examples of two back-to-back complete early psychoanalytic sessions are given below:

Session #35.
SEP2012.
P [patient]: Yesterday after I left here, I went and just stayed at home.
It helped not being around anybody.
I did a few things at the motor pool.
It's been quieting down.
But, I have my GI appointment. [Note his symptoms and their relationship to his psychiatric condition.]
And, I was so angry yesterday.
T [therapist]: What led to that?
P: Not sure.
I know that I did want the appointment, but I want to be by myself.
I want to be by myself, but I Skyped my wife and kids. [They lived about an hour away, and the patient would commute there on weekends.]
That's all I did yesterday.
I didn't want to do anything yesterday. It was a mood swing toward the bad.
T: Maybe there's a connection between what was going on and your mood. What do you think?
P: I don't know. What would it be?
T: Maybe one of the ways that you deal with the bad feelings is to isolate and withdrawal.
P: I want to be relaxed and not worried.
T: How is that connected?
P: It's the same thing.
Because I'm not worried, I'm more relaxed. More comfortable
T: Would you be more specific about the worries?
P: It's when I'm not alone. People around me.
I am watching their hands. I keep on guard.
It's about that they may be there to hurt me or my family.
It's just that being in a group; I'm worried.
I'm worried about myself.
Am I going to hurt somebody, when I don't need to?
T: Would you describe more about the worries about hurting somebody?
P: I might have another flashback.
I'm going to freak out.
I'm going to smash them.
Things I was trained to do downrange or as a police officer.
I'm uneasy.
When I'm by myself, I'm in control.
Otherwise in crowds, it's chaos.
T: You mentioned throwing people down, what do you mean?
P: Well, in the villages, while deployed, they would keep getting closer.
Sometimes you had to force them off, to the ground.
I don't want that to happen again, especially stateside.
I want to forget that part of my life.

I now have issues with trust due to the patrols.
T: Would you be more specific?
P: It was a lot of different things.
A couple of times we needed space.
[Local police] would be pushing them back. They would throw things, even without being attacked.
They couldn't do that.
It was so crowded in the villages: narrow passages, mud bricks, people lined in the alleys.
You would look up and there would be guys with guns on the roof—right above your head.
On the vehicle patrols, they would throw stuff at us.
We would sometimes give bags of chips and that sort of thing, but they would still be angry.
One time, some in the platoon left on foot patrol. There were just four of us left behind to guard the vehicles—hundreds of villagers.
And, we had another incident in the mountains.
Our lead truck slammed into something.
We needed parts.
But, all we saw was a cloud of smoke.
I didn't know if it was an IED [improved explosive device] or what. One guy got banged up and broke some ribs. The gunner was thrown around in the turret.
We had to wait on the QRF. [Quick Reaction Force]
I was in an open truck.
Then, they started to throw rocks.
I wanted to just start shooting. I didn't know if they would start escalating.
And, I can't keep track. And, they're gathering.
I don't like talking more about this, and people and the crowds.
[silence]
T: What feelings are being stirred?
P: Then, I had to stay calm.
I just tried to forget, and I would tell myself to stay strong.
Before you mentioned tears, but if I cry, then I would be giving up.
I'm not going to lose control.
I just want to forget.
It's in the past.
T: What do you mean by lose control?
P: I'm trying to keep control of myself.
I told myself that I would be strong during deployment.
If I had a problems, I told myself that I could make it through it without breaking down.
T: Yes, but, you're not on deployment now.
P: Yes, but I won't lose control.
T: I wonder about how showing emotion would necessarily mean losing control.
P: It means that to me.

T: How so?
P: Because I told myself that I wouldn't break down and crying is breaking down and breaking down is losing control.
T: Where, then, do all the emotions go?
P: I just want peace and quiet
T: Yes, we've been learning that the ways you deal is to be in a quiet place. But, I wonder if there are other ways?
P: For me, it's just quietness.
T: We have just a few more minutes in the session. Any other thoughts or questions?
P: No
T: Ok, see you tomorrow.

This session highlighted the themes of anger and his fears of getting overwhelmed by his anger. It also demonstrated his fears of his other emotional impulses. Both of these were dealt with, psychologically, by isolation, both in affect and interpersonally. The analyst's technique was significant for basically assisting the patient elaborate verbally on his thoughts and feelings. Technically, it did seem notable that there was a lack of transferential work in this session, other than the general containing and holding transferences of a patient sharing his emotional experience in the presence of the therapist. The lack of transference, in the traditional sense, where a patient relates to the analyst as a way similar to early relationships, and the internal conflict which gets lived out in this relationship with the analyst (transference neurosis) were never significantly clearly present in this case. Despite lack of transference interpretation, there is emerging evidence that non-transference interpretation may be just as helpful as transference interpretation [36]. Another notable technical point is how the patient's telling of his combat exposure resembled imaginal exposure (recounting combat memories in a controlled way) consistent with behavioral exposure therapies.

The next session:

Session 36.
SEP2012.
P: I have the scope scheduled.
He says it's straightforward [diagnosis of his GI condition].
He said mental things affect this.
And, that's probably the reason for my having more issues.
He suggested more fiber and to stay on the Bentyl.
It was a quick appointment—30 min.
T: What do you make of the statement about mental disorders affecting the body and your GI track?
P: My stomach is more screwed up, the more upset I get.
He also said to drink 8 glasses of water.
T: What do you mean by the more upset you get the more it affects your stomach?
P: It applies. I get stressed and worked up.
Regular people don't get upset like this. It's the stuff from deployment.

T: Yes, coping with deployment has affected your body.
P: The more upset I get the more pains in my stomach.
But it stays. It won't go away.
I go to the bathroom; nothing happens. No relief.
Sometimes I can't stop or it's diarrhea.
I don't know how it's going to happen.
It hurts.
The more stress, the worse it comes on.
I could even be at home, and I'm still in pain. But, it doesn't hurt as bad there.
T: It does seem that the more intense the upset feelings are, the more it affects your gut.
[pause]
How is it to talk about this?
P: I'm alright.
I've been dealing with it.
I watched my mom go through stomach issues.
I'm not afraid to talk about it. It's different from talking about deployment.
T: Yes, you've had some experience something similar in your family, with your mother.
[silence]
T: With the recent GI appointment, how did you make the decision to get the colonoscopy?
P: It's been since 2010. I need one every two years until I'm 40.
I'm uncomfortable about the colonoscopy but I have to do it.
My mom had a colostomy bag.
I go through it to avoid that. I had to go ahead and schedule one.
T: They're screening for the condition you mom had?
P: Yes, familial polyps.
And I take the Bentyl and fiber pills, that are over-the-counter.
I want it to be clean.
T: Do you have any hesitance with the colonoscopy and all of this?
P: Nobody looks forward to it, but it's got to get done.
I don't know of anybody who wants a camera up their butt.
I hope the results come back clean.
T: You have mentioned that before: "clean"?
[silence]
T: Have you finished the bowel prep?
P: I haven't eaten.
If it's not in the bottom, then it's not familial. They told me that it would be carpeted. [Referring to familial polyposis.]
The results should be in be Friday.
[pause]
T: Is your wife involved?
P: Not this time, but she normally is.
I took the laxative to clean it out.

I've been going.
It doesn't take much to get me going: black tea; apple juice.
I just need the enemas.
They're not giving me anesthesia.
T: No anesthesia?
P: Yes, I'm not happy.
I would rather not remember it.
With anesthesia, someone would need to take me home. And, I don't trust anyone, in my unit.
I've been made fun of. I don't want to be the butt of jokes.
I'll go in afterwards.
T: You won't get quarters?
P: Don't know.
T: Have you thought about asking the doctor?
P: I'm not that kind of person.
T: What do you mean?
P: I know I have a job to do.
And, they make you bring in the slip.
You still have to go in anyway.
T: Is it possible to call them and say that you bring the slip in tomorrow?
P: I don't want to tell them [his unit/chain-of-command].
They would make fun of me.
I'm not going there. They talk about me and my shakes and my PTSD.
T: Could you just tell them you had a doctor's appointment and that the doctor told you to be off?
P: I understand the chain-of-command. I can't tell my supervisor what to do. I don't want to be disrespectful. They will take it out on me.
I try to be polite, to step around it.
It seems to help out.
I'm not going to be disrespectful.
I'm polite, respectful; not a dick.
T: Maybe there's a middle ground.
[pause]
T: We have just a few minutes left in today's session. Any other thoughts or questions?
P: No.
T: Ok.

The themes of the content of this session were centered on how he could appreciate the psyche affecting his soma. Once again, the somatic seemed uncontrolled for him, and he significantly feared the lack of control. The presence of his military unit is noted in this material, but as a shaming and not supportive entity. His reporting lack of support from the unit was contrasted with his own beliefs in how he was striving to do the right things for the military. The idea of a bowel problem is especially noted in the context of this patient, with a primary relative who had died of gastrointestinal (GI) cancer. Additionally, the closeness and potential intimacy of the internal probes seem to be not considered but taken instead, by the patient, as simply a sterile medical procedure, which, to this author, seems related to the way he often approached the analysis. The lack of transference work, in a specific sense, was highlighted by the inability to address the question of how it might be to speak of these issues in the relationship with the analyst.

8.2.1 Outcomes/Resolution

The following chart indicates the PTSD Checklist—Military Version (PCL-M) scores during the course of the psychoanalysis (scores were obtained naturalistically, every few weeks, throughout the course of treatment; Fig. 8.1).

The following chart indicates the course of the Outcome Questionnaire 45 (OQ45) scores during the course of the psychoanalysis (scores were obtained naturalistically, every few weeks, throughout the course of treatment; Fig. 8.2).

In both cases of measurements, after 88 sessions of classical couch 4 ×/week psychoanalysis (not including pre-analytic psychotherapy and assessment), there was a general trend toward improvement. With a 20-point start-to-finish change, there was "reliable change" on the OQ45 [37]; with a 10-point change on PCL-M, there was "meaningful change" on PCL-M [38]. The one outlier higher score, on both measures, toward the end of the course of analysis was obtained directly after he had a meeting with his command, and this likely represented the anxiety related to his conflicts concerning authority figures. Given the conversion comorbidity and since this was a treatment-resistant case, in that he remained symptomatic despite initial psychotherapy and several medication trials, it was notable that there was

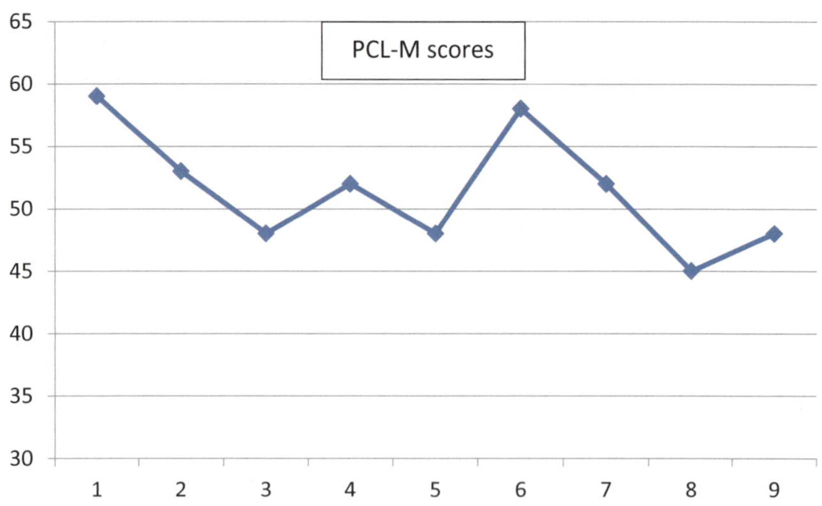

Fig. 8.1 Posttraumatic Checklist Military version (PCL-M) scores. (The x axis is the iteration of the scale administration, approximately every 3-4 weeks. The y axis is the PCL-M score value.)

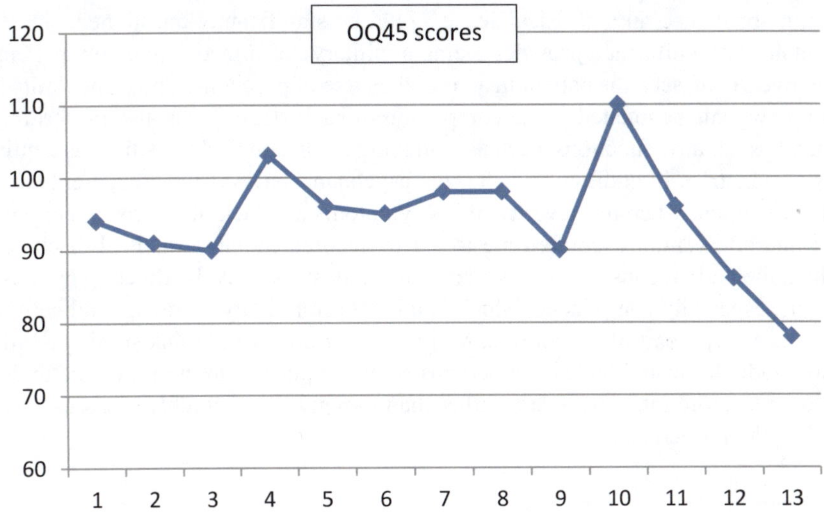

Fig. 8.2 Outcomes Questionnaire (OQ45) scores. (The x axis is the iteration of the scale administration, approximately every 2-3 weeks. The y axis is the OQ45 score value.)

any improvement whatsoever. The improvement seemed to have persisted, since at 1-year follow-up after treatment termination and leaving the military, he did report that his tremor "shakes" had diminished to basically not noticeable and that he was looking for a job but had not found one yet. He also remained married and had a new child. Additionally, after termination, he went for approximately 6 months with no treatment at all. So, in addition to the measures reported, the traditional psychoanalytic measure of health as the capacity to love and work demonstrated improvement or, perhaps, just turning the Freudian "hysterical misery into ordinary unhappiness" [39].

With regard to traditional psychoanalytic formulation, it might be suggested that the conversion symptom would be a compromise between his impulse to strike out and the reality of the dangers of doing so, which would make sense from the history and the material, though speculative for this short analysis. Specifically, he was extremely angry (out of his awareness/unconscious) with what he perceived was a self-interested company-level leadership, rather than believing his command showed genuine concern for his welfare during combat. In this case, he was unable to appropriately express his anger, for several reasons, including the reality of the hierarchy in military organization and his own parts of identity (mostly out of his awareness/unconscious) which valued compliance with authority. With regard to psychoanalytic technique, the patient worked in line with the "fundamental rule of psychoanalysis" [40]. Specifically, he came on time to four or five 45-min appointments per week, lay on the couch, and said what came to mind (or usually answered my questions, punctuated by silences). More importantly, I offered a safe place offering psychological "holding" [41] and containment for his experiences [42]. Some unique aspects of the analytic situation, due to the military environment, were that he always called me by my military rank. Additionally, my neutrality and abstinence, in a classical sense, could be significantly questioned, since I was a military uniformed provider seeing a military uniformed active duty patient. Moreover, I had seen the patient in an initial course of psychotherapy (time limited) with new goals negotiated at the completion of each stage. I was also performing general psychiatric functions, such as managing medication. My position, as a military psychiatrist, in addition to being his psychoanalyst, was most apparent early in his treatment when the severity of his symptoms and lack of improvement with first-line interventions required me to act by recommending a medical discharge (which the patient consciously favored). The analysis was likely affecting by these aspects, especially compliance, which is inherent in military hierarchy and culture and was a major part of his conflict. Moreover, in retrospect, I think starting a little more gradually would have been perhaps a better option to let him more naturally build up to more intensive work, rather than moving from monthly visits to twice weekly, then psychoanalysis.

8.3 Conclusions

This is the "talking cure," as first voiced by Anna O., the famous analytic patient of Freud's original collaborator, the internist Dr. Breuer [39], which is to say the treatment gave meaning in the midst of unmetabolized impulse, affect, and reaction to trauma. As I think about the case, it was somewhat a guided exploration of his unrepresented affects and bringing that material to verbal symbolization. Though this was an analysis, with the patient invited to "say what comes to mind" in free association, I found myself trying to gently guide the patient encouraging him to verbalize by asking questions, or having him elaborate, seeking clarification, or gently confronting, or occasionally making links. However, what makes psychoanalysis unique is the "remembering" in the form a transference and the ability to understand that and change in the present [43], which seemed minimal in this case.

For psychoanalytic treatment of PTSD, some of the healing is likely a very slow titration, in a mitigated form, with microlevels of anxiety from exposure, like behavioral treatment. In the PE protocol, the imaginal exposure is the retelling, and this is similar to analysis. Additionally, the in vivo element comes alive in the treatment frame in that the patient is coming to the office daily and the behavioral experiments become coming in and sitting in the waiting room. It seems to me that psychoanalysis is holistic and noninterventionist in a medical sense. It opens up the possibility of the patient using the psychological holding and containment of the treatment to heal naturally.

Beyond general efficacy, the cost-effectiveness of treatment-resistant PTSD is another area for future study. Economically, the cost of treatment is astounding as many treatment-resistant PTSD cases go to partial hospital or specialized inpatient treatment centers. The inpatient may cost up to US$1000 per day, with partial approximately US$500 per day (personal communication, 2014). The typical 30-day inpatient program for complex, comorbid, resistant PTSD can run upwards of US$30,000. My treatment is estimated to cost less than one third of that, with the added benefit of more naturalistic environment, such as staying in the milieu of the primary supports and no concerns for decompensation upon discharge from the hospital environment. In conclusion, it seems psychoanalysis is a valuable approach (combined with other interventions, such as SSRIs) in treatment-resistant combat PTSD cases.

8.4 Clinical Pearls

Although not rigorously researched as an independent treatment modality, psychoanalysis in the treatment of combat PTSD may include evidence-based elements such as narration, cognitive restructuring, exposure, and education.

Despite the patient being classified as being treatment-resistant, psychoanalysis can provide measureable relief to the patient.

Psychoanalysis can allow the possibility of the patient using the psychological holding and containment of the treatment to heal naturally.

The psychoanalytic approach can be cost-effective in comparison with inpatient programs for complex, comorbid, resistant PTSD.

References

1. Adams C. Millions went to war in Iraq, Afghanistan, leaving many with lifelong scars. McClatchy Newspapers. http://www.mcclatchydc.com/2013/03/14/185880/millions-went-to-war-in-iraq-afghanistan.html. Accessed 12 Jan 2015.
2. Hoge CW, Castro CA, Messer SC, McGurk D, Cotting DI, Koffman RL. Combat duty in Iraq and Afghanistan, mental health problems, and barriers to care. N Engl J Med. 2004;351(1):13–22.
3. Hoge CW, Auchterlonie JL, Milliken CS. Mental health problems, use of mental health services, and attrition from military service after returning from deployment to Iraq or Afghanistan. JAMA. 2006;295(9):1023–32.
4. Milliken CS, Auchterlonie JL, Hoge CW. Longitudinal assessment of mental health problems among active and reserve component soldiers returning from the Iraq War. JAMA. 2007;298(18):2141–48.
5. Hoge CW, Grossman SH, Auchterlonie JL, Riviere LA, Milliken CS, Wilk JE. PTSD treatment for soldiers after combat deployment: low utilization of mental health care and reasons for dropout. Psychiatr Serv. 2014;65(8):997–1004.
6. Gay P. Freud: a life for our time. New York: Norton; 2006.
7. Freud S. Beyond the pleasure principle. In: Strachey J (Ed. and Trans.), editor. The standard edition of the complete psychological works of Sigmund Freud. Vol. 18. London: Hogarth Press; 1955. p. 1–64. (Original work published 1920).
8. Freud S. Inhibition, symptoms, and anxiety. In: Strachey J (Ed. and Trans.), editor. The standard edition of the complete psychological works of Sigmund Freud. Vol. 20. London: Hogarth Press; 1959. p. 77–176. (Original work published 1926).
9. Freud S. Introduction to psychoanalyis and the War neuroses. In: Strachey J (Ed. and Trans.), editor. The standard edition of the complete psychological works of Sigmund Freud. Vol. 17. London: Hogarth Press; 1955. p. 205–16. (Original work published 1919).
10. Ferenczi S, Abraham K, Simmel E, Jones E. Psychoanalysis and the War neuroses. Int Psycho-Anal Lib. 1921;2:1–59. (London: The International Psycho-Analytic Press).

11. Plant RJ. William menninger and American psychoanalysis, 1946–48. Hist Psychiatry. 2005;16(2):181–202.
12. Harrison T. Bion, Rickman, Foulkes and the Northfield experiments: advancing on a different front. London: Jessica Kingsley Pub; 2000.
13. Fairbairn WRB. Psychoanalytic studies of the personality. London: Tavistock/Routledge; 1952.
14. VA/DoD Clinical Practice Guideline. Management of Posttraumatic Stress. October 2010.
15. American Psychiatric Association (APA). Ursano R, Chair. Practice Guideline For The Treatment of Patients With Acute Stress Disorder and Posttraumatic Stress Disorder. 2004.
16. Foa EB, Hembree EA, Rothbaum BO. Prolonged exposure therapy for PTSD: emotional processing of traumatic experience. Oxford: Oxford University Press; 2007.
17. Resick PA, Monson CM, Chard KM. Cognitive Processing Therapy, Veteran/Military Version (manual). Boston: National Center for PTSD; 2006.
18. Shapiro F. Eye movement desensitization and reprocessing (EMDR). 2nd ed. New York: 2001. Guilford.
19. Hoge CW. Interventions for war-related posttraumatic stress disorder: meeting veterans where they are. JAMA. 2011;306(5):549–51.
20. Wilk JE, West JC, Duffy FF, Herrell RK, Rae DS, Hoge CW. Use of evidence-based treatment for posttraumatic stress disorder in army behavioral healthcare. Psychiatry. 2013;76(4):336–48.
21. Milrod B, Leon AC, Busch F, Rudden M, Schwalberg M, Clarkin J, et al. A randomized controlled clinical trial of psychoanalytic psychotherapy for panic disorder. Am J Psychiatry. 2007;164(2):265–72.
22. Bateman A, Fonagy P. Effectiveness of partial hospitalization in the treatment of borderline personality disorder—a randomized controlled trial. Am J Psychiatry. 1999;156:1563–9.
23. Bateman A, Fonagy P. Treatment of borderline personality disorder with psychoanalytically oriented partial hospitalization: an 18-month follow-up. Am J Psychiatry. 2001;158:36–42.
24. Bateman AW, Fonagy P. 8-year follow-up of patients treatment for borderline personality disorder: mentalization-based treatment versus treatment as usual. Am J Psychiatry. 2008;165(5):631–8.
25. Bateman AW, Fonagy P. Randomized controlled trial of outpatient mentalization-based treatment versus structured clinical management for borderline personality disorder. Am J Psychiatry. 2009;166(12):1355–64.
26. Clarkin JF, Levy KN, Lenzenweger MF, Kernberg OF. Evaluating three treatments for borderline personality disorder: a multiwave study. Am J Psychiatry. 2007;164(6):922–8.
27. Gunderson J. Handbook of good psychiatric management for borderline personality disorder. APPI; 2014.
28. Leichsenring F, Rabung S. Effectiveness of long-term psychodynamic psychotherapy: a meta-analysis. JAMA. 2008;300(13):1551–65.
29. Gerber AJ, Kocsis JH, Milrod BL, Roose SP, Barber JP, Thase ME, et al. A quality-based review of randomized controlled trails of psychodynamic psychotherapy. Am J Psychiatry. 2011;168(1):19–28.
30. Shedler J. The efficacy of psychodynamic psychotherapy. Am Psychol. 2010;65(2):98–109.
31. Plakun E, editor. The Austen Riggs reader: treatment resistance and patient authority. New York: Norton; 2011.
32. Phillips SH. Trauma and War—a fragment of an analysis with a Vietnam veteran. Psychoanal Study Child. 1991;46:147–80.
33. Carr RB. Combat and human existence: toward an intersubjective approach toward combat-related PTSD. Psychoanal Psychol. 2011;28:471–96.
34. Carr RB. Two war-torn soldiers: combat-related trauma through an intersubjective lens. Am J Psychother. 2013;67(2):109–33.
35. Carr R. Authentic solitude: what the madness of combat can teach us about authentically being-with our patient. Int J Psychoanal Self Psychol. 2014;9:115–30.
36. Hoglend P, Amlo S, Marble A, Kjell-Petter B, Oystein S, Sjaastad MC, et al. Analysis of the patient-therapist relationship in dynamic psychotherapy: an experimental study of transference interpretations. Am J Psychiatry. 2006;163:1739–46.

37. Lambert MJ, Kahler M, Harmon C, Burlingame GM, Shimokawa K. Administration & scoring manual for the Outcome Questionnaire-45.2. Salt Lake City: OQMeasures; 2011.
38. VA. National Center for PTSD. Using the PTSD Checklist for DSM-IV (PCL). http://www.va.ptsd.gov. Accessed 14 Jan 2015.
39. Breuer J, Freud S. Studies in Hysteria. In: Strachey J (Ed. and Trans.), editor. The standard edition of the complete psychological works of Sigmund Freud. Vol. 2. London: Hogarth Press; 1955. p. 1–323. (Original work published 1895).
40. Freud S. On beginning treatment. In: Strachey J (Ed. and Trans.), editor. The standard edition of the complete psychological works of Sigmund Freud. Vol. 12. London: Hogarth Press; 1958. p. 121–44. (Original work published 1913).
41. Winnicott DW. The maturational processes and the facilitating environment. Int Psycho-Anal Lib. 1965;64:1–276. (London: The Hogarth Press and the Institute of Psycho-Analysis; 1965).
42. Bion WR. Learning from experience. London: Tavistock; 1962.
43. Freud S. Repeating, remembering, and working through. In: Strachey J (Ed. and Trans.), editor. The standard edition of the complete psychological works of Sigmund Freud. Vol. 12. London: Hogarth Press; 1958. pp. 145–56. (Original work published 1914).

Part III
Emerging Treatments

Accelerated Resolution Therapy

9

Wendi M. Waits, Kevin E. Kip and Diego F. Hernandez

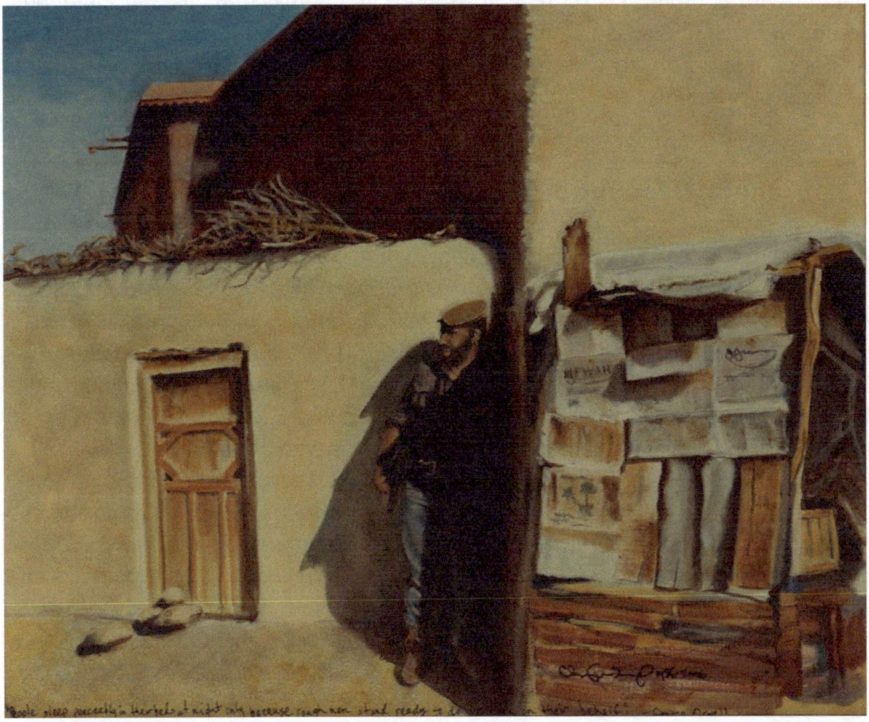

Masters of Chaos, by MSG Christopher Thiel, courtesy of the Army Art Collection, US Army Center of Military History.

W. M. Waits (✉)
Directorate of Behavioral Health, Fort Belvoir Community Hospital, Fort Belvoir, VA, USA
e-mail: wendi.m.waits.mil@mail.mil

K. E. Kip · D. F. Hernandez
College of Nursing, University of South Florida, Tampa, FL, USA

E. C. Ritchie (ed.), *Posttraumatic Stress Disorder and Related Diseases in Combat Veterans,* DOI 10.1007/978-3-319-22985-0_9

Accelerated resolution therapy (ART) is a relatively new therapy that includes many techniques for resolving the traumatic memories associated with posttraumatic stress disorder (PTSD). Preliminary evidence to date suggests that ART is highly effective, requires fewer sessions, and has a much greater completion rate than traditional PTSD therapies. A key difference between ART and other therapies for PTSD is that ART is an *internal process* that focuses on *images* rather than cognitions or feelings. This aspect is particularly important in a military population, since veterans are often not comfortable or legally permitted to share the details of their combat traumas due to their graphic intensity, potential association with war crimes, or inclusion of classified information. Herein, we provide a general description of the therapy, a summary of relevant clinical investigations, and present two cases that highlight the use of ART in resolving combat-related and early childhood traumas. The first case is of a fairly typical Iraq/Afghanistan veteran with complex PTSD related to multiple combat traumas and childhood abuse. The second case is of a different veteran's first ART session, demonstrating ART's unique ability to resolve long-standing, painful emotions such as shame and guilt very rapidly.

9.1 General Description

ART is an emerging, trauma-focused approach to addressing traumatic memories, as well as difficult and conflicted feelings that may be based on past experience. ART employs imagery, metaphors, and Gestalt techniques to help patients achieve reduction of their emotional symptoms and a self-directed resolution to their problems. Developed in 2008 by Laney Rosenzweig, it has primarily been studied at the University of South Florida for symptoms related to PTSD [1–3]. A summary of published literature on ART may be found later in this chapter.

ART is both therapist-directed and patient-driven. It consists of a basic protocol to address specific memories and events, as well as an advanced protocol to address more psychologically complex issues that arise within the context of the basic protocol. ART interventions are carefully scripted and designed to help the patient symbolically separate from a troubling past and advance toward a more positive future. While ART foundationally addresses traumatic memories, its design and structure permit its application in a number of other psychiatric syndromes and conditions, including generalized anxiety, depression, bereavement, and addictions.

9.2 Protocols

The basic ART protocol is designed to address singular traumatic experiences, as well as more basic fears and phobias, such as fear of public speaking and fear of flying. It combines imaginal exposure (IE) with smooth-pursuit eye movements to rapidly facilitate desensitization, imagery rescripting (IR), and stress inoculation [3]. Like more widely studied therapies for PTSD—including eye movement desensitization and reprocessing (EMDR), prolonged exposure (PE), and cognitive processing therapy (CPT)—ART relies on psychotherapy elements carrying an A-level recommendation in the 2010 Department of Defense and Veterans Affairs (DoD/VA) Clinical Practice Guidelines for PTSD [4]. The basic protocol is designed for discrete experiences and has the potential to resolve a traumatic event in a single session. Even particularly intense memories can be virtually disassembled and reorganized into a meaningful narrative in 1–5 sessions, with each session focusing on different scenes or concerns as they relate to the presenting problem.

The advanced protocol allows for a more detailed exploration of complex past events, unresolved developmental issues, and conflicted feelings, such as dreading the loss of a critically ill parent while simultaneously craving the relief one might expect at that parent's passing. It incorporates the use of metaphors and Gestalt techniques into the basic protocol, allowing deeper exploration of past experiences in relation to current affective and cognitive states. Rosenzweig describes these advanced techniques as ways to engage a patient's creative energies in more of a dreamlike state, where individuals are able to imagine and freely address thoughts, feelings, and sensations without the limitations of traditional talk therapies, and often in a less traumatic way [5].

9.3 Procedure

The ART protocol begins with exposure and desensitization. The patient is asked to identify the targeted memory and provide a score on a Subjective Unit of Distress (SUD) scale. Discussion of the trauma may be as detailed or as brief as necessary to establish rapport while generating a moderate degree of somatic distress. The patient is given permission to share as many or as few details as desired about the event, making ART particularly useful for memories involving classified, criminal, or intensely disturbing material. Focusing internally on the targeted event, the patient evokes the images, sensations, cognitions, and emotions he or she initially recalled from the event, or those that were generated by the exposure process. Once desensitized, the patient is able to explore the traumatic content more deeply, often yielding impressive new understandings and insights.

Initial exposure begins with the patient visualizing the targeted event (referred to in ART as a *scene*) while simultaneously being guided by the therapist in sets of eye movements. The exposure and desensitization process typically lasts between 5 and 20 min. During this period, any distressing images, sensations, thoughts, or emotions are targeted with the protocol to reduce their intensity. Simple and less complex experiences may resolve quickly, while memories that are rooted in earlier experiences may require additional interventions to resolve.

One such intervention is known as the *scene match*. Scene match addresses an earlier event that evokes thoughts, feelings, sensations, or images that are similar or somehow related to the targeted event. Any distressing component of the earlier event that is evident during IE is addressed using the ART protocol until the individual can recall the details of the event without experiencing distress. The IE and resolution of the patient's distress as related to the earlier scene is key to moving forward in the protocol.

The next procedural segment is called the *Director's Intervention*. The Director's Intervention accomplishes the critical process of rescripting the traumatic event. The procedure is directed by the therapist, but the new scene is self-selected by the patient, creating a very personalized resolution of the event. Rosenzweig calls this process "Voluntary Image Replacement," which refers to the imagining of a preferred, alternative version of the event in place of the original event [5]. This rescripting exercise allows patients to imagine themselves in a way that emphasizes a sense of mastery within or over the event. In other words, patients are able to metaphorically express their true wishes by visualizing a preferred scenario in place of the original targeted memory.

The subsequent procedural segment begins after the Director's Intervention, when the patient has finalized his or her preferred version of the targeted memory and is able to imagine the event differently while recalling the original narrative without distress. The images are changed while the actual memory of the event is retained in a narrative form. This segment starts with a test exposure to the original event (scene). Any remaining images, sensations, cognitions, or emotions are addressed until they are fully resolved, including scene matches to past or related events. The patient then processes future triggering events in a similar fashion. The emotions, sensations, images, and cognitions that arise when the patient visualizes future triggers are addressed using the same ART tools, permitting the patient to visualize positive but realistic outcomes.

The closing segment of a typical session includes a series of metaphorical interventions intended to help the patient completely resolve any lingering distress. The symbolic imagery evoked during this segment permits patients to visualize themselves taking charge of the past and consciously disposing of negative life experiences. The process helps generalize the resolution achieved during the session to previously untargeted stressors and traumatic memories. The patient often elects to bring significant individuals from their past or present life to a future in which they envision themselves no longer burdened by their present problem. This segment also provides a final opportunity for the therapist to identify lingering issues or alternatively for the patient to solidify a newfound sense of mastery over past traumas.

9.4 Description Summary

Through the use of IE and IR, ART targets the original memory in its entirety and promotes resolution of the associated sensations, cognitions, images, and feelings within a singular period of reactivation. However, ART goes beyond basic exposure therapies by attaching more positive, empowering, self-directed images, sensations, feelings, and cognitions to the event within the reconsolidation window, which bench research suggests may contribute to lasting change [6, 7]. The event's original content and narrative remains intact, but without the affective valence previously assigned to it, and often with more detail than the patient was initially able to recall.

9.5 Current Evidence Base for ART

9.5.1 Funding History

As of this publication, there have been seven funded research efforts related to ART. Of these, two have been federally funded and the remaining five studies are from a range of funding sources. Three of the funded studies are completed and four are in progress, but manuscripts and scientific presentations are being developed across all studies. Solicitation for additional funded research is ongoing and includes federal, nonfederal, and foundation sources. Table 9.1 below summarizes the funded ART research studies including purpose, sponsor, and a brief description.

9.5.2 Completed Study Results

For the three completed studies of ART, two have resulted in a total of five peer-reviewed publications to date (four data based and one case report). In the first prospective cohort study to evaluate the efficacy and safety of ART as a brief treatment modality for symptoms of PTSD, a total of 80 adults aged 21–60 years with symptoms of PTSD (mostly civilians) were enrolled, of whom, 66 (82.5 %) completed treatment and 54 of 66 (81.8 %) provided 2-month follow-up data [1]. ART was delivered in a median of three treatment sessions. Mean scores pre- and post-ART and at 2-month follow-up were: PTSD checklist-civilian version (PCL-C): 54.5 ± 12.2 versus 31.2 ± 11.4 versus 30.0 ± 12.4, Brief Symptom Inventory: 30.8 ± 14.6 versus 10.1 ± 10.8 versus 10.1 ± 12.1, Center for Epidemiologic Studies Depression Scale (CES-D): 29.5 ± 10.9 versus 11.8 ± 11.1 versus 13.5 ± 12.1, Trauma-Related Growth Inventory-Distress scale: 18.9 ± 4.1 versus 7.4 ± 5.9 versus 8.2 ± 5.9 ($p < 0.0001$ for all pre-ART versus post-ART and 2-month comparisons). No serious adverse events were reported. While this study did not include a control group, it provided empirical evidence of ART as a potential brief treatment modality for symptoms of PTSD and related comorbidities.

In a subgroup analysis of the above study, which consisted of 28 adults with high levels of comorbid symptoms of PTSD and major depressive disorder, subjects underwent a mean of 3.7 ART treatment sessions (range 1–5) [8]. For the 17-item PCL-C (PTSD checklist), the pre-ART mean score (standard deviation) was 62.5 (8.8) with mean changes of −29.6 (12.5), −30.1 (13.1), and −31.4 (14.04) at post-ART, 2-month, and 4-month follow-up, respectively ($p \leq 0.0001$ for comparisons to pre-ART score). Compared to pre-ART status, this corresponded to standardized effect sizes of 2.37, 2.30, and 3.01, respectively. For the 20-item CES-D measure of depressive symptoms, the pre-ART mean was 35.1 (8.8) with mean changes of −20.6 (11.0), −18.1 (11.5), and −15.6 (14.4) at post-ART, 2-month, and 4-month follow-up, respectively ($p < 0.0001$ compared to pre-ART score). This corresponded to standardized effect sizes of 1.88, 1.58, and 1.09, respectively. Strong correlations were observed at 2-month and 4-month follow-up for posttreatment changes in PTSD and depression symptom scores ($r = 0.79$, $r = 0.76$, respectively, $p \leq 0.0002$).

In the controlled trial of ART, 29 service members or veterans with symptoms of military PTSD were randomly assigned to receive ART, and 28 service members

Table 9.1 Summary of the funded ART research studies

Title	Sponsor	Status	Population	Brief description
Accelerated resolution therapy (ART) for rapid resolution of symptoms of psychological trauma	Substance Abuse and Mental Health Services Administration	Completed	Adults (mostly civilians) with symptoms of PTSD (n=80)	Prospective cohort study to evaluate efficacy and safety of ART as a brief treatment modality for symptoms of PTSD
ART for psychological trauma	Telemedicine & Advanced Technology Research Center (TATRC)	Completed	US Service members and veterans with symptoms of PTSD (n=57)	Randomized controlled trial of ART versus an attention control (AC) regimen for treatment of symptoms of PTSD and related comorbidities, with 3-month follow-up evaluation
Psychophysiological assessment of PTSD before and after treatment with ART	Charles Stark Draper Laboratory	Completed	Adults (principally civilians) with diagnosed PTSD (n=13)	Pilot investigation that applied psychophysiological assessment before and after treatment with ART to a selected sample of civilians and veterans with PTSD
Pilot study of delivery of ART by Scottish registered nurses in mental health for treatment of military psychological trauma	University of South Florida and University of Stirling	Ongoing	Veterans of the British Armed Forces with symptoms of PTSD (n=24)	Prospective pilot study to evaluate efficacy and safety of ART as a brief treatment modality for symptoms of PTSD among British veterans
Use of ART for women veterans experiencing posttraumatic stress disorder (PTSD) secondary to military sexual trauma (MST)	University of South Florida	Ongoing	Female veterans with MST and symptoms of PTSD (n=10)	Pilot study to evaluate efficacy and safety of ART as a brief treatment modality for PTSD secondary to MST
ART for PTSD and sleep dysfunction	American Psychiatric Nurses Association	Ongoing	Veterans with symptoms of PTSD and sleep dysfunction (n=15)	Pilot study to examine efficacy of ART for treatment of symptoms of comorbid PTSD and sleep disturbance
Prospective cohort study of ART for treatment of military psychological trauma	Chris T. Sullivan Foundation	Ongoing	Service members and veterans with symptoms of PTSD (n=200)	Prospective cohort study (n=200) to evaluate efficacy and cost-effectiveness of ART for treatment of symptoms of PTSD, with oversampling of MST and refractory PTSD

or veterans were assigned to an attention control (AC) regimen that consisted of two sessions of either fitness counseling or career counseling [2]. After random assignment, those assigned to the AC regimen were offered crossover to ART, with 3-month follow-up on all subjects. Mean age was 41 ± 13 years with 19% female, 54% Army, and 68% with prior PTSD treatment. The ART was delivered in 3.7 ± 1.1 sessions with a 94% completion rate. Mean reductions in symptoms of PTSD, depression, anxiety, and trauma-related guilt were significantly greater ($p < 0.001$) with ART compared to AC. Favorable results for those treated with ART persisted at 3 months, including reduction in aggression ($p < 0.0001$). Adverse treatment-related events were rare and not serious. This trial provided controlled evidence indicating that ART is a brief, safe, and effective treatment for symptoms of combat-related PTSD, including refractory PTSD.

In a secondary analysis of the above-described controlled trial of ART, type and magnitude of comorbid pain was assessed among 45 service members/veterans with symptoms of combat-related PTSD (24 assigned to ART and 21 assigned to the AC regimen) [9]. Mean age was 41.0 years, 20% were female, and most subjects (93%) reported at least some level of current pain. The majority (78%) used descriptive terms indicative of neuropathic pain, with 29% reporting symptoms of a concussion or feeling dazed. Mean pre-/post-change (standard deviation) on the pain outcomes questionnaire (POQ) was −16.9 (16.6) in the ART group versus −0.79 (14.2) in the AC group ($p = 0.0006$). Among POQ subscales, significant treatment effects with ART were reported for pain intensity (effect size = 1.81, $p = 0.006$), pain-related impairment in mobility (effect size = 0.69, $p = 0.01$), and negative affect (effect size = 1.01, $p = 0.001$). This secondary analysis provided controlled evidence of ART being able to acutely reduce concomitant pain among service members and veterans treated for symptoms of combat-related PTSD.

9.5.3 Ancillary Analyses (in Progress)

As listed in Table 9.1, there are multiple studies of ART in progress in addition to further analyses of existing data. At present, data collection and results are being compiled for future dissemination of the following outcomes in relation to treatment with ART for symptoms of PTSD:

- Comparison of pre- versus posttreatment response for psychophysiological measures of heart rate, skin conductance, and pupil diameter.
- Comparison of pre- versus posttreatment response for neuromarkers of sleep quality including electroencephalogram (EEG) measures of coherence and sleep fragmentation. In addition, actigraphy measures of sleep quality are being collected and will be reported in future publications.
- Assessment of ART treatment response in key military sample subgroups, including those with a history of military sexual trauma (MST), refractory PTSD, as well as handedness (strongly right, strongly left, mixed).
- Cost effectiveness analysis of ART versus current first-line evidence-based treatment for PTSD, including PE therapy.

9.6 Case 1

9.6.1 Presentation and History

The patient was a 44-year-old former Army E-6 infantryman who had completed one combat tour in Afghanistan in 2004, during which he was exposed to numerous battlefield traumas. He had never been seen before by behavioral health, citing concerns about stigma. At the time of evaluation, he was employed as a tattoo artist and lived with his wife, an active duty Army soldier. They had no children. The patient was referred for ART by his treating psychiatry resident.

9.6.2 Diagnosis and Assessment

The patient presented with classic signs and symptoms of PTSD: nightmares; intense physiological and psychological distress upon exposure to reminders of trauma; efforts to avoid people, places, and conversations reminding him of trauma; persistent self-blame about the loss of one of his soldiers; a persistently negative emotional state; a persistent inability to feel positive emotions; frequent angry outbursts; hypervigilance, exaggerated startle response; and extreme sleep problems.

On mental status examination, he appeared older than his actual age and wore casual attire that revealed extensive tattoos on all exposed skin except for his face. His muscles were tense, especially those in his jaw, and he appeared tired and agitated. However, his eye contact was good and he was polite and expressed motivation for treatment. He denied recent suicidal or homicidal ideation and had no history of suicide attempts.

9.6.3 Treatment and Management

The patient underwent a total of four ART sessions during a 5-week period. A summary of each session is as follows:

9.6.3.1 Session 1

The patient's presession PCL-C score was 72. A score of 50 is generally accepted as the cutoff, predicting PTSD with a sensitivity of 82 % and a specificity of 83 % [10]. He rated his anxiety at the start of the session as a 9 on a 1–10 SUD scale. He identified "guilty" as the prominent emotion he was feeling. He elected to process a combat scene in which he had been leading an allied patrol ordered to search a building for a "high value" enemy target. He had sent six squad members around to the rear of the building and had approached the front of the building with a seventh soldier. As the soldier stepped forward into the building, the patient had a bad feeling. When he tried to pull his comrade back, the latter was shot in the neck from above and died instantly.

While picturing this scene during the initial desensitization process, the patient became visibly upset. He was crying and breathing heavily, and at one point even shouted out loudly. In accordance with the basic ART protocol, the therapist then shifted the patient's attention to his bodily sensations, including muscle tightness, a "pounding" heart, a clenched jaw, and a feeling of "adrenalin" in his chest and hands. Following some basic instructions and sets of eye movements, the patient looked and reported feeling "calm."

Pearl A unique and critical aspect of ART is the requirement to extinguish strong physical sensations before pressing forward with processing a difficult scene. The therapist directs the patient's attention to either sensations or the scene in an alternating fashion, maintaining the patient's exposure to traumatic recollections at a tolerable level while minimizing distress.

The patient rescripted this scene by visualizing all of his squadmates enjoying a relaxing time at a "beautiful oasis" that included palm trees, a beach, and lawn chairs. To further inoculate himself against his typical triggers (e.g., facing his agitated wife after a long day at work), he also envisioned himself driving home and seeing his squad at the oasis, then arriving home calm and in a good mood. His SUD score at the end of session # 1 was 3 out of 10.

9.6.3.2 Session 2 (14 Days after First Session)

The patient's presession PCL-C score was 62. He identified "anger" as his prominent emotion and elected to process a recent intense argument with his wife, after which he had smashed his head through their bathroom door.

With the therapist's assistance, the patient successfully eliminated muscle tightness from his back, chest, and shoulders, replacing it with a sense of "calmness and relaxation." During the rescripting process, he chose to maintain the setting of the argument scene, but replaced the screaming match with a regular conversation. He saw himself using positive self-talk to stay calm and rational when his wife made accusations against him. No argument ensued; they took a shower together, made breakfast, and went shopping as they had planned. The patient reinforced this image by seeing it twice, then envisioned future interactions with his wife as being much more positive. He appeared very relaxed and reported feeling "pretty calm" at the end of the session. A SUD score was not elicited.

9.6.3.3 Session 3 (21 Days after First Session)

The patient's presession PCL-C score was 55, and he again identified "anger" as his prominent emotion at the start of the session. He elected to process another combat scene.

The scene involved a vehicle-borne improvised explosive device (VBIED) that was detonated by the vehicle's driver at a checkpoint in Afghanistan. The patient reported that "car parts and shrapnel went everywhere," and as the dust cleared, he encountered a young boy with a dark complexion who appeared to be dead but also seemed to be mouthing the word "Mama."

In changing the scene, the patient took control of the situation, sending his squad out to investigate the vehicle well outside of the gate, where they apprehended the driver before he could detonate himself. He also included women and children in his new scene. His squad mates moved them aside to a safe location and the young boy clung securely to his mother's skirt.

As commonly happens, image and sensory fragments or "crumbs" of the initial scene remained vivid. The patient had two crumbs during this session—the approaching vehicle and the dying child. He replaced the image of the vehicle with that of an American convoy and attempted to replace the child's image with a smiley face and the words "have a nice day." However, this somehow seemed insufficient, so he used another set of eye movements to give the child legs and see him standing confidently on the side of the road. An SUD score was not elicited.

Pearl This is an excellent example of how the most powerfully rescripted scenes involve the patient self-directing an alternative scenario and essentially "fixing" the problem as opposed to just putting a bandage (or in this case, a smiley face) over it. The patient applied this solution to future triggers by seeing himself walking around the ethnic neighborhood near his work studio without feeling anxious, and realizing that the dark-complected children who liked to wander into his tattoo parlor were not dangerous and were "just looking for candy."

9.6.3.4 Session 4 (37 Days after First Session)

The patient decided to process a scene involving childhood sexual abuse for his fourth ART session. He had suspected it would be his most difficult scene, and his presession PCL-C score of 77 reflected this anticipatory anxiety. He rated his distress at the start of the session as a 7 out of 10 on the SUD scale and identified "distrustful," "confused," and "powerless" as the emotions he experienced when thinking about the event.

The patient elected to share very little about the scene, only disclosing that his head was being forced into a pillow. He became quite tearful, experiencing tightness and "sadness" in his chest, pain in the back of his head, jaw tightness, and a feeling of "disgust" throughout his body. These sensations and feelings were decreased to a tolerable level using several sets of eye movements, which nearly eliminated all discomfort except the jaw tightness. At the therapist's suggestion, the patient was able to resolve this remaining sensation by using a metaphorical needle "with relaxing medicine in it" to help relax his jaw, and this relaxation persisted throughout the remainder of the session.

Pearl Suggestions, such as the one mentioned above, are a critical component of ART; they stimulate creativity and widen the breadth of solutions available to a patient. The therapist will typically provide one or two suggestions at a time, always ending with the phrase "or anything else you like," to emphasize the patient's control over the therapeutic process.

While envisioning his original trauma a second time, the patient realized that he had never told anyone about the abuse because the perpetrator had threatened to kill his mother and sister if he did so. This insight appeared to bring him significant relief. Later, the therapist used a Gestalt-style technique to ascertain if the patient had anything to say to his younger self, and the patient calmly related, "I told him I understand now." His SUD score at the end of the session was 2.5 and he reported feeling "calm."

9.6.4 Outcomes and Case Resolution

Shortly after session 4, the patient left his wife, moved halfway across the country, and was essentially lost to follow-up. However, 5 months after his first ART session, he emailed his therapist an update. He had been through a difficult time with his wife and their marriage was essentially over, but the patient was doing well. He wrote:

> On a brighter note, I am hanging in there. I have had ZERO PTSD issues since I arrived [here]. Even when [my wife] was screaming at me, hitting me, pushing me down a flight of stairs, and mocking me for attempting to get healthy… I stuck to the tools I was taught and maintained myself. Even as she was lying about me in court and on post, I maintained my behavioral health progress. I've had no PTSD incidents with my family or friends as well. I'm not saying it has been easy. I work hard every single day to avoid my triggers and stay positive no matter what is/has been thrown at me. I weaned myself off the meds [the psychiatry resident] prescribed about three weeks ago….I have had some minor issues sleeping but nothing I haven't been able to overcome…. Anyhow, I am alive and well. My life has been a complete nightmare until recently but I am persevering, surrounding myself with only healthy people, and staying optimistic.

He agreed to complete and return a final PCL-C inventory. His score was 26.

9.7 Case 2

9.7.1 Presentation and History

The patient was a 38-year-old married, mixed ethnicity male marine corps officer with 19 years' time in service (including 12 years of duty as an enlisted marine). He had heard about ART five months earlier while participating in a 28-day residential treatment program for alcohol dependence. However, treatment with ART had been deferred to maximize his participation in other planned therapies, beginning in the residential treatment program and continuing through a four-week partial hospitalization program, a three-week comprehensive traumatic brain injury (TBI) evaluation program, and intermittent weeks of individual outpatient therapy.

9.7.2 Diagnosis and Assessment

The patient's PTSD symptoms began as impatience and anger that emerged as he was recovering from a severe rocket injury to his left forearm three and a half years prior to evaluation. Over time, his symptoms developed into the full-blown PTSD syndrome, including intrusive memories of various combat traumas and traumatic losses, psychological distress upon exposure to reminders of these events, active avoidance of triggers, inappropriate self-blame, a sense of disconnection from family, irritability, difficulty sleeping, exaggerated startle response, and hypervigilance. He was also diagnosed with alcohol use disorder and mild TBI, but had been sober for more than five months at the time of his ART intake and was performing adequately in his job as a military school faculty member.

9.7.3 Treatment and Management

The patient had no formal behavioral health treatment until he self-referred for alcohol rehabilitation. During the ensuing five months, he participated in various substance abuse and trauma-focused treatments, including individual supportive therapy and EMDR, as well as group-based psychoeducation, peer support, relapse prevention, and graphic narrative therapies. Upon initial evaluation for ART, he expressed motivation to participate, but felt he had worked through most of his PTSD issues except for disrupted sleep and profound guilt regarding one of his marines who was severely wounded after the patient left theater. His PCL-5 score was 5. He rated his level of distress as a 1 on a 1–10 SUD scale.

9.7.3.1 Session 1

The patient chose to process a scene in which he hosted this marine—now a medically retired double amputee—at a marine corps ball. The feelings he identified at the start of the session were "shameful," "anxious," "insecure," and "confused." While thinking about this event, the patient reported having a slight headache and pain in the area of his injured left forearm. The therapist helped the patient eliminate both sensations successfully using the basic ART protocol.

As the patient "saw" his scene the first time, he reported feeling pain in his sternal area. With eye movements, this pain "moved up to the back of [his] throat." When subsequent sets of eye movements failed to decrease this sensation any further, the therapist performed a scene match.

Pearl Scene match is a powerful ART tool that permits rapid access to earlier life memories which may be contributing to present-day feelings and sensations. Using eye movements, the therapist helps the patient look back at his or her earlier life for another event in which that same sensation(s) may have occurred.

Following the scene match, the patient responded, "I'm feeling like I felt many times as a child, like I did something wrong." He then related a childhood scene in which his father came home, hit his mother, then broke a mirror over her head while the patient and his brother sat on the stairs, watching.

Pearl This example highlights the rapid speed with which ART can help connect and address early childhood memories that may be at the core of the more recent distressing experience. The patient recalled this childhood event within minutes of starting his first ART session with a new therapist.

The therapist then switched from processing the initial scene involving the double amputee to this nested childhood scene. When the sensation in the patient's throat persisted further, the therapist asked the patient if he could envision a metaphor to describe the feeling.

Therapist: "What does the pain in the back of your throat feel like? Can you think of a metaphor to describe it?"

Patient: "It feels like a cloud of smoke."

Therapist: "O.K. Picture that cloud of smoke and I want you to see if you can come up with a solution to get rid of it while you follow my hand with your eyes. Maybe you can blow it out, vacuum it out, or maybe someone can help you. I don't know. You can use my suggestions or anything else you like. Here we go."

Patient (after a set of eye movements): "I tried to grab it and pull it out, but it got stronger… more intense."

Therapist: "No problem. Maybe you need a tool or device to help you get it out of there. See if you can find a tool to help you remove it."

Patient (after another set of eye movements): "I put a chain around it and hooked it up to a van. It came partly out."

Therapist: "Good! It's moving! Let's see if you can get it completely out."

Patient (after another set of eye movements): "It's stubborn. It's still stuck to my lips."

Therapist: "Maybe you need someone to help you. Maybe the cloud is someone who has control over you and doesn't want to let you go. See what you can do to take care of this."

Pearl The therapist has suggested to the patient that the sensation may represent something deeper—a connection to a figure from the past. ART is unique in its ability to permit this testing of interpretations so quickly in the therapeutic relationship. Notice also that the therapist phrased the suggestion in the form of a hypothesis, allowing the patient to maintain full control over whether or not to accept or reject it, allowing for a self-directed solution that promotes a sense of mastery.

Patient (after another set of eye movements): "It was my dad; he tried to push it back in my throat. I used a machete to hack him up, but he just kept laughing, so I used a baseball bat to beat him but he just kept laughing. Finally I gave him a hug and told him I loved him and he went away."

Pearl Consider the rich psychodynamic material that emerged from this simple exploration of a bodily sensation. The use of metaphor and imagery helped the patient simultaneously express and resolve persistent and even conflicting feelings without a lengthy analysis. The therapist now has the option to explore many more hypotheses about the patient's primitive drives, traumatic experiences, and primary attachments if he or she deems it appropriate.

Having helped the patient resolve this sensation, the therapist returned to the nested domestic violence scene. In reviewing this scene, the patient reported feeling pain in his chest again, which he described as feeling "like an old wooden vise."

Therapist: "Let's see if you can get rid of that pain like you did with the pain in your throat."
Patient (after another set of eye movements): "It's partly reduced."
Therapist: "Do you need help?"
Patient: "No."
Patient (after another set of eye movements): "It's almost gone."
Therapist: "Great! Go ahead and open that vise up wide."
Patient (after another set of eye movements): "The pain is gone."

Pearl Once patients learn how to use the eye movements to process bodily sensations, they are often able to rapidly eliminate pain, tightness, and other discomfort.

The therapist then instructed the patient to see his childhood scene a second time.

Patient: "This time I noticed that my mom had tried to hold open the front door. I also realized I had my feet between the railings because I could see my hands and feet and realized how small they were."

As is commonly found with the second viewing of the traumatic scene, the patient reported no additional physical sensations and appeared to be in no distress. He was then directed through the rescripting process.

Patient: "My dad came in smiling. He gave my mom a hug and a kiss and said 'hi' to me and my brother. Mom went into the kitchen to get dinner out of the oven. Dad gave her a friendly swat on the behind and we all laughed."

Pearl The ART protocol allows patients to envision preferred scenarios that often resolve unmet needs from early childhood. The virtual fulfillment of these needs changes the emotional valence they attach to the original scene, thereby reducing present-day distress. Research and anecdotal experience to date suggests that ART patients will retain the narrative memory of their original scenes and could report these events in detail if asked to do so, but they will no longer be burdened by the negative emotions formerly associated with them.

When asked to see the new scene again to reinforce it, the patient reported that he now saw *himself* coming through the door as an adult, giving his wife a big hug and hugging his kids. He stated that he could not wait to go home and hug his family.

Pearl This example nicely demonstrates the generalizability of insights developed during ART. On presentation, one of the patient's chief complaints was the fact that he did not feel close to his kids. Having now "seen" both his father and himself modeling affectionate paternalistic behavior, the patient can now imagine himself interacting with his children in a positive, more nurturing way.

The therapist then directed the patient back to the original scene involving him escorting his double-amputee marine comrade at the ball. The patient started seeing his scene without difficulty, but got "stuck" at the point where his buddy had asked for a chair to use in the shower and the true realization of his disability struck the patient for the first time.

Patient: "It feels like there's a thumb on my heart."
Therapist: "See what you can do to remove that sensation."
Patient (after another set of eye movements): "The thumb is gone, but now there are fingers there."
Therapist: "Do the fingers feel good or bad?"
Patient: "They feel good."
Therapist: "See if you can spread the sense of security afforded by the fingers throughout your whole body."
Therapist (after another set of eye movements): "Were you able to spread that sense of security?"
Patient: "Yes."

The patient finished his scene, saw it a second time, then rescripted it to a scene in which he and his buddy (the latter on prosthetic legs) were each running the Marine Corps Marathon independently but kept bumping into one another along the way. At the end, his buddy raced ahead, beating the patient to the finish line. The therapist asked the patient if his buddy had anything to say to him after they finished the race. After a set of eye movements, the patient reported that his friend had told him, "I'm alright [patient's name], I'm alright." The patient then felt a pleasant, warm sensation, which the therapist helped him spread throughout his body.

Pearl This vignette highlights the use of a Gestalt-style technique to enhance the basic ART protocol, which can be particularly useful for patients struggling with grief and bereavement. While following the protocol, patients are often able to "see" earlier or better versions of themselves, as well as to "hear" positive interactions between themselves and others.

The therapist then directed the patient to see himself during a future event that would have been stressful before ART, and to make this scene as positive as possible. The patient saw himself meeting his fellow marine at the next Tunnel to Towers run in New York City. Instead of awkwardly shaking his hand as he would have done previously, he hugged his buddy and told him that he loved him. The marine hugged him back and said the same.

At the end of the first session, the patient's SUD score was "a solid zero" and he reported that his initial feelings of shamefulness, anxiety, insecurity, and confusion were gone.

9.7.4 Outcomes and Case Resolution

Seven weeks after his initial ART session, the patient reported that his guilt regarding his marine buddy was significantly reduced. He stated, "I don't think about it much… I have no real feelings about it… I look at my relationship with [that Marine] just like the relationship I have with the rest of my Marines." The PCL-5 was not repeated due to his low initial score. Overall, he was doing very well. He had remained sober, he and his wife were in the process of purchasing a house, his relationship with his children had improved, and he was very hopeful about the future.

9.8 Conclusion

ART constitutes an efficient and effective therapy for PTSD that packages A-level psychotherapy elements in a novel format. Capitalizing on the memory reconsolidation window, the experienced ART therapist can eliminate negative images and sensations, while helping the patient rescript distressing memories and positively envision future events. Meanwhile, the patient remains in control—alert, aware, and at liberty to share as many or as few details of the experience as he or she deems comfortable.

Although research on ART to date has been limited, the number of trained ART therapists in the DoD community is growing. Interest in research to explore and further validate ART's clinical utility is also expanding. Future clinical trials are planned to evaluate the effectiveness of ART as compared to established trauma therapies, and researchers are also hoping to investigate the use of ART in specific clinical populations, such as victims of MST, first responders, patients with TBI, and children and adolescents. It will also be important to explore potential contraindications and the risk of adverse effects. However, should future research efforts yield results as promising as those that have been published to date, ART could one day become the preferred PTSD therapy for combat veterans.

Acknowledgments We humbly acknowledge Ms. Laney Rosenzweig and Dr. Megan Marumoto for their valuable editorial input on this chapter.

References

1. Kip KE, Elk CA, Sullivan KL, Kadel R, Lengacher CA, Long CJ, Rosenzweig L, Shuman A, Hernandez DF, Street JD, Girling SA, Diamond DM. Brief treatment of symptoms of Post-traumatic stress disorder (PTSD) by use of accelerated resolution therapy (ART). Behav Sci. 2012;2(2):115–34.
2. Kip KE, Rosenzweig L, Hernandez DF, Shuman A, Sullivan KL, Long CJ, Taylor J, McGhee S, Girling SA, Wittenberg, T, Sahebzamani, FM, Lengacher CA, Kadel R, Diamond DM. Randomized controlled trial of accelerated resolution therapy (ART) for symptoms of combat-related Posttraumatic stress disorder (PTSD). Mil Med. 2013;178:1298–309.
3. Kip KE, Shuman A, Hernandez DF, Diamond DM, Rosenzweig L. Case report and theoretical description of accelerated resolution therapy (ART) for military-related Posttraumatic stress disorder. Mil Med. 2014;179:31–7.
4. The Management of Posttraumatic Stress Working Group. VA/DoD clinical practice guideline for the management of posttraumatic stress. Department of Veteran's Affairs and Health Affairs, Department of Defense. 2010.
5. Personal communication with Ms. Rosenzweig.
6. Monfils MH, Cowansage KK, Klann E, LeDoux JE. Extinction-reconsolidation boundaries: key to persistent attenuation of fear memories. Science. 2009;324:951–5.
7. Schiller D, Monfils MH, Raio CM, Johnson DC, LeDoux JE, Phelps EA. Preventing the return of fear in humans using reconsolidation update mechanisms. Nature. 2010;463:49–53.
8. Kip KE, Sullivan KL, Lengacher CA, Rosenzweig L, Hernandez DF, Kadel R, Kozel FA, Shuman A, Girling SA, Hardwick MJ, Diamond DM. Brief treatment of co-occurring Posttraumatic stress and depressive symptoms by use of accelerated resolution therapy. Front Psychiatry. 2013;4(article 11):1–12.

9. Kip KE, Rosenzweig L, Hernandez DF, Shuman A, Diamond DM, Girling SA, Sullivan KL, Wittenberg T, Witt A, Lengacher CA, Anderson B, McMillan SC. Accelerated resolution therapy (ART) for treatment of pain secondary to combat-related Posttraumatic stress disorder (PTSD). Eur J Psychotraumatol. 2014;5:24066.
10. Conybeare D, Behar E, Solomon A, Newman MG, Borkovec TD. The PTSD checklist—civilian version: reliability, validity, and factor structure in a nonclinical sample. J Clin Psychol. 2012;68(6):699–713.

Meditation for Combat-related Mental Health Concerns

10

Marina Khusid

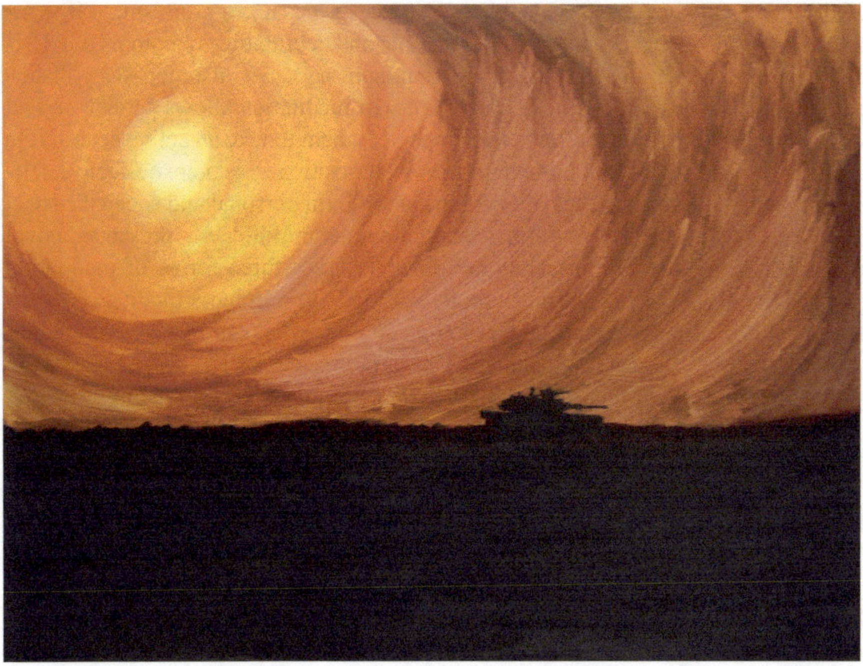

Twilight Warrior, Darrold Peters, courtesy of the Army Art Collection, US Army Center of Military History.

M. Khusid (✉)
Deployment Health Clinical Center, Defense Centers of Excellence for Psychological Health and Traumatic Brain Injury, Silver Spring, MD, USA
e-mail: khusid.marina@gmail.com

E. C. Ritchie (ed.), *Posttraumatic Stress Disorder and Related Diseases in Combat Veterans,* DOI 10.1007/978-3-319-22985-0_10

The evidence base for mind–body interventions has been rapidly expanding, as reflected in the 2011 systematic review [1]. Although the 2010 Veterans Administration (VA)/Department of Defense (DoD) clinical practice guideline for management of PTSD does not recommend any mindfulness approaches as first-line treatments for posttraumatic stress disorder (PTSD), they were found to be viable adjunctive treatments to reduce hyperarousal symptoms. Mind–body interventions reduce intrusive memories, avoidance, anger, and increase self-esteem, pain tolerance, energy and ability to relax, and cope with stress [2–4]. Among various mind–body approaches, meditation is one of the most accepted among veterans and appropriate for PTSD management. Meditation-based approaches are being widely implemented across the VA and DoD [5, 6]. A 2012 survey of 125 VA-specialized PTSD treatment programs indicated that 88 % offered sitting meditation practices, or movement meditation practices like yoga.

Meditation is safe, portable, easy to learn, affordable, with steadily increasing evidence of effectiveness as an adjunct to standard care. It is a promising self-management approach that can alleviate the chronic and debilitating symptoms of PTSD and comorbid conditions such as depression, substance use disorder, sleep disturbance, and chronic pain. This self-care quality of meditation allows patients to feel more in control of their symptoms and empowers them to take an active central role in their own healing process. Meditation is well positioned as a cost-effective self-management approach that may help reduce long-term personal and societal costs.

In this chapter, the author defines meditation and mindfulness, presents a novel classification of meditation techniques, and discusses three forms of meditation practice that offer the most promise in PTSD care—mindfulness meditation, mantram repetition program, and compassion meditation. The neurobiology of meditative practice and the role of meditation in emotion regulation, addressing PTSD symptoms, and promoting well-being are also presented. Neuroimaging research and clinical trials for each meditation technique are followed by instructions for each practice, and illustrated through clinical case discussions.

10.1 Meditation Defined

Meditation has been practiced since antiquity, and embedded in different cultures, worldviews, and traditions. Each meditative practice is rooted in spiritual and health beliefs of its unique culture of origin. The distinctness usually lies in the body position assumed during practice (sitting or in motion), eyes being open or closed, and the particular focus (i.e., breath and sensation) during meditation practice. To better appreciate the vastness and diversity of meditation traditions, and get familiar with specific terminology, we propose a novel classification based on body position and attention focus and give examples of common techniques in Table 10.1. Although meditation may take different shapes and forms, the common denominator is that each practice represents a form of mental training.

In contrast to the view of traditional cultures, neuroscientists describe meditation as "mental training consisting of complex emotional and attentional regulatory

Table 10.1 Meditation classification according to posture and focus

1. *Sitting meditations*	
1A *Focus on automatic physiologic process of breathing*	
Traditional Buddhist mindfulness meditations	
	For example, Shambhala, Zen, and Vipassana focus on the breath
Contemporary group-based mindfulness meditation protocols	
	For example, mindfulness-based stress reduction (MBSR), mindfulness-based cognitive therapy (MBCT), and mindfulness-based relapse prevention (MBRP) also use breath as their main object of attention
1B *Focus on specific sensation or object*	
Focus on sensations associated with positive emotions	
	For example, compassion meditation is also known as loving–kindness meditation and has two main traditional variations—*Metta* and *Tonglen.* When practicing compassion meditation, the attention is focused on the sensation in one's heart to guide the emotional experience of compassion
Focus on sensations in different body parts	
	For example, progressive muscle relaxation (PMR), body scan, or tantric meditation direct their respective focus to a specific body part or a tantric center
Focus on energy centers described in various Eastern healing traditions	
	For example, central channel meditation, chakra meditation, qigong with focus on dantian, and kundalini meditation
Visual focus on a given object	
	For example, one-pointed meditation, mandala meditation
1C *Focus on experience of meditation procedure itself*	
Focusing on the repetition of a word, phrase, or chant with the purpose of quieting the mental process	
	For example, mantram repetition program, chanting meditations, and transcendental meditation focus on the procedure of repeating a mantra
1D *Multiple focus*	
	For example, relaxation response (RR) training uses breath, mantra, and progressive muscle relaxation to guide focus and physiologic relaxation
2. *Movement meditations*	
	Yoga and Tai Chi are common examples of movement meditations; they also utilize breath to assist in the flow of movement

regimens developed for cultivation of well-being and emotional balance" [7]. A recent quantitative meta-analysis of ten neuroimaging studies illustrates that different meditative traditions share the same central process underlying this phenomenon of emotion regulation and attention training, and involves activation of basal ganglia (caudate body), limbic system (enthorinal cortex), and medial prefrontal cortex (mPFC) [8]. The aim of such training is to reduce or eliminate maladaptive thought processes, leading to physical and mental relaxation, stress reduction, psycho-emotional stability, and enhanced concentration [9].

Table 10.2 Meditation classification according to EEG signature and cognitive process

1. *Focused attention (FA) or concentrative meditation*
a. *EEG waves and corresponding cognitive process:*
i. Gamma (30–50 Hz) activity reflects highly active mental process responsible for problem-solving and object recognition, great for learning and long-term memories
ii. Gamma synchronization helps to gain control of mental processing and to integrate various sensory stimuli into unified perception. Voluntary and sustained attention on a given object is a resulting outcome
iii. Beta 2 (20–30 Hz) is characteristic of normal awake and alert state and has been reported during focused executive processing, such as highly focused attention to a specific object
b. *Object of attention:* specific internal sensation or emotion
c. *Examples:* compassion or loving–kindness meditation, Qigong, diamond way Buddhist meditation
2. *Automatic self-transcending (AST) meditation*
a. *EEG waves and corresponding cognitive process:* Alpha 1 pattern (8–10 Hz) results in a very relaxed state. It appears to reflect the level of internally directed attention, alertness, expectancy, helps group isolated elements into the unity of experience, and is associated with problem solving by intuition or insight
b. *Object of attention:* specific meditation procedure (such as mantra repetition) used until the attention no longer needs to be consciously directed and the mind is free of thought
c. *Examples:* transcendental meditation and other mantra meditations
3. *Open monitoring (OM) meditations*
a. *EEG waves and corresponding cognitive process:* Theta wave (4–7 Hz) or frontal midline theta (originating from medial prefrontal and anterior cingulated cortices) is characteristic of deep relaxation, and involved in tasks requiring self-control, internal timing, assessment of reward, working memory, memory retention, and mental imagery
b. *Object of attention:* breath and moment-to-moment experience
c. *Examples:* mindfulness meditations such as Vipassana, Zen, and Sahaja

EEG electro-encephalogram

Lutz [7] and Travis [10] proposed another way to categorize meditation practices; that way is based on their neural mechanism, specific brain wave patterns, cognitive processes used, and the object of attention during the practice of meditation. They identify three distinct categories of meditation techniques: open monitoring (OM), focused attention (FA), and automatic self-transcending (AST) meditations. The details for each category are outlined in Table 10.2, with examples and observed overlap with the first classification in Table 10.1. It is important to note that several meditation practices may utilize more than one of these mechanisms.

OM meditation uses breath to practice nonreactive nonevaluative moment-to-moment awareness without attempt to control or manipulate the content of ongoing experience. *FA* meditation, also called *concentrative meditation,* is characterized by sustained voluntary attention on a chosen object or experience, such as creating a vivid emotion or a strong visual image, concentrating on specific body part sensations. In FA, the attention is brought back to the object of attention when the mind has wondered. The goal of *AST* meditation is the absence of focus or mental control, which is obtained through the use of self-transcending procedures that are automatic, effortless, and require minimal cognitive control, such as repeating a mantra. The rate of transcending may vary person to person, one meditation session to another, and depends on years and frequency of practice [10].

Three meditation traditions that have the most emerging scientific evidence for PTSD to date are mindfulness meditation, mantram repetition, and compassion meditation. They differ in the spectrum of their effects on PTSD and co-occurring conditions; this allows providers to custom-tailor treatment to each unique case and achieve the most therapeutic benefit. Patients are encouraged to choose a technique that resonates with them, and that they are most likely to adopt as regular practice.

These three practices are also evidence-based, free, simple to practice, and therefore accessible. These meditations are quick to teach in a treatment room or as part of a group visit, easy for patients to learn and adopt as their daily routine, can be practiced anywhere, and do not require significant time commitment. Mantram repetition and loving–kindness meditation can be tailored to an individual's beliefs and needs. All of these considerations are important for establishing a sustainable self-management regimen for PTSD and other mental health conditions, and for making a successful lifestyle change for overall well-being.

10.2 Mindfulness Meditation

10.2.1 Definition

Mindfulness meditation is a practice to achieve open, acceptant, nonjudgmental awareness (i.e., mindfulness) of the present moment by focusing the person's attention on their breathing. Jon Kabat-Zinn is the pioneer of clinical applications of mindfulness in the West. He describes mindfulness as "the ability to maintain moment by moment, open, acceptant, non-judgmental awareness" [11]. Segal further describes four characteristics of this type of attention to present experience as curiosity, openness, acceptance, and love (COAL) [12]. He suggests that curiosity and ability to simply observe our feelings, thoughts, and reactions with openness lie at the heart of mindfulness and help generate self-acceptance and self-love.

To explore neural underpinnings of mindfulness, Farb used functional magnetic resonance imaging (fMRI) to trace two distinct forms of awareness [13]. The first type, *awareness of the self across time,* engages mPFC and results in cognitive attempts to control negative emotions. The second type is what we refer to as *mindful awareness,* directed to the self in the present moment, which focuses on somatosensory experience of the present by recruiting right lateralized network [13]. Voluntary regulation of prefrontal cortex and directing attention toward the transitory nature of a present somatosensory experience provides an alternative to cognitive efforts to control negative emotion and cultivates conscious, open, and receptive attitude rooted in the now [14, 15].

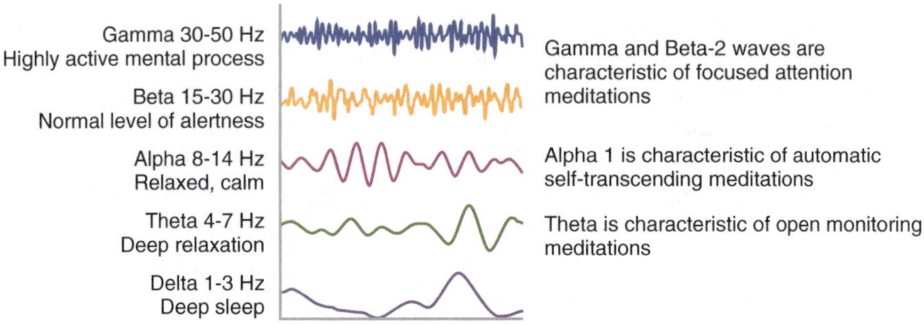

Fig. 10.1 EEG patterns characteristic for different types of meditation

Since neural mechanisms show that mindful awareness activates the somatosensory cortex, it is not surprising that most meditation techniques (Fig. 10.1) involve focus on a particular somato-visceral sensation (e.g., breathing, vibration, muscle relaxation/heaviness) or rely on a sensory organ perception (e.g., vision in mandala meditation and hearing in chanting meditation). Based on this observation and the neural mechanism of mindful awareness described by Farb, it is fair to assume that although mindfulness meditation was specifically developed to cultivate mindfulness, other meditation traditions are likely to do the same to a certain degree. When Buddhist mindfulness meditation sees the development of mindful attitude toward life as a final goal, other meditation traditions may pursue additional aims. Loving–kindness meditation, for example, seeks to cultivate compassion, and transcendental meditations aim to free the mind of thought and achieve a more peaceful level of consciousness [16].

10.2.2 Types of Mindfulness Meditation and Mindfulness-based Group Interventions

There are several types of mindfulness meditation that originated from different Buddhist monastic traditions, for example, Zen, Vipassana, and Shambhala meditations [17]. All universally involve the person sitting still and observing the breath, but may differ slightly in posture, eyes being open or closed, or hand and leg position. When thoughts inevitably arise, a meditator is instructed to nonjudgmentally acknowledge and accept them, and then bring her attention back to the simple sensation of air going in through her nostrils, into the chest and out again, in a natural and relaxed way. This process of repeatedly returning one's attention back to the essential process of respiration, gradually trains the brain the mindful art of staying in the present, and offers significant benefits of controlling one's otherwise automatic stress response to thoughts, negative emotions, and memories of PTSD [16, 18].

Several modern group-based meditation protocols have been developed in an attempt to standardize care delivery, target unique mechanisms of a specific condition, and help replicate research findings. These modern 6–8 weeks meditation programs are mindfulness-based stress reduction (MBSR), mindfulness-based cognitive therapy

Table 10.3 Mindfulness meditation instructions

1. Choose a time of day when you are the most awake and alert. Sit upright on the floor or a chair, keeping the spine straight and maintaining a relaxed but erect posture so you do not get drowsy. Depending on your comfort, you can keep your eyes open or closed during this practice
2. Now focus on your breathing, on the sensations it triggers throughout your body. Notice how your abdomen moves with each inhalation and exhalation
3. Focus on the tip of the nose, noticing the different sensations that arise with each breath
4. When you notice that you have been distracted by unrelated thoughts or feelings that have arisen, simply return your focus to your breathing
5. Try this for 5–10 min at a sitting, once or twice a day. As you feel more comfortable, you can increase the length of your practice sessions

(MBCT), mindfulness-based relapse prevention (MBRP), and mind–body bridging (MBB). Although most research studies use one of these structured programs, it is important to recognize that they were created to make it easier to standardize clinical programs, and replicate research protocols. The common active ingredient to all of these mindfulness-based group interventions is mindfulness meditation (Table 10.3). Therefore, if MBSR or MBCT is cost- or time-prohibitive or not available locally, a patient can start by following simple instructions for mindfulness meditation home practice. The following provides an example of such instructions adapted from Richard J. Davidson, one of the most prominent researchers of neurobiological basis of meditation [19].

10.2.3 Mindfulness-based Stress Reduction (MBSR) Program

MBSR was originally developed at the University of Massachusetts Medical School [20]. Below is the description of the 8-week MBSR program Kearney et al. used in the randomized controlled pilot in veterans with PTSD [21]. The MBSR groups usually meet for 2 h once per week for 8 weeks, in addition to a daylong retreat. MBSR instruction emphasizes bringing a curious, kind, and nonjudging attitude to the present moment, including any difficult or unpleasant experiences.

During each class, participants receive instructions on mindfulness meditation and have an opportunity to ask questions and practice newly learned skills. Homework assignments include daily meditation or yoga for 45 min per day, and bringing mindful attention to experiences in daily life. Attention training includes developing the ability to place and sustain attention on the breath, as well as maintaining flexibility of attention (e.g., the ability to let go of ruminative cycles of thought and return attention to the breath). The "body scan" and gentle yoga are two additional mindfulness exercises taught. The body scan exercise is a 45-min exercise in which attention is systematically directed to each part of the body. During the daylong mostly silent retreat, participants practice mindfulness exercises more intensively.

10.2.4 Mindfulness-based Cognitive Therapy (MBCT) Program

MBCT is a group program integrating cognitive behavioral therapy (CBT) and mindfulness meditation. It was initially developed by Teasdale, Segal, and Williams to prevent relapses of depression currently in remission [22]. The program teaches individuals to become more aware of thoughts and to view thoughts as "mental events" rather than as aspects of the self or accurate reflections of reality. Adopting this "mindful" mode of neutral nonjudgmental observation empowers patients to recognize and disengage from their dysfunctional ruminative negative thought patterns and prevent habitual reactive emotional responses that would otherwise fuel the relapse process. Unlike CBT, there is little explicit emphasis on changing the content or specific meanings of negative automatic thoughts. Teasdale states that the MBCT program "involves facilitation of an aware mode of being, characterized by freedom and choice of response, in contrast to a mode dominated by habitual, overwhelmed, automatic patterns of cognitive-affective processing" [22].

An MBCT program is usually delivered by an instructor in 8-week 2-h group training sessions with daily homework exercises. Homework consists of some form of awareness exercises, directed at increasing moment-by-moment nonjudgmental awareness of bodily sensations, thoughts, feelings, and integrating application of awareness skills into daily life. Specific relapse/recurrence prevention strategies are also explored. Most programs offer up to four, monthly follow-up meetings upon completion of the initial 8-week program, thus extending guided support of this therapeutic intervention for up to 6 months.

10.2.5 Neurobiology of Mindfulness Meditation

To better understand the neural mechanisms responsible for the therapeutic effect of mindfulness meditation in PTSD, it is important to recognize the abnormalities in the prefrontal cortex (PFC)—amygdala neurocircuit that are associated with PTSD. Amygdala, the brain structure responsible for memory and emotion processing, is overactivated in PTSD resulting in persistent negative emotions that are difficult to control. In healthy individuals, activation in the PFC inhibits the amygdala. In individuals with PTSD, the PFC is under-responsive, and therefore generates insufficient negative feedback on the hyperactive amygdala. Symptomatically, this manifests as persistent fear, phobic avoidance, hyperarousal, impulsivity, reexperiencing of painful memories, and depressive rumination. Coincidently, this very same neural mechanism is a shared neuropathology of PTSD, depression, poor impulse control in addictions, and aggressive outbursts.

Creswell, in his 2007 fMRI study, was able to show that mindfulness training is associated with greater PFC activation and reduced amygdala activity [23], the exact effect desired to normalize neural circuitry implicated in PTSD and comorbid disorders. A systematic review by Chiesa in 2010 confirmed that MM practice activates the PFC and the anterior cingulate cortex (ACC) [15]. Through PFC inhibition of the amygdala, mindfulness redirects attention from cognitive control of negative emotions to the transitory nature of momentary experience. This redirection of

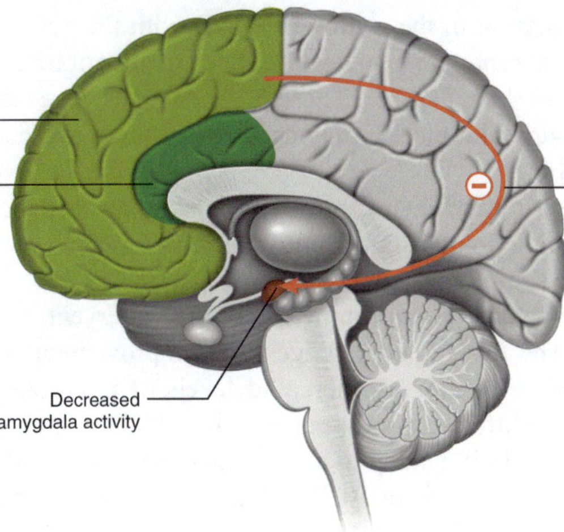

Fig. 10.2 Effect of mindfulness meditation on PFC-Amygdala neurocircuit

awareness helps people with PTSD to increase tolerance for negative emotions, such as fear, shame, guilt, and pain, to reduce automatic negative self-evaluation, and to engage in self-compassion [24]. Figure 10.2 illustrates the effect of mindfulness meditation on PFC-amygdala neurocircuit.

In another landmark study, anatomical MRI was done pre and post an 8-week MBSR program (N=26) and illustrated that reported reduction in perceived stress positively correlated with decrease in right basolateral amygdala gray matter density. By decreasing amygdala activity these MBSR-mediated neuroplastic changes could help decrease the negative consequence of chronic stress [25]. MBSR also increased gray matter volume in areas of learning, attention and memory process, emotion regulation, and self-referential processing [26].

Mindfulness meditation exhibits positive effect on emotional symptomatology of PTSD. It has been shown to increase positive mood, reduce distractive ruminative thoughts and behaviors [27], reduce emotional reactivity [28, 29], and improve impulse control [30]. One study showed that MBSR may influence the hypothalalmic-pituitary-adrenocortical (HPA) axis, resulting in adjustment of cortisol levels [23]. Higher plasma melatonin levels were also shown in advanced meditators and may be helpful in mitigating PTSD-related sleep difficulties [31]. These multifaceted neural, endocrine, and psychological effects of mindfulness and mindfulness meditation suggest its versatile clinical utilization for a variety of mental health conditions and warrants further investigation.

10.2.6 Clinical Trials of Mindfulness Meditation for PTSD

Limited number of randomized controlled trials on mindfulness meditation for PTSD exists to date. Several nonrandomized studies have assessed the efficacy of mindfulness meditation in the setting of PTSD with the evidence of improved PTSD symptoms, depression, mental health-related quality of life, as well as acceptance and mindfulness skills [32, 33]. These improvements were largely maintained at 6 months follow-up, with most pronounced reduction in avoidance, depression, and emotional numbing.

In two consequent randomized controlled trials in cancer patients ($N=71$), an 8-week MBSR training course significantly decreased perceived stress and post-traumatic avoidance symptoms and increased positive affect and mindfulness compared to a wait-list control group, immediately post-intervention and at 6-month follow-up [3, 34]. The investigators suggest that improvements in psychological well-being are likely explained by increased levels of mindfulness as measured with the five-facet mindfulness questionnaire. In 2013 Kearney et al. conducted a randomized controlled pilot study to assess outcomes associated with an 8-week MBSR program for veterans with PTSD. They randomized participants to treatment as usual (TAU, $N=22$), or MBSR plus TAU ($N=25$) [21]. More veterans randomized to MBSR reported enhanced levels of mindfulness and had clinically significant improvement in health-related quality of life, but not PTSD symptoms. These changes were noted immediately post-intervention and at 4-month follow-up.

The largest and most rigorous RCT was completed by Polusny et al. It compared adjunctive MBSR and present-centered group psychotherapy in veterans with PTSD diagnosis (n=116). Study participants did not use any other psychotherapeutic treatment during the study, but some were on psychoactive medications used at stable doses for at least 2 months prior to entering the study. MBSR resulted in a greater decrease of PTSD symptoms, and showed improvement of depressive symptoms, mindfulness, and quality of life. This therapeutic improvement was sustained during the 9-week intervention administration, and at 2-months follow-up.

Although, there were no neuroimaging studies done on meditation effects for PTSD, two fMRI studies confirmed that MBSR diminishes negative emotions, avoidance behaviors, automatic emotional reactivity, and engages attention regulation of distorted habitual self-views in patients with anxiety [35, 36]. It is thought to reduce negative emotions by enhancing emotional regulation and reducing reactivity through suppressing amygdala activity [36, 37]. Negative self-beliefs are also monitored through attention regulation in the parietal cortex neural networks [37]. Thus, MBSR employs both emotion and attention regulation to control anxiety-related symptoms.

In 2013, a nonrandomized pilot study investigated the feasibility, acceptability, and clinical outcomes of an 8-week MBCT group program ($N=20$) in comparison to TAU ($N=17$). Pre- and post-therapy assessments through clinician-administered and self-report PTSD measures suggest that group MBCT is an effective adjunctive therapy for combat-related PTSD, well accepted by patients, with good treatment compliance, and the potential for a reduction in the avoidance and numbing symptom cluster, and PTSD cognitions, such as self-blame [38]. No randomized controlled studies on use of MBCT for PTSD were done.

Several quasi experimental studies examined more traditional mindfulness meditation techniques. A mindfulness meditation intervention was used in a pilot study of mental health workers with PTSD who, 10 weeks after Hurricane Katrina, re-

Table 10.4 Utility of adjunct mindfulness meditation for PTSD

Cognitive and emotional processes	Utility in PTSD management
Encourages nonjudgmental observation of the moment-to-moment experience [10, 16, 41]	Decreases cognitive appraisal of intrusive thoughts, memories, feelings of shame, guilt or anger, and allows for more effective access and processing of emotions
Increases self-control, internal timing, and assessment of reward [10]	Improves emotional control and tolerance of negative affect, pain, unpleasant thoughts and memories, decreases reactivity and automatic negative self-view
Reduces negative emotions of PTSD and depression [33]	Reduces worry and depressive rumination, and avoidance [33]
Focuses on the present [10, 16]	Promotes resilience and reintegration into civilian life by shifting attention to more productive coping strategies, such as problem-solving

ceived 4 h of mindfulness training, followed by an 8-week home study. Participants reported good treatment adherence, significant improvements in well-being, and a decrease in PTSD and anxiety symptoms; the improved results were correlative with the total number of minutes of daily meditation practice [39]. A small Vipassana meditation study among incarcerated individuals showed no significant difference in PTSD symptom severity between Vipassana and treatment as usual groups; however, participation in the Vipassana course was associated with significantly greater reductions in comorbid substance use [40].

Further randomized controlled studies of sufficient sample size are needed to establish efficacy of mindfulness meditation as adjunct for PTSD. Preliminary findings suggest that mindfulness meditation is safe, well accepted by patients, effective adjunctive therapy with good treatment adherence, and meditation practice compliance at up to 6 months follow-up. Research findings are consistent in showing increased levels of mindfulness, improved health-related quality of life and well-being, and reduced avoidance, depression, and numbing symptoms (Table 10.4) [41].

10.2.7 Mindfulness Meditation for Conditions Commonly Co-occurring with PTSD

10.2.7.1 Mindfulness Meditation for Depression

MBCT offers a valuable cost-effective [42] self-management treatment option that shows reproducible reduction in depression relapse rate to 36 % [43], comparable to maintenance antidepressant medications in stable patients with remitting depression [42, 44] , and lasting 2–3 years post-intervention with ongoing mindfulness practice [45]. MBCT was more effective than maintenance antidepressants in reducing residual depressive symptoms and psychiatric comorbidity and in improving mental and physical quality of life [42]. MBCT was also found helpful in retaining a balanced pattern of prefrontal asymmetry in previously suicidal patients, associated with decreased depression vulnerability [46].

There are three main mechanisms explaining the therapeutic advantage of mindfulness meditation in depression. First, MBCT reduces dysfunctional ruminative thought process exacerbating depressive moods [45, 47]. Second, sustained mindfulness training can reduce emotional reactivity and the likelihood of depressive symptom development [28, 48]. Last, mindfulness meditation helps cultivate self-compassion, which in turn fosters positive affect and decouples the relationship between reactivity and the likelihood of relapse [48–50]. Neurally, mindfulness breathing meditation and MBCT demonstrate increase in left PFC activation on EEG, associated with reduced vulnerability to depression [46, 51]. The self-care nature of mindfulness practice empowers the patient to take an active role in achieving health, managing chronic illness, and is associated with decreased healthcare costs [52].

10.2.7.2 Mindfulness Meditation for Substance Use Disorder (SUD)

According to Chiesa et al.'s 2013 systematic review, the evidence from 24 studies suggests that mind–body interventions reduce the consumption of several substances, including alcohol, cocaine, amphetamines, marijuana, cigarettes, and opiates to a significantly greater extent than wait-list controls, educational support groups, and specific control groups [53]. Another systematic review evaluated 25 eligible studies specific to mindfulness meditation and similarly suggested efficacy and safety of mindfulness meditation for SUD [54]. MBRP was specifically designed for SUD, and integrates cognitive-behavioral relapse prevention skills with mindfulness meditation. It targets cravings, a significant predictor of substance use and relapse following treatment for SUD [55].

Participants of mindfulness meditation report reduction in cravings [53], better acceptance of uncomfortable states or challenges without reacting automatically [56, 57], and lessening of the conditioned response to craving in the presence of depressive symptoms, strong emotional states and mood fluctuations [58], and much improved impulse control [59]. The review of neuroimaging literature, suggests that MBRP affects numerous brain systems associated with craving, negative affect, impulse control, and relapse, and may reverse, repair, or compensate for the neuroadaptive changes associated with addiction and relapse [56]. These research findings suggest MBRP is a viable aftercare self-management approach for individuals who have recently completed an intensive treatment for substance use disorders.

10.2.7.3 Mindfulness Meditation for Sleep Disturbance

In a 2007 systematic review, Winbush et al. describe the findings of four uncontrolled trials suggesting that MBSR can significantly improve sleep quality, duration, and decrease sleep-interfering cognitive processes, such as worry and racing thoughts [60]. A recent randomized controlled pilot ($N=57$) investigated the effects of mindfulness meditation and mind–body bridging (MBB) on sleep in cancer survivors. Both interventions improved sleep more effectively than the sleep hygiene education control and showed reductions in self-reported depression symptoms, improvements in overall levels of mindfulness, self-compassion, and well-being post-intervention [27].

10.2.7.4 Mindfulness Meditation for Chronic Pain

In the 2011 systematic review, Chiesa identified ten eligible studies that showed that mind–body interventions could have nonspecific effects for the reduction of chronic pain [61]. Independent neuroimaging research findings by Grant, Zeidan, and Gard additionally demonstrated that meditative practices are associated with reduction in chronic pain intensity and unpleasantness, decreased sensitivity to pain, and improved ability to observe and not react to pain [62–65]. Meditators report better pain management compared to controls with reduction in pain intensity between 22–50% [64–66], decrease in pain unpleasantness by 57% [65], and decrease in anticipatory anxiety by 29% [64]. Additionally, more experienced meditators modulate their perception and response to pain more effectively [62, 67].

10.3 Mantram Repetition Program

10.3.1 Definition

Mantram repetition belongs to a group of mantra meditations. The other two well-known practices in this group are transcendental meditation (TM) and relaxation response training, and both use a similar technique of repeating a word, phrase or sound, silently or aloud to create a sense of peace and relaxation [68]. Mantra means "to cross the mind" in Sanskrit and has a purpose of bringing mental clarity, calmness, and inner peace. It is present in all major spiritual traditions with a sacred phrase handed down for generations. The term mantram, rather than mantra, is used to differentiate the mantram repetition program from TM and to acknowledge its originator, Eknath Easwaran [69].

Mantram repetition is a portable practice of meditation where the individual silently repeats a word or phrase which carries a spiritual significance (i.e., Mantram) [70]. A mantram is chosen by the individual and is meant to be a source of inspiration, comfort, peace, or inner truth. It can be used intermittently throughout the day or night, whenever symptoms arise, to interrupt unwanted thoughts and elicit the relaxation response. It is thought to redirect the person's attention from ruminating or maladaptive thought patterns and allow time for decision-making by slowing down the thought process [71]. It also helps to increase existential spiritual well-being and decrease hyperarousal symptoms, anxiousness, and fear by facilitating physiologic relaxation response [40, 72]. The spiritual meaning of the words selected by the individual could be powerful in eliciting feelings of well-being, self-confidence [16, 73], and mitigating self-reported feelings of guilt and shame, important in the process of reintegration and recovery.

Table 10.5 Utility of adjunct mantram repetition program for PTSD

Cognitive and emotional processes	Utility in PTSD management
Reduces physiologic hyperarousal [16, 74], produces a very relaxed state [10]	Rapidly reduces symptoms of hyperarousal, stress, anxiety, unwanted thoughts and can be used as needed to improve emotion regulation in a particular situation [70, 74]
Increases spiritual well-being [70, 73]	Improves life satisfaction [40, 70], reduces PTSD symptoms [40, 73] likely through mediation of anger [70], guilt, shame, moral injury and encouragement of self-compassion and forgiveness

Table 10.6 Mantram repetition instructions. (Courtesy of Dr. Jill Bormann)

1. Choose your mantram. A mantram is a spiritual word, phrase, or brief prayer that we repeat silently to ourselves to calm the body, quiet the mind, and improve concentration to restore the spirit. We recommend using a word or phrase that has spiritual connections and has been handed down for generations—it has passed the "test of time." If you do not have one in mind, you can try examples from Table 10.6. Pick one that has a positive feeling, meaning, or even sound. Try it out and see how it feels to you
2. Use it simply by repeating it to yourself as often as you can—silently, aloud, or in writing
3. At first, use it at times when you are calm and relaxed, before sleep, while walking, etc. Later, you can repeat your mantram when symptoms of distress arise—anytime, anyplace, and intermittently throughout the day
4. Make it a daily habit. With practice and persistence, you will be able to feel less stress, sleep better, and improve quality of life. The more you use it, the better you will feel, think, and be. Build the mental muscle of your mind

10.3.2 Clinical Trials

Mantram repetition has been shown to reduce the severity of PTSD symptoms in veterans with combat-related trauma [40, 73]. An initial randomized trial of mantram repetition for combat veterans with PTSD was conducted by Bormann et al. in 2012 [73]. Those who completed six group sessions of the mantram repetition program plus usual care ($n=71$) as compared with controls receiving usual care only ($n=75$) demonstrated significantly greater reduction of PTSD and depression symptoms, and improvement in mental health-related quality of life. Change in PTSD symptoms was mediated by levels of spiritual well-being, highlighting the importance of the spiritual aspect of the practice. The study had very few dropouts (7%), and showed no safety concerns with mantram repetition use.

Mantram repetition is highly practical (Table 10.5). It is free, portable, immediate, safe, easy to use, private, and allows for creating individual spiritual meaning [70, 74]. Although, the preliminary results are promising, additional research studies are needed to establish reproducibility and efficacy. Future study designs should include an active comparison group and parallel investigation of underlying neural effects. In the meanwhile, using mantram repetition as a self-management strategy

Table 10.7 List of common mantrams. (From [72], with permission)

Mantrams	Meaning
Buddhist	
Om Mane Padme Hum (Ohm mah-nee pod-may-hume)	An invocation to the jewel (Self) in the lotus of the heart
Namo Butsaya (Nah-mo boot-sie-yah)	I bow to the Buddha
Christian	
My God and My All	St. Francis of Assisi's mantra
Maranatha (Mar-uh-naw-tha)	Lord of the Heart (Aramaic)
Kyrie Eleison (Kir-ee-ay Ee-lay-ee-sone)	Lord have mercy
Christe Eleison (Kreest-ay Ee-lay-ee-sone)	Christ have mercy
Jesus, Jesus	Son of God
Hail Mary or Ave Maria	Mother of Jesus
Hindu/Indian	
Rama (Rah-mah)	Eternal joy within
Ram Ram Sri Ram (Rahm rahm shree rahm)	Gandhi's mantra (variation on Rama)
Om Namah Shivaya (Ohm Nah-mah Shee-vy-yah)	An invocation to beauty and fearlessness
Om Prema (Ohm Pray-Mah)	A call for universal love
Om Shanti (Ohm Shawn-tee)	An invocation to eternal peace
So Hum (So Hum)	I am that Self within
Jewish	
Barukh Atah Adonoi (Bah-ruke Ah-tah Ah-don-aye)	Blessed are Thou O Lord
Ribono Shel Olam (Ree-boh-noh Shel Oh-lahm)	Lord of the Universe
Shalom	Peace
Sheheena (Sha Hee-nah)	Feminine aspect of God
Muslim	
Allah	
Bismallah Ir-rahman Ir-rahim (Beese-mah-lah ir-rah-mun ir-rah-heem)	In the name of Allah, the merciful, the compassionate
Native American	
O Wakan Tanka	Oh, Great Spirit

in adjunct to standard care and with regular follow-up visits could be empowering for individuals with PTSD. Tables 10.6 and 10.7 offer simple mantram repetition instructions and a list of common mantrams from six different spiritual traditions. Both of these tables are generously provided by Dr. Jill Bormann, the principal investigator of recent studies on mantram repetition for PTSD [70].

10.3.3 Transcendental Meditation

TM is a form of mantra meditation that originates from the Vedic tradition of India. Although, the studies of TM for PTSD are very small and methodologically limited, it has been widely publicized in the media and, therefore, warrants mentioning. Maharishi Mahesh yogi described TM in 1969 as a technique designed to transcend its own activity by directing one's attention to silently repeating a mantra until the repetition no longer needs to be consciously directed and the mind is free of thought [68, 75]. The goal of TM is a state of no thought, physiologic relaxation, and mental alertness. EEG studies categorize TM as an AST technique that produces alpha 1 brain wave pattern and results in a very relaxed but alert state [10]. This mental state is often referred to as "restful alertness" or "pure consciousness."

TM is a registered trademark and can be learned only through personal instruction for a fee from a certified TM instructor who assigns a mantra to a student. This presents a unique research challenge especially related to independence of scientific investigation and ability to reproduce research findings, since specific TM technique protocols are either omitted or not well described in the literature. There are only two very small poorly designed uncontrolled studies investigating TM effectiveness for PTSD. One was a randomized prospective study of 18 veterans comparing TM ($n=9$) with individual psychotherapy ($n=9$) administered for 3 months in the treatment of post-Vietnam adjustment. TM group experienced clinically significant reductions in PTSD symptoms and anxiety compared to psychotherapy group [76]. The second was a very small ($n=5$) uncontrolled pilot of TM in Iraq and Afghanistan veterans and showed PTSD symptom and quality-of-life improvement on clinician-rated and self-reported measures [77]. In conclusion, the studies of TM for PTSD are very small with significant methodological issues, and therefore, provide insufficient data to draw any meaningful clinically relevant conclusions at this time. The fee associated with learning the technique may also limit TM's accessibility.

10.4 Compassion Meditation

10.4.1 Definition

Compassion meditation takes roots in Buddhism and involves allowing one's mind to be filled by feelings of compassion or of loving–kindness to self, close ones, and eventually all beings [19]. It is interesting that Buddhism differentiates between compassion and loving–kindness. Compassion involves wishing oneself or another freedom from suffering and results in desire to help. Loving–kindness is wishing well-being or feeling altruistic love toward self or another [19]. The goal is that with continued practice these feelings of compassion arise more readily, effortlessly, and accompanied by a desire to act to benefit others [16].

There are several variations of this practice. The terms commonly used in the West include compassion, loving–kindness, self-compassion meditation, and a structured program called cognitively based compassion training (CBCT). The two

Table 10.8 Instructions for tonglen. (From [19], with permission)

1. Visualize as vividly as you can as someone who is suffering. It can be a friend or relative who is ill, a colleague who is struggling at work, or a neighbor whose marriage is ending. The closer the person is to you, the stronger and clearer the visualization will be. This person can also be yourself, or a generic person you do not know
2. On each inhalation, imagine the suffering leaving her each time you inhale. As you breathe in, conjure an image of pain and anguish leaving her body like fog dissipating under a bright sun
3. On each exhalation, imagine that her suffering is transformed into compassion. Direct this compassion toward her, a gift of empathy and love that will envelop and enter her, assuaging her pain
4. Try this exercise for 5–10 min up to five times a week

original Buddhist practices are *metta* and *tonglen*. Sharon Salzberg's work describes these practices in great detail. In Table 10.8, we provide modified instructions for tonglen: a practice based on the Tibetan Buddhist tradition and is a visualization exercise of transforming another person's suffering into compassion [19].

10.4.2 Mechanistic and Clinical Research

There is no published research evaluating compassion meditation specifically for PTSD or any other anxiety disorder. However, there is newly sparked research interest due to preliminary neuroimaging and empirical findings related to stress response, positive emotions, and social connectedness. Several randomized controlled trials in veterans with PTSD are currently registered at clninicaltrials.gov, and investigate neural and clinical effects of compassion meditation on PTSD and depressive symptoms immediately after intervention, and at 3–6-month follow-up. While we are anxiously awaiting their results, let's consider preliminary research findings that placed compassion meditation back on the research map.

Recent research by Lamm, Bernhardt, Singer, and Klimecki is brilliant at differentiating neural mechanisms and core networks of compassion vs. empathy. It suggests that empathy is related to "feeling" someone's pain that can result in the negative emotions and activate actual neural pathways of pain (bilateral anterior insular cortex and medial/anterior cingulate cortex) in the observer [78, 79]. Compassion, on the other hand, allows one to witness suffering without being negatively affected, and instead to experience a positive desire to help [79]. Compassion training elicits activity in a distinct neural network including the medial orbitofrontal cortex, putamen, pallidum, and ventral tegmental area—brain regions previously associated with positive affect [50]. This ability to deliberately foster positive outlook even when confronted with the distress of others may offer a new coping strategy to mitigate recurrent overwhelming negative memories and emotions of PTSD, and instead promote engagement and meaning creation in present life.

Both clinical and neuroimaging studies show that compassion meditation increases positive emotions and decreases negative emotions [80, 81]. It activates

Table 10.9 Utility of adjunct compassion meditation for PTSD

Cognitive and emotional processes	Utility in PTSD management
Increases positive emotion [16, 50, 83]	Improves outlook and life satisfaction, increases motivation, hope, sense of purpose in life, and resilience [81, 84]
Reduces negative affect [16, 86]	Decreases fear, anger, shame, depression, dysphoria, and anhedonia [81]
Increases social connectedness [16, 80]	Improves family relationships and builds social support important for reintegration and recovery [80]
Reduces hyperarousal [16]	Increases coping, decrease reactivity [16]

specific areas of the brain associated with positive affect and empathy, and strengthens their connections to the left mPFC [16, 19, 49, 50, 82, 83]. Fostering positive emotions and outlook may result in a profound clinical benefit by decreasing a whole cluster of negative emotions of PTSD (i.e., fear, anger, guilt, shame, depression, and dysphoria), building resilience [84], reducing symptoms of autonomic hyperarousal, and increasing coping [16]. Compassion meditation also encourages pro-social behavior and social connectedness [16, 80, 85], essential for building social support, family relationships, resilience, and reintegration during the recovery process in individuals with PTSD [16, 19].

Several small trials on compassion meditation for stress, chronic pain, and mental illness show positive effects that may be of interest in future research on PTSD. Johnson et al. studied loving–kindness meditation in individuals with schizophrenia-spectrum disorders and persistent negative symptoms ($n=18$ pilot) [86]. Their findings suggest that loving–kindness meditation may improve factors associated with psychological recovery such as increased positive emotion, life satisfaction, hope and purpose in life, while simultaneously reducing negative symptoms, anhedonia, and asociality [86, 87]. Carson demonstrated similar results in patients with chronic low back pain ($N=43$), suggesting that the loving–kindness meditation can be beneficial in reducing anger, hostility, psychological distress, and pain [88]. Finally, Pace et al. showed improved neuroendocrine (cortisol), immune (IL-6), inflammatory (C-reactive protein), and behavioral markers of stress with practice of compassion meditation [89, 90].

Overall, preliminary data suggest that compassion meditation may offer a valuable adjunct to standard PTSD care. It may help increase positive emotions, reduce negative affect, improve resilience, and help facilitate recovery and reintegration process through fostering social connectedness (Table 10.9). Future well-designed randomized controlled trials specific to PTSD and co-occurring conditions are warranted and should include simultaneous investigation of neuroimaging correlates and at least a 6-month follow-up.

10.5 Clinical Cases

10.5.1 Mindfulness Meditation Case

10.5.1.1 Clinical Presentation

A 42-year-old service member presents to a primary care provider with a history of two tours in Iraq and a diagnosis of combat PTSD and moderate depression for the past 4 years. He is a 1-pack-a-day smoker but denies misuse of any other illicit substances or alcohol. He has no other past medical or surgical history. His family history is significant for alcohol abuse in his father and major depressive disorder in his older sister.

The patient has been on fluoxetine 40 mg daily for 3 years and has been seeing a psychologist every 2 weeks for trauma-focused psychotherapy for a year. He reports noticeable improvements in both his PTSD and depression symptoms, but admits to being "emotionally reactive," having difficulty controlling his impulses, and sometimes loosing and responding to his children in a harsh and aggressive manner. He also desires to quit smoking but reports it to be hard to control cravings and his impulse to smoke, especially when he is under stress. He asks if there is something he can do at home to help him gain better control of his emotions, and self-manage symptoms of PTSD and depression.

10.5.1.2 Assessment

Diagnoses: (1) PTSD—controlled, (2) moderate MDD—controlled, in remission, (3) tobacco use disorder—uncontrolled. Impression: the patient is proactive and motivated to quit smoking and explore self-management options to improve his psychological health. His wife is supportive and eager to help.

10.5.1.3 Management

In this case, mindfulness meditation is an excellent adjunct self-care option for the patient himself or practiced as a family activity. Mindfulness meditation instructions, related evidence, required training, and time commitment were discussed. A sample 3-min mindfulness meditation demonstration was offered to the patient and his wife during this consultation. Instructions for home practice and additional resources were offered through appropriate referrals to a local community MBCT classes. Since the patient was ready to try a mindfulness meditation practice, a start date for this lifestyle change was determined and documented, and a 6-week follow-up visit was scheduled. The patient was instructed not to discontinue fluoxetine or psychotherapy and to contact his physician if he has any questions before the next visit.

10.5.1.4 Outcome

After 6 weeks, the patient reports that he is practicing mindfulness meditation every morning with his 9-year-old son. His wife joins them on weekends and enthusiastically comments how much she enjoys this family time together. He reports a better control over his residual depressive and PTSD symptoms (e.g., rumination, intrusive negative thoughts), decreased cigarette cravings, improved impulse control related to smoking, and occasional aggressive outbursts. Most importantly, mindfulness meditation equipped and empowered this service member with tools to gain better control of his emotional state and mental health. The follow-up visit should address continued compliance with psychotherapy and pharmacotherapy, and any questions about the practice of the chosen mindfulness technique.

10.5.2 Mantram Repetition Program and Compassion Meditation Case

10.5.2.1 Clinical Presentation

A 45-year-old Operation Enduring Freedom (OEF) veteran presents with a history of combat PTSD. He recently retired and reports having difficulty reintegrating back into civilian life, a lot of anxiety about his future path, and the ability to provide for his family. He commonly catches himself worrying and getting easily overwhelmed. The patient also reports having a hard time reconciling the "brutality and destruction of war," blaming himself, and feeling guilty "for surviving, when so many have fallen." He reports feeling isolated and not being able to share these feelings with anyone. When questioned about experiencing joy, he states that he feels numb, unmotivated, and indifferent in his family life and at work. The patient is not on any medication but is seeing a psychologist and reports that his PTSD is otherwise well controlled. He has no other past medical or surgical history, and no family history of mental illness. He is married with two teenage children.

10.5.2.2 Assessment

Diagnosis: PTSD—controlled. Impression: The patient's reintegration into work and family life is inhibited due to his feelings of guilt. It is complicated by decreased capacity to experience positive emotions, emotional numbing, avoidance, isolation, and anxiousness.

10.5.2.3 Management

In this case, a combination of mantram repetition and compassion meditation may be the best approach. Choosing a mantra that carries a personal spiritual significance and practicing mantram repetition can help increase spiritual well-being, reduce shame, guilt, and cope with moral injury of war. It will also reduce hyperarousal symptoms and anxiousness. Compassion meditation in addition to decreasing negative emotions has a unique ability to increase positive affect (e.g., motivation and joy), promote a sense of connectedness, improve family relationships, and decrease a sense of isolation.

Both interventions were described and demonstrated for the patient, including related evidence, and key benefits. Additional resources and instructions for home practice were given, a start date was determined, and a 4-week follow-up visit was scheduled. The patient was instructed not to discontinue psychotherapy without discussing with his physician first.

10.5.2.4 Outcome

After 4 weeks the patient reports decreased anxiousness, feeling more grounded, comforted, and connected during his meditation practice. He practices compassion meditation daily and mantram repetition situationally at the time of increased stress or a wave of anxiety. He likes that this new tool is available to him anytime anywhere, and can now feel more confident with this new found sense of control. The veteran also reports that it is becoming more natural for him to experience positive emotions such as love and joy and easier to be social at work, and connect with his wife and children. He has made plans to spend time with the extended family and is excited about an upcoming fishing trip with his friend.

10.6 Clinical Pearls and Conclusions for Clinical Practice

The evidence of the meditation effectiveness as an adjunct to standard PTSD care is rapidly growing. Brewer et al. discuss overlaps in common neural pathways of PTSD and comorbid conditions, and how potential mechanisms of mindfulness training may offer unique promise for their treatment [91]. This wide-spectrum potency of meditation and established safety make it a versatile, valuable, and cost-effective self-management addition to standard care of PTSD and co-occurring mental health conditions. The self-care nature of meditation practice allows patients to feel more in control of their symptoms and empowers them to take an active central role in their own healing process. The physician's role is to educate the patient about the benefits of different meditation techniques as it relates to a specific clinical presentation, and encourage a patient to choose the technique that resonates with him/her to assure compliance and successful long-term adoption of meditation practice. As the benefits of meditation accrue over time, selecting a method that motivates sustained practice is a critical objective if therapeutic effects are to be achieved [92]. It is critical to emphasize the importance to continue medications and psychotherapy while using meditation adjunctively, and to schedule regular follow-up visits to monitor compliance. Patients should be advised not to discontinue their usual care without consulting with their physician.

References

1. Strauss J, Coeytaux R, McDuffie J, Nagi A, Williams JJ. Efficacy of complementary and alternative medicine therapies for posttraumatic stress disorder [Internet]. VA-ESP Project 2011;090(010).
2. Kim S, Schneider S, Kravitz L, Mermier C, Burge M. Mind-body practices for posttraumatic stress disorder. J Investig Med. 2013;61(5):827–34.
3. Bränström R, Kvillemo P, Brandberg Y, Moskowitz J. Self-report mindfulness as a mediator of psychological well-being in a stress reduction intervention for cancer patients–a randomized study. Ann Behav Med. 2010;39(2):151–61.
4. Strauss JL, Lang A. Complementary and alternative treatments for PTSD. PTSD Res Q. 2012;23(2):1–3.

5. Libby D, Pilver C, Desai R. Complementary and alternative medicine in VA specialized PTSD treatment programs. Psychiatr Serv. 2012;63(11):1134–6.
6. Libby D, Reddy F, Pilver C, Desai R. The use of yoga in specialized VA PTSD treatment programs. Int J Yoga Therap. 2012;22:79–87.
7. Lutz A, Slagter H, Dunne J, Davidson R. Attention regulation and monitoring in meditation. Trends Cogn Sci. 2008;12(4):163–9.
8. Sperduti M, Martinelli P, Piolino P. A neurocognitive model of meditation based on activation likelihood estimation (ALE) meta-analysis. Conscious Cogn. 2012;21(1):269–76.
9. Rubia K. The neurobiology of meditation and its clinical effectiveness in psychiatric disorders. Biol Psychol. 2009;82(1):1–11.
10. Travis F, Shear J. Focused attention, open monitoring and automatic self-transcending: categories to organize meditations from Vedic, Buddhist and Chinese traditions. Conscious Cogn. 2010;19(4):1110–8.
11. Kabat-Zinn J. Bringing mindfulness to medicine: an interview with Jon Kabat-Zinn, PhD. Interview by Karolyn Gazella. Adv Mind Body Med. 2005;21(2):22–7.
12. Segal Z. Finding daylight: mindful recovery from depression. Psychotherapy networker. January/February 2008; 1–6.
13. Farb N, Segal Z, Mayberg H, Bean J, McKeon D, Fatima Z, et al. Attending to the present: mindfulness meditation reveals distinct neural modes of self-reference. Soc Cogn Affect Neurosci. 2007;2(4):313–22.
14. Farb N, Anderson A, Mayberg H, Bean J, McKeon D, Segal Z, et al. Minding one's emotions: mindfulness training alters the neural expression of sadness. Emotion. 2010;10(1):25–33.
15. Chiesa A, Serretti A. A systematic review of neurobiological and clinical features of mindfulness meditations. Psychol Med. 2010;40(8):1239–52.
16. Lang A, Strauss J, Bomyea J, Bormann J, Hickman S, Good R, et al. The theoretical and empirical basis for meditation as an intervention for PTSD. Behav Modif. 2012;36(6):759–86.
17. Chiesa A, Malinowski P. Mindfulness-based approaches: are they all the same? J Clin Psychol. 2011;67(4):404–24.
18. Khusid M. Self-care mindfulness approaches for refractory posttraumatic stress disorder. Psychiatric Annals. 2013;43(7):340–4.
19. Davidson RJ, Begley S. The emotional life of your brain: how its unique patterns affect the way you think, feel, and live—and how you can change them. USA: Plume Book; 2012.
20. Kabat-Zinn J. An outpatient program in behavioral medicine for chronic pain patients based on the practice of mindfulness meditation: theoretical considerations and preliminary results. Gen Hosp Psychiatry. 1982;4(1):33–47.
21. Kearney D, McDermott K, Malte C, Martinez M, Simpson T. Effects of participation in a mindfulness program for veterans with posttraumatic stress disorder: a randomized controlled pilot study. J Clin Psychol. 2013;69(1):14–27.
22. Teasdale J, Segal Z, Williams J, Ridgeway V, Soulsby J, Lau M, et al. Prevention of relapse/recurrence in major depression by mindfulness-based cognitive therapy. J Consult Clin Psychol. 2000;68(4):615–23.
23. Creswell J, Way B, Eisenberger N, Lieberman M. Neural correlates of dispositional mindfulness during affect labeling. Psychosom Med. 2007;69(6):560–5.
24. Bränström R, Kvillemo P, Akerstedt T. Effects of mindfulness training on levels of cortisol in cancer patients. Psychosomatics. 2013;54(2):158–64.
25. Hölzel B, Carmody J, Evans K, Hoge E, Dusek J, Morgan L, et al. Stress reduction correlates with structural changes in the amygdala. Soc Cogn Affect Neurosci. 2010;5(1):11–7.
26. Hölzel B, Carmody J, Vangel M, Congleton C, Yerramsetti S, Gard T, et al. Mindfulness practice leads to increases in regional brain gray matter density. Psychiatry Res. 2011;191(1):36–43.
27. Nakamura Y, Lipschitz D, Kuhn R, Kinney A, Donaldson G. Investigating efficacy of two brief mind-body intervention programs for managing sleep disturbance in cancer survivors: a pilot randomized controlled trial. J Cancer Surviv. 2013;7(2):165–82.

28. Barnhofer T, Duggan D, Griffith J. Dispositional mindfulness moderates the relation between neuroticism and depressive symptoms. Pers Individ Dif. 2011;51(8):958–62.
29. Taylor V, Grant J, Daneault V, Scavone G, Breton E, Roffe-Vidal S, et al. Impact of mindfulness on the neural responses to emotional pictures in experienced and beginner meditators. Neuroimage. 2011;57(4):1524–33.
30. Kozasa E, Sato J, Lacerda S, Barreiros M, Radvany J, Russell T, et al. Meditation training increases brain efficiency in an attention task. Neuroimage. 2012;59(1):745–9.
31. Solberg E, Holen A, Ekeberg Ø, Østerud B, Halvorsen R, Sandvik L, et al. The effects of long meditation on plasma melatonin and blood serotonin. Med Sci Monit. 2004;10(3):CR96–C101.
32. Kimbrough E, Magyari T, Langenberg P, Chesney M, Berman B. Mindfulness intervention for child abuse survivors. J Clin Psychol. 2010;66(1):17–33.
33. Kearney D, McDermott K, Malte C, Martinez M, Simpson T. Association of participation in a mindfulness program with measures of PTSD, depression and quality of life in a veteran sample. J Clin Psychol. 2012;68(1):101–16.
34. Bränström R, Kvillemo P, Moskowitz J. A randomized study of the effects of mindfulness training on psychological well-being and symptoms of stress in patients treated for cancer at 6-month follow-up. Int J Behav Med. 2012;19(4):535–42.
35. Goldin P, Ziv M, Jazaieri H, Gross J. Randomized controlled trial of mindfulness-based stress reduction versus aerobic exercise: effects on the self-referential brain network in social anxiety disorder. Front Hum. Neuroscience. 2012;6:295.
36. Goldin P, Gross J. Effects of mindfulness-based stress reduction (MBSR) on emotion regulation in social anxiety disorder. Emotion. 2010;10(1):83–91.
37. Goldin P, Ziv M, Jazaieri H, Hahn K, Gross J. MBSR vs aerobic exercise in social anxiety: fMRI of emotion regulation of negative self-beliefs. Soc Cogn Affect Neurosci. 2013;8(1):65–72.
38. King A, Erickson T, Giardino N, Favorite T, Rauch S, Robinson E, et al. A pilot study of group mindfulness-based cognitive therapy (MBCT) for Combat Veterans with posttraumatic stress disorder (PTSD). Depress Anxiety. 2013;30(7):638–45.
39. Waelde L, Uddo M, Marquett R, Ropelato M, Freightman S, Pardo A, et al. A pilot study of meditation for mental health workers following Hurricane Katrina. J Trauma Stress. 2008;21(5):497–500.
40. Bormann J, Thorp S, Wetherell J, Golshan S. A spiritually based group intervention for combat veterans with posttraumatic stress disorder: feasibility study. J Holist Nurs. 2008;26(2):109–16.
41. Farb N, Anderson A, Segal Z. The mindful brain and emotion regulation in mood disorders. Can J Psychiatry. 2012;57(2):70–7.
42. Kuyken W, Byford S, Taylor R, Watkins E, Holden E, White K, et al. Mindfulness-based cognitive therapy to prevent relapse in recurrent depression. J Consult Clin Psychol. 2008;76(6):966–78.
43. Ma S, Teasdale J. Mindfulness-based cognitive therapy for depression: replication and exploration of differential relapse prevention effects. J Consult Clin Psychol. 2004;72(1):31–40.
44. Segal Z, Bieling P, Young T, MacQueen G, Cooke R, Martin L, et al. Antidepressant monotherapy vs sequential pharmacotherapy and mindfulness-based cognitive therapy, or placebo, for relapse prophylaxis in recurrent depression. Arch Gen Psychiatry. 2010;67(12):1256–64.
45. Mathew K, Whitford H, Kenny M, Denson L. The long-term effects of mindfulness-based cognitive therapy as a relapse prevention treatment for major depressive disorder. Behav Cogn Psychother. 2010;38(5):561–76.
46. Barnhofer T, Duggan D, Crane C, Hepburn S, Fennell M, Williams J, et al. Effects of meditation on frontal alpha-asymmetry in previously suicidal individuals. Neuroreport. 2007;18(7):709–12.
47. Teasdale J, Moore R, Hayhurst H, Pope M, Williams S, Segal Z, et al. Metacognitive awareness and prevention of relapse in depression: empirical evidence. J Consult Clin Psychol. 2002;70(2):275–87.

48. Kuyken W, Watkins E, Holden E, White K, Taylor R, Byford S, et al. How does mindfulness-based cognitive therapy work? Behav Res Ther. 2010;48(11):1105–12.
49. Lutz A, Greischar L, Perlman D, Davidson R. BOLD signal in insula is differentially related to cardiac function during compassion meditation in experts vs. novices. Neuroimage. 2009;47(3):1038–46.
50. Klimecki O, Leiberg S, Lamm C, Singer T. Functional neural plasticity and associated changes in positive affect after compassion training. Cereb Cortex. 2012;23(7):1552–161.
51. Barnhofer T, Chittka T, Nightingale H, Visser C, Crane C. State effects of two forms of meditation on prefrontal EEG asymmetry in previously depressed individuals. Mindfulness (N Y). 2010;1(1):21–7.
52. Hibbard J. Engaging health care consumers to improve the quality of care. Med Care. 2003;41(1 Suppl):I61–70.
53. Chiesa A, Serretti A. Are mindfulness-based interventions effective for substance use disorders? A systematic review of the evidence. Subst Use Misuse. 2014;49(5):492–512.
54. Zgierska A, Rabago D, Chawla N, Kushner K, Koehler R, Marlatt A, et al. Mindfulness meditation for substance use disorders: a systematic review. Subst Abus. 2009;30(4):266–94.
55. Witkiewitz K, Bowen S, Douglas H, Hsu S. Mindfulness-based relapse prevention for substance craving. Addict Behav. 2013;38(2):1563–71.
56. Witkiewitz K, Lustyk M, Bowen S. Retraining the addicted brain: a review of hypothesized neurobiological mechanisms of mindfulness-based relapse prevention. Psychol Addict Behav. 2012;27(2):351–65.
57. Bowen S, Chawla N, Collins S, Witkiewitz K, Hsu S, Grow J, et al. Mindfulness-based relapse prevention for substance use disorders: a pilot efficacy trial. Subst Abus. 2009;30(4):295–305.
58. Witkiewitz K, Bowen S. Depression, craving, and substance use following a randomized trial of mindfulness-based relapse prevention. J Consult Clin Psychol. 2010;78(3):362–74.
59. Skanavi S, Laqueille X, Aubin H. Mindfulness based interventions for addictive disorders: a review. Encephale. 2011;37(5):379–87.
60. Winbush N, Gross C, Kreitzer M. The effects of mindfulness-based stress reduction on sleep disturbance: a systematic review. Explore (NY). 2007;3(6):585–91.
61. Chiesa A, Serretti A. Mindfulness-based interventions for chronic pain: a systematic review of the evidence. J Altern Complement Med. 2011;17(1):83–93.
62. Grant J, Courtemanche J, Duerden E, Duncan G, Rainville P. Cortical thickness and pain sensitivity in Zen meditators. Emotion. 2010;10(1):43–53.
63. Grant J, Rainville P. Pain sensitivity and analgesic effects of mindful states in Zen meditators: a cross-sectional study. Psychosom Med. 2009;71(1):106–14.
64. Gard T, Hölzel BK, Sack AT, Hempel H, Lazar SW, Vaitl D, et al. Pain attenuation through mindfulness is associated with decreased cognitive control and increased sensory processing in the brain. Cereb Cortex. 2011;22(11):2692–702.
65. Zeidan F, Martucci K, Kraft R, Gordon N, McHaffie J, Coghill R, et al. Brain mechanisms supporting the modulation of pain by mindfulness meditation. J Neurosci. 2011;31(14):5540–8.
66. Kabat-Zinn J. An outpatient program in behavioral medicine for chronic pain patients based on the practice of mindfulness meditation: theoretical considerations and preliminary results. Gen Hosp Psychiatry. 1982;4(1):33–47.
67. Grant J, Courtemanche J, Rainville P. A non-elaborative mental stance and decoupling of executive and pain-related cortices predicts low pain sensitivity in Zen meditators. Pain. 2011;152(1):150–6.
68. Ospina M, Bond K, Karkhaneh M, Tjosvold L, Vandermeer B, Liang Y, et al. Meditation practices for health: state of the research. Evid Rep Technol Assess (Full Rep). 2007;155:1–263.
69. Easwaran E. The mantram handbook. Tomales: Nilgiri Press; 2008.
70. Bormann J, Smith T, Becker S, Gershwin M, Pada L, Grudzinski A, et al. Efficacy of frequent mantram repetition on stress, quality of life, and spiritual well-being in veterans: a pilot study. J Holist Nurs. 2005;23(4):395–414.
71. Vujanovic AA, Niles B, Pietrefesa A, Schmertz SK, Potter CM. Mindfulness in the treatment of posttraumatic stress disorder among military veterans. Prof Psychol: Res Pract. 2011;42(1):24–31.

72. Bormann J. Frequent, silent mantram repetition: a Jacuzzi for the mind. Top Emerg Med. 2005;27(2):163.
73. Bormann J, Liu L, Thorp S, Lang A. Spiritual wellbeing mediates PTSD change in veterans with military-related PTSD. Int J Behav Med. 2012;19(4):496–502.
74. Bormann J, Oman D, Kemppainen J, Becker S, Gershwin M, Kelly A, et al. Mantram repetition for stress management in veterans and employees: a critical incident study. J Adv Nurs. 2006;53(5):502–12.
75. Maharishi M. Maharishi Mahesh Yogi on the Bhagavad Gita. New York: Penguin; 1969.
76. Brooks J, Scarano T. Transcendental meditation in the treatment of post-Vietnam adjustment. J Couns Dev. 1985;64:212–5.
77. Rosenthal J, Grosswald S, Ross R, Rosenthal N. Effects of transcendental meditation in veterans of operation enduring freedom and operation Iraqi freedom with posttraumatic stress disorder: a pilot study. Mil Med. 2011;176(6):626–30.
78. Lamm C, Decety J, Singer T. Meta-analytic evidence for common and distinct neural networks associated with directly experienced pain and empathy for pain. Neuroimage. 2011;54(3):2492–502.
79. Bernhardt B, Singer T. The neural basis of empathy. Annu Rev Neurosci. 2012;35:1–23.
80. Hutcherson C, Seppala E, Gross J. Loving-kindness meditation increases social connectedness. Emotion. 2008;8(5):720–4.
81. Fredrickson B, Cohn M, Coffey K, Pek J, Finkel S. Open hearts build lives: positive emotions, induced through loving-kindness meditation, build consequential personal resources. J Pers Soc Psychol. 2008;95(5):1045–62.
82. Engström M, Söderfeldt B. Brain activation during compassion meditation: a case study. J Altern Complement Med. 2010;16(5):597–9.
83. Lutz A, Brefczynski-Lewis J, Johnstone T, Davidson R. Regulation of the neural circuitry of emotion by compassion meditation: effects of meditative expertise. PLoS ONE. 2008;3(3):10.
84. Cohn M, Fredrickson B, Brown S, Mikels J, Conway A. Happiness unpacked: positive emotions increase life satisfaction by building resilience. Emotion. 2009;9(3):361–8.
85. Leiberg S, Klimecki O, Singer T. Short-term compassion training increases prosocial behavior in a newly developed prosocial game. PLoS ONE. 2011;6(3):e17798.
86. Johnson D, Penn D, Fredrickson B, Kring A, Meyer P, Catalino L, et al. A pilot study of loving-kindness meditation for the negative symptoms of schizophrenia. Schizophr Res. 2011;129(2–3):137–40.
87. Johnson D, Penn D, Fredrickson B, Meyer P, Kring A, Brantley M, et al. Loving-kindness meditation to enhance recovery from negative symptoms of schizophrenia. J Clin Psychol. 2009;65(5):499–509.
88. Carson J, Keefe F, Lynch T, Carson K, Goli V, Fras A, et al. Loving-kindness meditation for chronic low back pain: results from a pilot trial. J Holist Nurs. 2005;23(3):287–304.
89. Pace T, Negi L, Adame D, Cole S, Sivilli T, Brown T, et al. Effect of compassion meditation on neuroendocrine, innate immune and behavioral responses to psychosocial stress. Psychoneuroendocrinology. 2009;34(1):87–98.
90. Pace T, Negi L, Dodson-Lavelle B, Ozawa-de S, Reddy S, Cole S, et al. Engagement with cognitively-based compassion training is associated with reduced salivary C-reactive protein from before to after training in foster care program adolescents. Psychoneuroendocrinology. 2013;38(2):294–9.
91. Brewer J, Bowen S, Smith J, Marlatt G, Potenza M. Mindfulness-based treatments for co-occurring depression and substance use disorders: what can we learn from the brain? Addiction. 2010;105(10):1698–706.
92. Burke A. Comparing individual preferences for four meditation techniques: Zen, Vipassana (mindfulness), Qigong, and Mantra. Explore (NY). 2012;8(4):237–42.)

Use of Transcranial Magnetic Stimulation for the Treatment of PTSD

11

Geoffrey G. Grammer, Jeffrey T. Cole, Cody J. Rall and Caroline C. Scacca

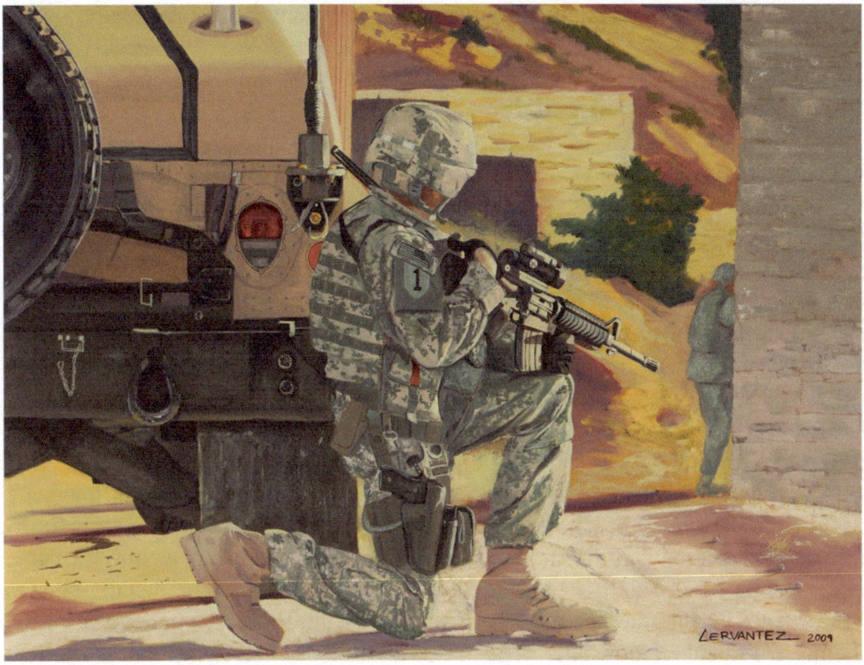

I Got Your Six, by MSG Martin J. Cervantez, courtesy of the Army Art Collection, US Army Center of Military History

G. G. Grammer (✉)
National Intrepid Center of Excellence, Walter Reed National Military Medical Center, 8901 Wisconsin Ave, Bethesda, MD 20889, USA
e-mail: geoffrey.g.grammer.mil@mail.mil

J. T. Cole
Department of Neurology, Booz Allen Hamilton, McLean, VA 22102, USA

E. C. Ritchie (ed.), *Posttraumatic Stress Disorder and Related Diseases in Combat Veterans,* DOI 10.1007/978-3-319-22985-0_11

Posttraumatic stress disorder (PTSD) is a complex illness that rarely occurs in isolation from other psychiatric morbidities, and often fails to remit with standard therapies. Traditionally, PTSD is treated with psychotherapy and/or pharmacotherapy, with treatment choices often based on availability, patient preference, and patient tolerance. One of the more commonly recommended psychotherapy treatment modalities is exposure-based therapy, where a patient recalls traumatic events, usually with some form of relaxation, with the hope of inducing extinction of the anxiety response to the stimulus [1]. In addition to treatment with psychotherapy, pharmacotherapy is also commonly administered, despite potentially adverse side effects and the risk of polypharmacy. Many patients are prescribed psychotropics to ameliorate symptoms, particularly if PTSD exists with other comorbid conditions. While psychotherapy and pharmacology may have utility for many patients, their limited efficacy promotes the need for novel treatment options. One possible alternative treatment option is transcranial magnetic stimulation (TMS), which is a noninvasive brain stimulation technique that has a broad range of therapeutic capabilities.

11.1 Care Presentation/History

A 35-year-old African American male with a history of recurrent depression since age 14 and PTSD symptoms resulting from two deployments to Afghanistan, self-referred for repetitive transcranial magnetic stimulation (rTMS) after hearing about the technology on the radio and investigating its features online. His depressive symptoms were characterized by depressed mood, anhedonia, low energy, fragmented sleep, hyperphagia with unintentional weight gain, guilt, a sense of worthlessness, and recurring thoughts of dying without suicidal ideations or intent. Since age 14, these had been present to varying degrees, without any complete resolution. For the past 9 years, he reported his symptom severity continually met criteria for a depressive episode with no periods of partial resolution.

Approximately 10 years prior to his presentation to the transcranial magnetic stimulation (TMS) clinic, the patient had deployed twice to Afghanistan with direct combat operational duties. Since that time, he admitted to feeling on edge, experiencing ease of startle, daytime intrusive recollections of combat, nightmares associated with the trauma, and efforts to avoid stimuli that reminded him of the trauma. He found relationships difficult due to a sense of disconnectedness and was profoundly socially isolated. There was also a sense of foreshortened future, which propagated a sense of hopelessness that his symptoms would not abate.

C. J. Rall
Department of Psychiatry, Walter Reed National Military Medical Center,
Bethesda, MD 20889, USA

C. C. Scacca
Department of Behavioral Health, Walter Reed National Military Medical Center,
Bethesda, MD 20889, USA
e-mail: caroline.c.sacca.mil@mail.mil

11.1.1 Developmental History

The patient denied any history of physical, emotional, or sexual abuse, with no history of legal troubles. He graduated high school on time and had earned a 4-year college degree. After serving in the military, he obtained work as a Department of Defense government employee. The patient had never been married and had no children. He had been without a sustained romantic relationship since returning from Afghanistan. His predominant recreational activity was weight training several hours each day.

11.1.2 Past Medical History

On presentation, there were no known medical illnesses and no history of seizures. He denied any metallic fragments or implants above the neckline. The patient had not received any surgical procedures to date. He took several supplements, including a daily multivitamin, Omega-3 supplements, probiotics, and amino acids. He did not report any allergies. He admitted to occasional 1–2 cigarette use when he was out with friends. There was no report of illicit drug use, including anabolic steroids.

Alcohol use was a concern. He admitted to daily use of alcohol, up to six drinks each night, over the past 10 years. He had developed a tolerance to alcohol, would have trouble limiting the amount he did drink, struggled to cut back his drinking, and admitted that it worsened his mood over time. Three months prior to presentation, he made a conscious effort to limit his intake on the advice of his therapist, drinking 3–4 drinks once a week, but he continued to struggle with strong alcohol cravings.

11.1.3 Family History

Both of his biological parents suffered from major depression. His sister was diagnosed with bipolar disorder type I and had been psychiatrically hospitalized once. There had been no suicides in the family.

11.1.4 Military History

The patient served a total of 7 years, achieving the rank of staff sergeant before an honorable discharge at the end of his enlistment period. During his deployment, he served with special operations units early in the Afghanistan campaign. He received several commendations for his service and never received any disciplinary actions.

Table 11.1 Drug, dose, and result of medication trials in which the patient participated

Trial date	Treatment (dose)	Result
2006	Lamictal starter pack	Rash
2006	Depakote (250 mg qday)	Tinnitus, sedation, dysarthria
2006–2008	Trazodone (100 mg qday)	Sedated during the day
2006–2009	Wellbutrin XL (300 mg qday)	Insomnia
2007–2013	Xanax (0.5 mg prn for anxiety)[a]	
2010–2013	Prozac (40 mg qday)	Weight gain and insomnia
2010–2013	Hydroxyzine (50 mg tid)	Ineffective

[a] Used several times a week for anxiety

11.1.5 Past Psychiatric History

No prior psychiatric hospitalizations were reported, and he had never attempted suicide. His psychiatric care was fragmented over the past 10 years. An attempt at exposure-based therapy several years prior was not tolerated. He was currently engaged in weekly cognitive behavioral therapy over the past 10 months. The patient had previously participated in several medication trials (Table 11.1).

11.2 Diagnosis/Assessment

Psychiatric review of systems was otherwise unremarkable for symptoms of obsessive-compulsive disorder, generalized anxiety, panic disorder, simple phobia, mania, psychosis, eating disorder, or other psychiatric conditions not already mentioned.

11.2.1 Mental Status Examination

The patient arrived wearing a suit and tie, having come straight from his workplace. He was an articulate male, obviously muscular, and remained well composed and professional during the interview. His speech was slightly decreased in volume, but was of normal rate. His motor activity was normal. The patient described his mood as depressed, and while his affect was congruent, he did display brief periods of levity before drifting back to an apathetic baseline. Thought content was without suicidal or homicidal ideation. He denied delusions but did admit to recurrent thoughts of his own mortality. The patient's thought process was goal directed, logical, and linear, with good insight, and intact judgment and impulse control. Cognition was intact as evidenced by a normal Montreal Cognitive Assessment (MoCA), ease of recall of his historical narrative, and varied vocabulary with appropriate low-frequency word use. The patient scored a 22 on the Patient Health Questionaire-9 (PHQ-9), which is indicative of severe depression. On the PTSD Checklist-Military version (PCL-M), the patient scored a 60, which is indicative of PTSD.

The patient's blood was analyzed as follows: Complete blood count (CBC), comprehensive metabolic panel, B12, folate, lyme, thyroid stimulating hormone, rapid plasma reagin, HIV, total and free testosterone, which were all normal or negative. Total cholesterol was 230 mg/dl (125–200). Triglycerides were 194 mg/dl (< 150), high-density lipoprotein (HDL) was 38 mg/dl (> or = 40), and low-density lipoprotein (LDL) was 153 mg/dl (< 130).

Genetic analysis by commercial genetic assay (Genecept™ Assay) showed no clinically significant variations of Ankyrin G (ANK3), Methylenetetrahydrofolate reductase (MTHFR), Cytochrome P450 2D6 (CYP2D6), and Cytochrome P450 3A4 and 3A5 (CYP3A4/5). SLC6A4 was L(G)/L(G) variant suggesting the likelihood of poor or slow response and greater side effects with Selective serotonin reuptake inhibitors (SSRIs) [2]. Catechol methyl transferase (COMT) was Val/Val variant suggesting a reduction in frontal lobe dopamine [3] Serotonin 5HT2C receptor (5HT2C) was C/C variant which may be associated with an increased incidence of weight gain with atypical antipsychotics [4]. Dopamine receptor D2 (DRD2) was INS/DEL, which is associated with reduced efficacy and increased incidence of side effects with antipsychotics [5, 6]. calcium channel, voltage-dependent, L-type, alpha 1C subunit (CACNA1C) was A/A variant, which is a common variation associated with altered function of brain calcium channels [7], altered neuronal excitability, and possible mood instability. Cytochrome P450 2C19 (CYP2C19) was the Ultrarapid Metabolizer variant [8].

11.2.2 Assessment

This 35-year-old male has a genetic predisposition for mood disorders, likely accounting for much of his early age of onset and persistent symptoms despite the absence of a childhood trauma or maladaptive personality function. His genetic profile showing a variant of the serotonin transporter gene Solute carrier family 6 (neurotransmitter transporter), member 4 (*SLC6A4*) suggests suboptimal response to SSRI's. COMT Val/Val variant resulting in decreased frontal lobe dopamine may have contributed to his depressive symptomatology. His historically heavy use of alcohol likely hindered his recovery, and he remained at risk of full relapse if this was not addressed adequately. The patient's admission of weight gain and hyperphagia associated with his depression were reflected with his hyperlipidemia, which also adds a risk of cardiovascular morbidity if not addressed.

Patients with preexisting psychiatric conditions remain at risk of development of PTSD, and many service members with direct combat exposure will endorse some degree of PTSD symptomatology [9]. The presence of PTSD raises the risk of comorbid depression and certainly will hinder recovery from the depressive episode.

The constellation of alcohol dependence, major depressive disorder, and PTSD form a self-perpetuating cycle, where each condition reinforces the others. Therefore, a treatment plan was developed to account for all three of these conditions to maximize the chance of full psychiatric recovery.

11.3 Treatment/Management

Patient preference should figure into any treatment plan, and for this case, the patient had indicated a wish to receive non-pharmacologic treatment for his psychiatric symptoms. The patient was also not interested in receiving electroconvulsive therapy due to stigma and fears of cognitive impairment.

The decision was made to pursue TMS with an off-label pulse sequence to attempt amelioration of both depressive and PTSD symptoms. The decision to use TMS and the pulse sequence selected was based on existing literature and theoretic constructs for the neurophysiologic consequences of both depression and PTSD.

TMS uses a pulsed magnetic field to create neuronal action potentials within areas of the cerebral cortex [10]. Delivery of TMS incorporates several variables including the type of coil utilized, frequency of stimulus delivery, duration of pulse sequence, interstimulation rest periods, strength of the magnetic field delivery, total number of pulses delivered, and regularity of scheduled treatment delivery during the week [11].

11.3.1 Physics of Biological-Modulation

TMS device discharges a strong current through a coil, which produces a rapidly changing magnetic field, with lines of flux perpendicular to the coil's ion flow [12]. As this magnetic field changes with respect to the current in the coil, an electric field is induced that is proportional to the time rate of change of the magnetic field; yet, opposite in direction from the original current in the coil [12, 13]. Since the coil is adjacent to the scalp, and the neuronal tissue of the brain is electrically conductive, the electric field will stimulate a change in the flow of the ionic current [13]. This leads to modulation of the release of neurotransmitters of neurons affected by the induced field. This effect on those proximal neurons creates effects on the downstream neural networks [14]. The overall affect can have broad effects on neural function resulting from focal stimulation.

Both the target area and the power level of the induced-electric field are dependent on the shape of the coil. This allows variation in the field depth and spatial resolution [10]. There are numerous coil designs with corresponding variations of magnetic field production affecting area of spread and depth of penetration of the field.

Frequency of pulse delivery refers to the number of pulses delivered over time. While debate remains over the precise effects of different frequencies, the literature often denotes pulses delivered at less than 1 Hz as promoting long-term inhibition and pulses delivered at greater than 5 Hz as having long-term potentiating effects [11].

When magnetic pulses are delivered, they are typically delivered in trains. For example, a 10 Hz-frequency would be administered over 4 s, for a total of 40 pulses in that train. A rest interval occurs between trains to allow for restoration of the resting state. Higher-frequency stimulation, longer-train sequences, or shorter-recovery interval increases the risk of secondary generalization of the stimulation and subsequent induction of seizure activity. International guidelines exist for these parameters to ensure safe delivery of TMS [15].

The strength of the magnetic field affects the propensity to depolarize cortical neurons. Motor threshold is the amount of the magnetic field needed to depolarize cortical neurons in the primary motor cortex with subsequent contralateral muscle contraction. This level varies by individual and is affected by medications and substances that impact neuronal excitability. Treatments are often referred to as a percentage of this motor threshold. Sub- and supra-threshold stimulations may contribute to long-term inhibition or potentiation, though the impact when coupled with frequency remains ill defined.

The optimal number of pulses per session remains uncertain and likely varies depending on the intended treatment effect. The frequency of delivery also likely impacts the total number of pulses needed to start the cascade of events needed for long-term network changes. Up to 18,000 pulses per day have been administered, sixfold greater than the Food and Drug Administration (FDA) clearance for the figure-8 coil device, and yet was found to be safe and well tolerated [16]. Any treatment sequence also needs to consider the labor intensity to the patient and to the clinic providing care, and sequences that require hours per day are likely to be met with noncompliance and clinical impracticality. While depression is typically treated five times a week for 4–6 weeks, it is unclear if that intensity is needed for other conditions such as PTSD.

Considerations of clinical delivery factored into the pulse sequence that would be used for this patient. Without definitive guidance on a treatment paradigm, understanding the pathophysiology would help guide a TMS treatment program.

11.3.2 Pathophysiology of PTSD

TMS had been used as a diagnostic technique to measure brain GABAergic and glutamatergic tone using paired pulses, whereby a conditioning pulse is followed rapidly by a stimulating pulse. The interval between the two pulses will result in a motor threshold stimulation that is dependent on a gamma-aminobutyric acid (GABA) and glutamate tone reflected in short-latency intracortical inhibition and long-latency intracortical inhibition, respectively. Using these techniques, Rossi et al. (2009) reported that 20 drug-naïve patients with PTSD had reduced GABAergic tone in bilateral hemispheres and increased glutamatergic tone in the right hemisphere [17]. Kim et al. (2014) demonstrated reduced GABA levels in chronic unpredictable mild stress rat model brain extracts, and that TMS reversed these neurochemical changes. These findings suggest a possible pulse sequence model with stimulation of the left dorsolateral prefrontal cortex (DLPFC) and inhibition of the right DLPFC [18]. An excellent review by Karsen et al. (2014) identified the right DLPFC as a potential target for treatment with TMS, but there is a lack of consensus in the literature to clarify which frequencies and motor threshold intensities are optimal [19].

Given all of the factors cited above, the patient was offered treatment with TMS using a figure-8 iron core coil. Each session would involve first treating the left

DLPFC at 10 Hz and 120 % MT for 3500 pulses, in 4 s trains and 20 s intervals. This was followed immediately by right DLPFC stimulation at 1 Hz, 120 % MT, in 26 s trains, 4 s rest intervals, for 1500 pulses. The total treatment time was slightly more than an hour, offered five times a week for 6 weeks, followed by a tapering phase of three times a week in week 7, twice a week in week 8, and once in week 9. The goal was to increase activity of the left DLPFC, capitalizing on known antidepressant properties of this treatment location. The following inhibitory sequence at 1 Hz over the right DLPFC was prompted by data suggesting increase in glutamatergic tone in this area as well as some literature supporting this target as discussed previously.

The TMS pulse sequence described above was designed to address the patient's depressive and PTSD symptoms. However, without addressing his alcohol dependence, complete recovery was less certain. The patient's admission of ongoing alcohol cravings was addressed with a trial of naltrexone (25 mg each day for a week, followed by 50 mg each day). Baseline and follow-up liver function tests were ordered. The patient was instructed to obtain and wear a medical alert bracelet and carry a medical alert card in his wallet to identify his use of naltrexone for consideration in cases of emergency medical care and a requirement for opioid administration.

Additional treatments included encouragement to remain in therapy, utilizing a cognitive behavioral therapy technique. Often patients with chronic psychiatric symptoms experience new challenges when faced with recovery. The therapeutic benefit of psychotherapy, when combined with biologic interventions, can assist with acceptance of recovery and the impact this has on the patient's dynamic relationships and interface with life circumstances.

The patient was adamant about avoiding psychotropics for depression, so no further biologic treatment was recommended outside of his TMS pulse sequence. He was encouraged to make lifestyle changes, including total abstinence from alcohol, efforts to engage in social contact, increase cardiovascular activity to compliment his heavy weight training, and to balance work and leisure activities.

Risks and benefits of his treatment plan were reviewed and informed consent was obtained. The off-label nature of his TMS sequence was specifically discussed, including a lack of FDA clearance for PTSD and relatively unknown risks inherent with this specific sequence.

11.4 Discussion

11.4.1 Limitations of Current Therapies

Psychotherapy is a commonly recommended treatment; however, this modality requires skilled therapists who have specific training, which is often the limiting step in availability to patients [1] This patient had attempted exposure-based therapy, but like many he was unable to tolerate the escalation in anxiety that can occur during sessions.

Pharmacotherapy is often another option for treating depression, despite the risk of polypharmacy and potentially adverse side effects. The SSRIs sertraline and paroxetine have FDA approval for the treatment of adults with PTSD. This patient's genetic profile would suggest a propensity for greater adverse effects from this class of medications and less likelihood of achieving a timely and adequate response. Prazosin is another medication that is often used for the treatment of PTSD, particularly to target nightmares. Though it lacks FDA approval, there is mounting evidence for efficacy of not only sleep disturbance symptoms, but also daytime symptoms of PTSD. Effective doses require careful titration and patient compliance, and can be limited by orthostasis, syncope, somnolence, and sexual dysfunction. This patient's past experiences with medication negatively influenced his enthusiasm for further pharmacologic trials, though one could make a valid argument for a trial of prazosin.

Due to issues of limited efficacy of traditional therapies, other off-label strategies are often attempted, including mood stabilizers, benzodiazepines, antihistamines, and antipsychotics. These agents can have significant toxicity and data on effectiveness for core PTSD symptoms are underwhelming [20]. This patient's experience with off-label therapies mirrors the concerns for poor tolerability and lack of effectiveness.

Continued insistence on previously failed modalities is likely to be met with patient resentment, noncompliance, and ultimately disengagement from care. This may prompt the need for novel treatment options. Caution should be exercised; however, since desperation for symptom relief may influence patient consent for ineffective, expensive, and potentially dangerous unproven therapies. Preliminary research and modalities steeped in valid scientific framework should influence provider recommendations for patients who had not experienced adequate relief with traditional therapies. TMS is one therapy with a sound scientific basis, proven safety, and sufficient preliminary data to suggest efficacy for PTSD, as well as FDA clearance for the treatment of depression.

11.5 Outcomes/Resolution

Baseline scores on PCL-M and PHQ-9 were obtained on the day of his first treatment and were 60 and 24 respectively, suggesting severe symptom severity. At the TMS center, great effort is expended to create a pleasant treatment atmosphere. The architectural design was specifically created for an aesthetically pleasing tone. Staff members were hired with priorities given to technical mastery of the TMS device and interpersonal sophistication. From the start of treatment and throughout his course, the patient had great satisfaction with the experience, the impact of which should not be discounted.

The patient tolerated the TMS procedure well and was compliant with all appointments. He filled his prescription for naltrexone and abstained from alcohol use except for 1 day during the July 4th weekend. He attended all therapy appointments.

Over the course of treatment, the patient had a very steady decline in both his PCL-M and PHQ-9.At the conclusion of the tapering phase, his PCL-M had decreased to 31, which suggested that he no longer met criteria for PTSD. His PHQ-9 decreased to 9, which ranks in the mild severity range for depression.

The patient's subjective reports mirrored his objective rating scales. His PTSD symptoms had resolved and he was able to engage in crowds, interact in social situations, and had a sense of hopefulness for the future. He was able to abstain from drinking alcohol and wanted to continue the naltrexone to maximize his chances of remaining abstinent. Though there were some residual symptoms of depression, the patient was quite satisfied with his recovery and attributed much of his remaining depression to a grief reaction for the loss of a decade of his life to PTSD. He agreed to meet with a psychiatrist to fill his naltrexone, and was open to the idea of single psychopharmacologic maintenance therapy with considerations taken for his genetic profile report. He also agreed to continue seeing his therapist weekly.

11.6 Clinical Pearl

While TMS is undergoing preliminary clinical trials for PTSD, it should be included in the therapeutic armamentarium.

11.7 Conclusion

PTSD is a complex illness, often does not occur in isolation from other psychiatric morbidity, and often fails to remit with standard therapies. Brain stimulation with TMS offers a novel mechanism for the treatment of this condition with theoretical scientific underpinnings coupled with preliminary clinical trials, and may offer an alternative to methodologies that promote polypharmacy and systemic side effects. Any TMS treatment plan should be part of a comprehensive clinical program tailored to maximize recovery and is best implemented by providers familiar with the bevy of modalities available to assist patient recovery. Further study is needed to clarify how best to utilize TMS for conditions such as PTSD, but preliminary work is quite promising. Most importantly, for some patients this modality may pave the road to recovery and should be considered as a potential option when clinical conditions are appropriate.

References

1. Taylor S. Clinician's guide to PTSD: a cognitive-behavioral approach. New York: The Guilford Press; 2006.
2. Staeker J, Leucht S, Laika B, Steimer W Polymorphisms in serotonergic pathways influence the outcome of antidepressant therapy in psychiatric inpatients. Genet Test Mol Biomarkers. 2014;18(1):20–31.
3. Egan MF, Goldberg TE, Kolachana BS, et al. Effect of COMT Val108/158 Met genotype on frontal lobe function and risk for schizophrenia. Proc Natl Acad Sci U S A. 2001;98(12):6917–22.

4. Reynolds GP, Zhang ZJ, Zhang XB. Association of antipsychotic drug-induced weight gain with a 5-HT2C receptor gene polymorphism. Lancet. 2002;359(9323):2086–7.
5. Lencz T, Robinson DG, Napolitano B, et al. DRD2 promoter region variation predicts antipsychotic-induced weight gain in first episode schizophrenia. Pharmacogenet Genomics. 2010;20(9):569–72.
6. Zhang JP, Lencz T, Malhotra AK. D2 receptor genetic variation and clinical response to antipsychotic drug treatment: a meta-analysis. Am J Psychiatry. 2010;167(7):763–72.
7. Bhat S, Dao DT, Terrillion CE, et al. CACNA1C (Cav1.2) in the pathophysiology of psychiatric disease. Prog Neurobiol.2012;99(1):1–14.
8. Samer CF, Lorenzini KI, Rollason V, Daali Y, Desmeules JA. Applications of CYP450 testing in the clinical setting. Mol Diagn Ther. 2013;17(3):165–84.
9. Hoge CW, Castro CA, Messer SC, McGurk D, Cotting DI, Koffman RL. Combat duty in Iraq and Afghanistan, mental health problems and barriers to care. U.S. Army Med Dep J. 2008:7–17.
10. Hallett M. Transcranial magnetic stimulation: a primer. Neuron. 2007;55(2):187–99.
11. McCann UD, Kimbrell TA, Morgan CM, et al. Repetitive transcranial magnetic stimulation for posttraumatic stress disorder. Arch Gen Psychiatry. 1998;55(3):276–9.
12. Horvath JC, Perez JM, Forrow L, Fregni F, Pascual-Leone A Transcranial magnetic stimulation: a historical evaluation and future prognosis of therapeutically relevant ethical concerns. J Med Ethics. 2011;37(3):137–43.
13. Bolognini N, Ro T Transcranial magnetic stimulation: disrupting neural activity to alter and assess brain function. J Neurosci. 2010;30(29):9647–50.
14. Boggio PS, Rocha M, Oliveira MO, et al. Noninvasive brain stimulation with high-frequency and low-intensity repetitive transcranial magnetic stimulation treatment for posttraumatic stress disorder. J Clin Psychiatry. 2010;71(8):992–9.
15. Wassermann EM. Risk and safety of repetitive transcranial magnetic stimulation: report and suggested guidelines from the International Workshop on the Safety of Repetitive Transcranial Magnetic Stimulation, June 5–7, 1996. Electroencephalogr Clin Neurophysiol. 1998;108(1):1–16.
16 George MS, Raman R, Benedek DM, et al. A two-site pilot randomized 3 day trial of high dose left prefrontal repetitive transcranial magnetic stimulation (rTMS) for suicidal inpatients. Brain Stimul. May-Jun 2014;7(3):421–31.
17. Rossi S, De Capua A, Tavanti M, Calossi S, Polizzotto NR, Mantovani A, Falzarano V, Bossini L, Passero S, Bartalini S, Ulivelli M. Dysfunctions of cortical excitability in drug-naïve posttraumatic stress disorder patients. Biol Psychiatry. 2009;66(1):54–61.
18. Kim SY, Lee DW, Kim H, Bang E, Chae JH, Choe BY. Chronic repetitive transcranial magnetic stimulation enhances GABAergic and cholinergic metabolism in chronic unpredictable mild stress rat model: (1)H-NMR spectroscopy study at 11.7T. Neurosci Lett. 2014;572:32–7.
19. Karsen EF, Watts BV, Holtzheimer PE. Review of the effectiveness of transcranial magnetic stimulation for Posttraumatic stress disorder. Brain Stimul. 2014;7(2):151–7.
20. Group TMoP-TSW. VA/DoD Clinical practice guideline for management of Posttraumatic stress. In: Defense DoVAaDo, 2010.

Adding a Face and the Story to the Data: Acupuncture for PTSD in the Military

12

Anita H. Hickey and Robert Koffman

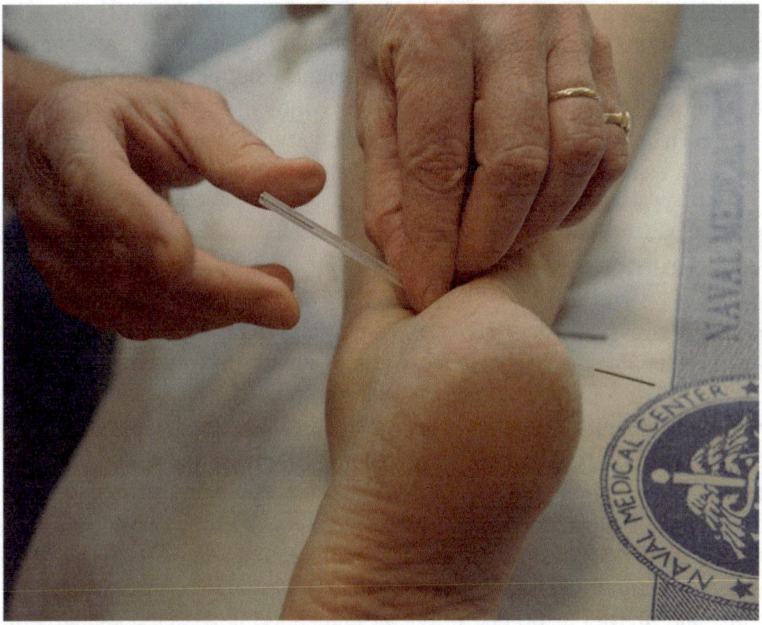

Courtesy of Anita Hickey, MD

A. H. Hickey (✉)
Integrative and Interventional Pain Medicine, Department of Anesthesiology, USNH Okinawa, PSC 482 BOX 173, FPO Okinawa 96362, Japan
e-mail: anihickey@gmail.com

R. Koffman
Integrative Medicine and Behavioral Health, National Intrepid Center of Excellence, Walter Reed National Military Medical Center, 8901 Rockville Pike, Bethesda, MD 20814, USA
e-mail: robert.koffman@semperfifund.org

E. C. Ritchie (ed.), *Posttraumatic Stress Disorder and Related Diseases in Combat Veterans*, DOI 10.1007/978-3-319-22985-0_12

Acupuncture is a holistic approach, which has been used since ancient times to treat physical, emotional, psychological, and spiritual disorders at a fundamental systemic level. This is in accordance with the current system's view of living systems, organizations and ecosystems, which recognize that the whole is greater than the sum of its parts due to the parts being in relationship [1].

Acupuncture has long been used for physical, emotional, psychological, and spiritual disorders in China, Korea, Japan, and other countries in the Far East. It utilizes thin, filament-like needles to treat more than 2000 points, which connect with 12 main and 8 secondary pathways called meridians. According to ancient texts, these channels conduct "qi" between the surface of the body and internal organs.

Qi is the circulating life force that regulates spiritual, emotional, and physical balance. The opposing forces of yin and yang influence qi. Imbalances of the flow of qi may be caused by illness, trauma, stress, and poor lifestyle choices. Acupuncture is believed to balance yin and yang, which keeps the normal flow of energy unblocked and restores harmony and health to the body and mind [2].

An acupuncture diagnosis is made after listening to the patient and performing an examination to determine the patient's mental, emotional, and physical condition. A treatment is then designed to treat both symptoms and the underlying imbalance. Just as in conventional Western medicine, varying amount of skill in diagnosis and treatment can result in differing outcomes.

12.1 Acupuncture for PTSD

Posttraumatic stress disorder (PTSD) is a complex syndrome, which affects mental, emotional, behavioral, and physical aspects of health. According to Otis and colleagues in a 2010 study, PTSD has been found to coexist in 34–50 % of veterans referred for treatment of chronic pain [3]. Persistent hyper arousal and activation of the fight or flight response in these patients results in dysregulation of the autonomic nervous system and other related neurophysiologic functions [4, 5]. Disruption of these systems in patients with PTSD has been shown to be associated with the multiple poor health outcomes including: metabolic disease, cardiovascular disease, asthma, cancer, back pain, peripheral vascular disease, gastrointestinal problems, and thyroid disorders. Polypharmacy and the risks associated with taking multiple medications are common in these patients because of their multiple comorbidities and symptoms, such as hypertension, headaches, sleep disorders, and nightmares [6].

James Reston, a New York Times reporter who accompanied President Nixon to China in 1971, introduced acupuncture to the public at large in the USA. Since then, awareness and use of acupuncture has increased throughout the US populace in general and among members of the military. In 2007, Smith et al. reported that active duty military members and veterans reported seeking treatment for acupuncture and other complementary and alternative therapies in order to avoid side effects from medications and to learn health strategies to prevent and treat the underlying cause of disease rather than focus on management of the symptoms of disease [7].

The growing use of complementary and alternative medicine (CAM) modalities was reflected in a 2013 article published in *The Journal of Complementary and Alternative Medicine,* which reported that the overall use of CAM, including acupuncture by active duty military members is higher (44.5 %) than in comparable civilian surveys (38.3 %), with the vast majority of treatments sought outside of the military health care system [8]. Simultaneously, research as to the mechanisms and effectiveness of acupuncture has grown both in quantity and quality [9].

A recent meta-analysis and systematic review on acupuncture for trauma spectrum response (a common symptomatic and functional spectrum of physical, cognitive, psychological, and behavioral effects seen in combat veterans who have experienced psychological and/or physical trauma), found acupuncture to be effective for headaches, and promising for chronic pain, sleep disturbances, anxiety and depression [10]. More specific to PTSD, a recent systematic review of randomized controlled trials (RCTs) and prospective clinical trials for PTSD, found that, based on one high-quality RCT and a meta-analysis, the effectiveness of acupuncture was statistically superior to waitlist control. No statistical difference was found between the effectiveness of acupuncture and cognitive behavioral therapy. Acupuncture plus moxibustion was shown to be superior to oral selective serotonin reuptake inhibitors (SSRI) therapy for PTSD in the meta-analysis [11].

Although high-quality controlled studies, meta-analysis and systematic reviews, are important in determining the effectiveness of a therapy, case reports help us to see the faces and stories of those who seek and benefit from the availability of acupuncture and other holistic therapies, which have been used since ancient time to treat wounds and disorders of the spirit as well as those of the body and mind.

Together with other military medical acupuncturists I have found that active duty military patients and veterans are very accepting of acupuncture [12]. Indeed, many of my patients have reported paying out of pocket for acupuncture prior to finding out that it was available in our pain management clinic.

It is well known that mental health disorders such as depression and anxiety are present in approximately 60 % of patients presenting for treatment of chronic pain [13]. Advanced imaging studies have revealed many commonalities in the neural processing of chronic pain and areas of the brain where emotional "suffering" is processed [14]. Because many of our pain patients present with a history of trauma and a diagnosis of PTSD, it is common to address this disorder in our pain patients (in addition to their chronic pain complaint) within the holistic approach afforded by acupuncture.

Although some patients request referral for acupuncture treatment to avoid medications, procedures, and surgery, the majority of our patients are referred for acupuncture after all the available and applicable conventional therapies have failed to significantly improve their condition(s). The latter is true for the patients in the following case reports.

12.2 Case 1: In-Patient with Severe Low Back Pain

A 21-year-old active duty female US Marine was referred to the pain clinic from orthopedics on a Friday afternoon with a complaint of severe low back pain and difficulty walking. Due to the severity of her complaints, she was admitted to the orthopedic service to rule out cauda equina syndrome. An urgent MRI showed no evidence of central spinal stenosis. Lumbar degenerative disc disease at the L4–5 and L5-S1 levels was mild with minimal neuroforaminal narrowing.

The patient had been brought to the pain clinic on a gurney. Pain medication consisted of intravenous (IV) morphine via a patient controlled analgesic device. Her history of present illness was significant for chronic remitting and relapsing low back pain since boot camp with no known trauma or initiating event. She had been seen in the pain clinic the previous year for an epidural steroid injection for right lower extremity leg pain and numbness in the L5-S1 distribution. Her leg pain had improved following the epidural steroid injection.

On physical exam, vital signs were within normal limits. Her pain was 9–10/10. The patient was 5 ft 4 in., and 120 lbs. She was able to move all of her extremities, but grimaced and moaned when asked to move her legs. Her back pain increased with any movement. Leg strength was 4/5 throughout all muscle groups both left and right with no asymmetry. Straight leg raises were negative for radicular pain but produced severe increase in her low back pain at 10–20 ° of elevation. Deep tendon reflexes were symmetrical. She had no sensory deficits.

The patient was unable to sit in the gurney or to roll to her side or abdomen. Three corpsmen were needed to assist in log rolling the patient to her side as any flexion or extension of her back resulted in cries of pain. No focal tenderness was found.

Initial conventional pain management treatment consisted of converting her IV morphine to oral long acting opioid equivalents, with short acting opioid for break through pain. A low dose of amitriptyline was started and given at bedtime both as a pain adjunct and to assist with sleep hygiene.

On the following Monday, a multidisciplinary meeting was convened to discuss the patient. Attendees included a pain management physician, an orthopedic surgeon, a psychiatrist, the health psychologist, a chaplain, a case manager, and a physical therapist. The psychiatrist proceeded to summarize the patient's social history, which included sexual molestation as a child, and gang rape as a teenager, with the latter resulting in pregnancy. She had kept the child, who was being reared by relatives. She had subsequently joined the US Marine Corps.

12.2.1 Subsequent Treatment

In addition to medication management, physical therapy, mental health counseling, and chaplain services and counseling, acupuncture was offered to the patient and she agreed to this. She was transported to the pain clinic Monday afternoon via gurney.

Due to her history of anxiety, insomnia, and general irritability the first treatment chosen was a "four gates" treatment consisting of LI 4 and LR 3 bilaterally. Although initially anxious, she tolerated the treatment well. After the 20 min treatment she was significantly calmer.

I then performed an "internal 7 dragon" treatment, which has been used since ancient times for patients with a history of severe emotional and/or physical trauma: CV 15, ST 25 bilaterally, ST 32 bilaterally, and ST 41 bilaterally placed top to bottom, right to left. After obtaining de qi sensation, the needles were dispersed and left in place for 15 min. The needles were then removed. The patient was then repositioned prone. A "7 external dragons" treatment was then performed: GV20, BL 11 bilaterally, BL 23 bilaterally, and BL 61 bilaterally. The needles were again placed from right to left, top to bottom, obtaining "de qi" sensation and dispersing (180 degrees counterclockwise) and left in place for 15 min. The needles were then removed. The patient appeared much more engaged and less anxious and fearful after the treatment.

The patient was seen the next afternoon for a second treatment. She was brought to the pain clinic by wheelchair, and was able to assist herself up onto the treatment table. Her pain was 4–5/10. She was able to lay prone and an NN+1 treatment was performed using the shao yin, tai yang meridians: KI 3, SP 6, HT 3, SI 3, and BL 60. A "mega mu shu" treatment was used: GB 25 (−) to BL 23X BL 52 (+) bilaterally at 4 Hz electrical stimulation. This was left in place for 30 min.

On Wednesday, the patient walked to the pain clinic in uniform for her third treatment. The same points as the day prior (shao yin, tai yang command points and "mega mu shu" treatment) with the addition of a percutaneous electrical nerve stimulation (PENS) treatment of the painful area of the lower back using inner and outer bladder lines from L3-S1 with crossed handles at each level in a daisy chain pattern (−), (+), (−), (+). The treatment was again left in place for 30 min. Her pain was 2–3/10 at discharge.

The patient was discharged to the barracks adjacent to the hospital the following day and by the end of the week had returned to her unit. Follow-up from the chaplain revealed that she had been able to return to working out at the gym and to remain on active duty status. He conveyed to us that she had experienced a profound benefit from the acupuncture.

The patient reported that in addition to helping her physical pain, the acupuncture helped her to feel that it was possible for her to recover emotionally and go on with living her life instead of reliving her past.

The chaplain requested to be treated with acupuncture using the "the same treatment which you used for her." When asked about history pertaining to PTSD, he said simply, "I was a chaplain in Vietnam and Korea." I treated him using the "7 internal dragons and 7 external dragon's" five-element acupuncture treatment. He returned to his work as a hospital chaplain. My follow-up consisted of a nod and a smile or a "thumbs up" when I later saw him on his rounds in the wards or walking the hospital passageways.

12.3 Case 2: Patient with Low Back Pain, Flat Affect with Pictures in Her Pocket

A 29-year-old female first class Petty Officer with chronic low back pain, refractory to other therapies, was referred to the pain management acupuncture clinic. Her low back pain of approximately 3 years began after she was injured in the bombing of the USS Cole in October of 2000.

Her lumbar spine MRI was significant for L4–5 and L5-S1 degenerative disease with no central or neuroforaminal stenosis. Her constant low back pain averaged 5–7/10 and limited her ability to run. It was worsened by bending, twisting, and lifting anything over 15 pounds. She denied radicular symptoms, leg weakness, and bowel or bladder incontinence. She had undergone chiropractic treatments, physical therapy, and other conservative treatment, including nonsteroidal anti-inflammatory medications, muscle relaxants and opioids which did not significantly alleviate her pain and caused intolerable side effects. She had also undergone trigger point injections and diagnostic medial branch blocks to rule out facet mediated low back pain without benefit.

She had been evaluated by neurosurgery and was not felt to be a surgical candidate. She gave a history of having suffered significant burns of the face and hands at the time of the blast. Although scarring from the burns was not visible, the patient produced pictures which had been taken of her at the time of her treatment for the burns at Landstuhl Regional Medical Center in Germany. The patient was also followed for chronic PTSD related to the blast.

On physical exam, vital signs were within normal limits. Her pain VAS 6–7/10. Her affect and speech were flat, but responses were appropriate and no cognitive deficits were appreciated. She was observed to have a normal gait and stance. She had tenderness to palpation over her lumbar paraspinous region bilaterally and pain was increased with flexion of the lumbar spine to 45° and lumbar spine extension to 25°. No sensory, motor, or deep tendon reflex abnormalities were observed and exam of all other systems was within normal limits.

12.3.1 Treatment Course

As no other treatment had been effective to date, the patient was eager to try any therapy which might offer her some relief of her physical and emotional symptoms. Her first treatment consisted of the "7 internal and external dragons" five-element acupuncture treatment (see detailed treatment description in text of first case history above). She did not note significant improvement in pain following the treatment, but did note significant improvement in mood. Due to complaint of lack of pleasure and depression together with low back pain, her second treatment consisted of a shao yin, tai yang N N+1 French energetic treatment in the prone position for 30 min with points: KI 10, SP 6, HT 3, SI 3, BL 60 together with a "mega mu shu" treatment: GV 4 and bilateral BL 23, BL 52, and GB 25 with electrical stimulation (e-stim) at 4 Hz. She noted a significant decrease in her pain from 6/10 to 2–3/10.

The following week, she returned with baseline low back pain lowered to 4/10. Her third treatment consisted of repeating the "7 internal and external dragons" five-element acupuncture treatment. Both her pain and her mood were significantly improved following her third treatment. The clinic staff noted that she now smiled and joked with them, displaying a much broader range of emotion and speech.

Her fourth treatment focused on her chronic low back pain and consisted of an NN+1 treatment using command points (−) KI 10 to (+) HT 3 and (−) SI 3 to (+) BL 40 together with a PENS treatment of the inner and outer bladder line points at the L4-S1 levels using a daisy chain pattern of e-stim at 30 Hz.

The patient returned approximately every 5–8 weeks for treatments to maintain improvement of her low back pain. Shao yin, tai yang meridian treatments were alternated with tai yin, yang ming meridian treatment using LU 7, LI4, LI11, ST 36 (*xiaqihai,* meaning lower sea of qi), and SP 6 together with CV 6 (The upper sea of qi, *qihai*) and ST 25 bilaterally to help irritable bowel symptoms, occasional headaches, and lack of energy.

Approximately 1 year after she began treatment, the patient's severe PTSD symptoms recurred, after she returned from testifying in the trial of the terrorists' accused of planning the bombing of the USS Cole. She again improved after repeating the "7 internal and external dragons" five-element treatment, on two occasions approximately 3 weeks apart. She continued to have improvement in her mood and returned approximately monthly for treatment of her low back pain.

After another 6 months, she again had a relapse in her PTSD symptoms when asked to tour the ship to which she was being transferred to for sea duty. The ship was of the same class as the USS Cole. The patient was again treated with the seven internal and external dragon treatments and on her second visit with LU7, LI4, LI 11, ST 36, SP 6, CV 6, and ST 25. After she once again improved in regard to mood, irritable bowel syndrome (IBS), sleep, back pain, and headaches, she decided to separate from the military in order to minimize the risk for reactivation of her PTSD. She indicated that she would continue to seek acupuncture treatment for both her emotional and physical well being.

12.4 Case 3: Combat Scarred Service Member Medevac'd from Theater

The patient is a 51-year-old officer. He reported last being well prior to his 2007–2008 Iraq deployment. During that deployment, the patient suffered a mild traumatic brain injury (mTBI) when a mortar barrage hit his base with about 10–15 rounds impacting near him. Diving for cover, the patient sustained shrapnel to his left knee but denied experiencing loss of consciousness (LOC) or posttraumatic amnesia. He did not seek immediate treatment.

Several other traumatic experiences occurred during that deployment, wherein the patient witnessed "death up close." Perhaps the most traumatic experience the patient described was losing his friend to an improvised explosive device (IED). The patient was supposed to be on the convoy which took the life of his good friend and subordinate. "That should have been me," the patient reported, noting that he asked his subordinate to attend the convoy so that he could go to lunch with a governmental organization.

Following his return home, the patient continued to experience marked guilt and recriminations. During the time when he was not at home, he worked nonstop, throwing himself into his work. To keep from thinking about things that he had seen during his deployment, the patient started drinking regularly, two or more drinks per night. He started to become depressed.

Symptoms of PTSD, chiefly, emotional numbing with memory loss, flashbacks, depersonalization and derealization, sleep disturbance, and hypervigilance, accompanied increasing guilt. He did not seek treatment and thought that by redeploying he might be able to make amends, particularly if he was killed in an act saving someone else. When the opportunity arose for another combat tour, this time to Afghanistan in 2012, the patient leaped at the chance.

Unable to drink (General Order #1 forbids all US military person from consuming alcohol in the area of the Central Command, for example, Afghanistan area of operations), the patient consumed himself with work, sleeping perhaps 2–4 h per night. Midway through the patient's deployment, "the wheels fell off the wagon." The patient became forgetful, distant, and "flashbacks" associated with his 2007 OIF deployment became more regular.

The flashbacks involved a bloody face of unknown identity in the bunker of unknown location. (The patient named the "flashback's principal" as "BFIB" or bloody-face-in-bunker). As noted by his coworkers, his sentences, often pressured and fraught with a flight of ideas, did not make sense. The member reported experiencing conversations which he was sure took place, however later learned were "all in his head."

Though not actively suicidal or homicidal, the patient did disclose that he felt that he should put himself in a situation wherein his life was in jeopardy for the good of his country and for the sake of turning off his unwanted thoughts. Witnessed to be acting bizarre, he surrendered his weapon to his staff and agreed to see mental health. He was flown to Bagram, then to Landstuhl, and ultimately to the continental US (CONUS).

On mental status exam (following medevac and stabilization with atypical antipsychotic medication), the patient was found to be a cooperative, albeit exhausted appearing male officer, dressed in gym clothes. He displayed a cordial demeanor with comfortable eye contact. Speech was fluid, with normal rate and rhythm. His stated mood was "better," and his affect was with full range and appropriate to expressed content. The patient denied suicidal or homicidal ideation. No evidence of hallucinations, delusions, or thought disorder. Thought processes were linear and logical. Memory was intact to recent and remote recall.

12.4.1 Treatment Course

Upon arrival to CONUS, the patient was placed on low dose Seroquel (quetiapine) at 50 mg nightly for sleep and for "disturbed thinking." The admitting diagnosis was

Chronic PTSD and mTBI, and rule out major depressive disorder. Over the course of the next 4 weeks of intensive outpatient treatment and follow-up care through the next several months, the patient was exposed to a number of integrative therapies. Whereas expressive art therapy, expressive writing, and animal assistance therapy were utilized, the individual received the greatest degree of relief from acupuncture, utilizing it as adjunctive therapy for his PTSD, to assist with pain management, and to facilitated return to normal sleeping patterns.

Excerpted from one of the sessions of expressive writing, is the following description of the patient's acupuncture treatment.

I was lost inside myself. When I arrived back in the Washington, DC area from Kabul via medical evacuation for symptoms, that ultimately were diagnosed as PTSD and mTBI, I was extremely depressed, ashamed, confused, cognitively impaired and I felt hopeless. My chief of staff had noticed anomalies in my behavior over a few months and knew I was getting very little sleep. A couple hours of sleep a day took its toll over the course of several years. I had relied on "self-medication" through alcohol to allow me to sleep and either avoid, or not remember my night terrors, morbid visions and day/nightmares. When in an alcohol free war zone, I relied on not sleeping and working 22/7. I would work out of my room often, until I was assigned a private office.

When I was first admitted to the hospital, I did not know what made me happy; I could not answer the question "who am I?" reasonably; I was paranoid of everyone and everything; I could not trust; I stayed on a couch, covered with a blanket, and avoided everyone for several months. I was prescribed mood stabilizing drugs, sleeping pills, tranquilizers, anti-anxiety medications, specific vitamins, and talk therapy. This clinical approach helped a great deal, but it was not until I embraced an integrated approach to healing, which included acupuncture, micro current brain stimulation, art therapy, meditation, heart math, audio calming techniques, animal therapy, cognitive exercises, and Reiki/massage therapies that I really began my full recovery.

Before my medical evacuation, I did not believe in alternative medicine. I thought acupuncture cures were fake and meditation/audio/Reiki/art/visual/animal therapies were for weirdoes and malingerers. During my time at the hospital, I began to see the benefits of some of these therapies, but it was after my discharge, when I began to work through these symptoms of my invisible injuries, that I truly found the value in them. I was fortunate to have many months where my primary focus was on recovery and I had amazingly strong support providers in my wife and my daughters."

Acupuncture

"I initially told the providers at the hospital that I did not need acupuncture, Reiki or the art, animal, music or meditation therapies. I was certainly not thinking very well when I arrived, and my paranoia made me think this was all somehow a trick since I was certain this stuff did not work and was just provided as a placebo. Then I had my first session with my acupuncturist.

My anxiety and corresponding cortisol levels were sky high. I was ultra-suspicious of everyone and everything and hyper-vigilant. The Doc recommended an acupuncture "cocktail" to ease my anxiety and stress level. I agreed. The next day he provided the treatment. I could not believe how it made me feel so much more relaxed. I also felt much more trusting of him. When I would return to my residence, I would curl up in a ball and cover myself with a blanket to hide. I was ashamed of leaving Afghanistan the way I did, I felt guilty leaving my troops behind and I felt utter failure for the first time in my life. I still had lots of trouble sleeping.

I had horrific visions of past war scenes, I repeatedly saw the man I sent on a mission in my place, in my seat, doing a part of my job so I could attend a lunch at the forward operating base (FOB). I would constantly see him looking at me as I watched him buckle up and gave me a thumbs-up. Then I would see him after the IED destroyed the vehicle and killed him and others. I would see a bloody face lying on the ground next to me in the bunker where I was wounded during a 2008 mortar attack on our compound. I saw many, many other horrors of war which would wake me and keep me awake to avoid the terrors of their re-appearance. I had been taking the medication Seroquel for nearly 3 weeks by then and even it did not allow me a full night's peace. When I covered myself up on the couch that evening and fell asleep, after taking the same dosages of all my medications, I did not have any visages or nightmares. I slept…and I slept well. The next morning I felt much less groggy and confused and I felt calmer and less threatened. Whether a placebo effect, or actual therapeutic benefit, I did not know…but I liked the effect it delivered and decided to try more. The next session was another anti-anxiety session, and it seemed to help, along with the lorazepam…I began to feel a bit less agitated. I then noticed that I was falling asleep faster than I used to (using only the Seroquel). After several months of continued anti-anxiety treatment, I found myself able to reduce the Seroquel dosage and still get to sleep…and stay asleep. Along with other acupuncture protocols, animal, art, meditation, breathing and white noise therapies would eventually fill the gap and I was eventually able to get off Seroquel all together.

I still had many more symptoms of PTSD and mTBI which I had to deal with. One day, the doctor suggested I have a "Dragons" session to identify the demons that plagued me. I agreed and encountered another therapy that would change my life forever.

The focused, compressed visions of my past that generate deep inside my head during dragon sessions are truly remarkable. The visages that are portrayed occur so rapidly, yet with such detail, that it takes me several days to comprehend and weeks to analyze through talk therapy. These sessions have provided me with the ability to gain a more comprehensive understanding of my memories, actions, and situations that have caused me survivor's guilt, shame, and depression.

Dragons. Death, attacks, threats, war. Then people that I felt were "out to get or kill" me. My deeply guarded inner most morbid thoughts. Wanting to get myself harmed, disassociation with the dearest things…family, myself, those that protected me. Confusion between exhilaration and fear, pain and exhaustion, life and death. A deep desire to make things right with (name withheld) and join him. I began to understand martyrdom. All these very complex feelings that were so strongly guarded by my psyche that even I did not know they existed. The hundreds of faces and battle scenes I saw in those few dragon minutes delivered a different type of explosion. This one was an explosion of emotion that provided me insight into the demons that plague me, and the issues I was working to overcome.

Some visions are delivered like an old fashioned flip picture show, but in color. Never smooth, a little out of focus, never perfect, yet vivid. Some seem like a short film loop...playing over and over again. Some are pictures which remind me of an elementary school film strip or a family slide show. Extraordinarily meaningful and filled with information. The bloody stump...is it (name withheld)? Sniper attack. Explosions...the noise...bright colors and deep vibrations that shake me to my core. The realization that now that I know what fear is, maybe I was afraid back then instead of being exhilarated. So much death, even though not directly caused by me, that I realize I had lost the value of life. Morbid thoughts of homicide and suicide, which I had in the past, return as hauntings...not good ideas. I realize I am confused about who I am and what really matters. I am reminded of mistakes I have made, professionally and with my family and friends. Hundreds of pieces of information are provided that I will have to categorize and sort in my brain.

I have many blank areas. Just when I think the answer to a question or another vision of the past is coming, a surprising blank pops in my mind. Seems like it lasts for hours, but it must only last a nanosecond. This releases a frustrating desire to pull what was coming into my mind out of my memory...but it is not there. I will later find that it will take me days and weeks to fully digest what when through my brain in just 30 min. Some things are missing and decide to try and find them. Through the help of my therapists, I would ultimately come to realize the bits of information I retrieved during dragons were like "dots" that would eventually be connected with other dots, my sub-conscious and conscious thoughts, memories of actions and decisions, as well as newly discovered deep seeded issues or desires. Going into the session, I am excited to find more dots to connect in an effort to see more detail in the picture that is emerging...the picture of who I am and how I got to be here. "

12.5 Discussion

PTSD is now characterized as a traumatic and stress-related disorder in the *Diagnostic and Statistical Manual 5* [15]. The hallmark features and triggers are: exposure to actual or threatened death, serious injury or sexual violation. The exposure must result from one or more of the following scenarios, in which the individual:

- Directly experiences the traumatic event;
- Witnesses the traumatic event in person;
- Learns that the traumatic event occurred to a close family member or close friend (with the actual or threatened death being either violent or accidental); or
- Experiences first-hand repeated or extreme exposure to aversive details of the traumatic event (not through media, pictures, television or movies unless work-related).

Chronic PTSD is perhaps the most apparent of disorders which affect all aspects of mind, body, and spirit and which require treatment of all of these aspects of the human being in order to restore health and balance to the individual who suffers from this disorder [16, 17]. A 2008 study by the Rand Corporation found that as many as 20 % of the US veterans who served in Iraq and Afghanistan suffer from PTSD or major depressive disorder [18].

Acupuncture and other integrative modalities offer Western medicine practitioners opportunities to expose their patients to interventions which may aid in patient engagement, and assist with the co-morbidities of pain and disturbed sleep. For this reason, acupuncture may be considered as treatment for patients with PTSD (Veterans Affairs and Department of Defense (VA/DoD) Clinical Practice Guidelines for Management of PTSD). Additionally, recently published research [19] further supports the use of acupuncture to help reduce the symptoms of PTSD.

Although acupuncture is thought of as a homogeneous treatment modality to those unschooled in its history and diversity, its history is complex with many different approaches and schools. The Nei Jing Su Wen Ling Shu, the classic of internal medicine and most famous of the ancient medical texts was written by Huangdi, the Yellow Emperor and is considered the basis for Chinese medicine. Written in two parts, the Su Wen (simple questions) and the Ling Shu (spiritual axis), compiled during the Han dynasty (206–220 CE), the Nei Jing describes the mental, emotional, and spiritual aspects of Chinese medicine [20].

The ancient masters of acupuncture are said to have gained their knowledge of acupuncture and other ways of ancient wisdom through deep meditation, fasting, and observation of the commonalities and relationships between heaven, (cosmology), earth, nature, and the human being. This knowledge was transmitted through pictographs with layers of meaning, which modern scientists have compared to our current scientific understanding of reality [21–23]. The meaning of the pictographs encompassed the levels of being to include undifferentiated energy, spirit, thoughts, emotion, and the denser physiological, functional and anatomical physical body aspects.

This understanding of life, health, and balance also included complex mathematical relationships, which revealed the order behind the cycles and transformations seen in living beings, the various levels of reality, and the creation and destruction of all things. This mathematical understanding of relationships was represented and taught through the use of trigrams and hexagrams, which resemble our modern computer binary language [24].

The most advanced practitioners, through this understanding, were said to be able to diagnose the presence of a disharmony through observation of subtleties such as the voice, skin color and temperature, the pulses, and emotional tendencies of the individual, prior to the appearance of advanced disease. Treatment included not only acupuncture but as in our multidisciplinary approach to treatment of complex disorders, the individual was treated with herbs (nutritional supplements), proper diet (nutrition), exercises such as Tai Chi and Qigong, and methods such as meditation (breathing and mindfulness) to calm and harmonize the nervous system.

Knowledge of the various aspects of qi or vital life energy was transmitted from teacher to student using symbolic language such as the five elements. The elements of wood, fire, earth, metal, and water represented energetic, physical, mental, emotional, and spiritual attributes of energy whose balance or imbalance could be assessed through the understanding of these interconnected attributes. The physician was then able, through proper selection of acupuncture points and adjunctive treatments to harmonize the subtle energy in the body in order to return the patient to a harmonious state of adaptation and function.

Dr. Charles, E. Moss, a leading teacher and practitioner of the five element style of acupuncture, quotes from Chap. 8 of the Ling Shu:

> The patient is the product and author of life's standards and of the control of the breaths and the meridians. The stability and firmness of life's lines, the permanent rooting in the spirits, are nothing more than a perpetual changing-a permanent process of adaptation.

Dr. Moss clarifies that the "spirits" in the context used here in the Ling Shu, refers to "the properties that are "stored" in each of the five elements." For example, the wood energy is associated with expansive energy associated with the rising sun, changing darkness to light and stimulating change and action. It corresponds to rebirth, renewal, and new ideas—the blueprint for growth, adaptability, and the ability to organize and make things happen. It is goal oriented and focused. It moves through the tendons and muscles as it rises from the lower extremities. It then supplies the visual system including the eyes and occipital cortex in the brain. In addition to its association with the physical sense of sight, it also governs our deeper "vision" which allows us to see clearly, be decisive, create and achieve goals. It is associated with the muscular system, flexibility, movement, and the ability to change direction as needed. It is also associated with the attributes of forgiveness and patience as well as the expression of emotions, including anger, to achieve goals.

Genetics or trauma were known to disrupt the balance of one of the five element types and hence the power to adapt. A more expansive and complete discussion of the history, traditional and scientific principles of five-element acupuncture treatment which is beyond the scope of this chapter, can be found in Dr. Moss's 2009 book, "Power of the Five Elements: The Chinese Medicine Path to Healthy Aging and Stress Resistance" [25].

Although acupuncture and traditional Chinese medicine in China were in decline by 1757, and banned by the health minister of the Chinese republic in 1914, due to the influence of Western missionaries and occupation of parts of China by European powers, they were revived by Chairman Mao Zedong after the Communists took power later in the twentieth century. However, this revival was based on governmental policy and philosophy with the aim of treating the maximum number of individuals with the greatest efficiency. Discussion of the spiritual and emotional aspects of health was forbidden.

The traditional use of acupuncture for treatment of mental, spiritual, and emotional disorders was transmitted through ancient texts and the ancient teachings were thus preserved in Japan, Korea, and other area of the Far East. Modern use of

Table 12.1 Indications for use of various acupuncture points for the treatment of numerous psychological disorders

Zusanli (ST-36)	*He* and earth point of the ST channel. Mania-depression, manic singing, raving, abusive talk, anger, fright, tendency to sadness, outrageous laughter
Fenglong (ST-40)	*Luo* point of the ST channel. Dizziness, plumpit qi, mania-depression, mad laughter, great happiness, desires to ascend to high places and sing, discards clothing and runs around, restlessness, seeing ghosts, indolence, epilepsy
Jiexie (ST-41)	*Jing* and fire point of the ST channel. Epilepsy, mania, agitation, sadness and weeping, fright palpitations, raving, seeing ghosts
Spleen channel (SP)	
Shangqui (SP-5)	Jing and metal point of SP channel. Mania-depression, agitation, excessive thinking, propensity to laughter, nightmares, melancholy, fright, stroke
Sanyinjiao (SP-6)	Meeting point of SP, LV, and KI channels. Heart palpitations, insomnia, fright, dizziness

acupuncture for these indications varies based on the training of the practitioner, however many traditional and modern texts contain lists of indications for use of various acupuncture points for the treatment of numerous psychological disorders as shown in Table 12.1 [26, 27].

12.6 Conclusion

In recent decades, advances in the quality of acupuncture research have been acknowledged by authoritative international scientific organizations [9]. Established research has documented neurobiological responses to acupuncture including release of endogenous opioids, modulation of serotonergic, noradrenergic, dopaminergic, and GABA neurotransmitters and effects on neurotrophins and cytokines. Additional publications have documented acupuncture's effects on the autonomic nervous system, neuroendocrine system, HPA, and immune system, all which are dysregulated in patients with chronic PTSD [27, 28]. The clinical effectiveness of acupuncture for various diseases, including PTSD and other psychological disorders has been more difficult to ascertain due to limitations such as study design, sample size, selection of appropriate controls, and non-standardized selection of points based on traditional methods of diagnosis and treatment [29].

Promising research has emerged in recent years, which cumulatively has the potential guide future clinical trial efforts due to a nascent understanding of acupuncture point specificity. A recently published meta-analysis of 82 fMRI studies, for example, reveals acupuncture effects in the brain through blood-oxygen-level dependent (BOLD) measurements with specific acupuncture points accessing brain networks which correspond to specific medical disorders. This is in contrast to sham points, which do not demonstrate similar specificity. Examples of acupoint cortical specificity noted by the researchers corresponded with traditional Chinese medicine point indications and included the following:

> Acupuncture at the three classical acupoints of Hegu (LI4), ST36, and Taichong (LV3) produced extensive deactivation of the limbic-paralimbic-neocortical brain network as well as activation of its anti-correlated activation network." Differentiation between the points was noted as the following, "LI4 was predominant in the pregenual cingulated and hippocampal formation, ST 36 response was predominant in the subgenual cingulate, and LV3 in the posterior hippocampus and posterior cingulated…." Taixi (KI3) mediated the executive network, Qiuxu (GB40) activated the auditory network, and "Jiaoxin (KI8) was associated with (the) insula and hippocampus in pain modulation. [30, 31].

The extensive activation of the limbic–paralimbic–neocortical brain network by Hegu (LI4) and Taichong (LV3) discovered in this research may explain the frequent treatment of patients with PTSD with protocols utilizing these points. Traditionally known as "The Four Gates" when used alone (LI 4 and LV3 bilaterally), and as "the Koffman Cocktail" when GV20 and GV 24.5 are added, these treatments are commonly used to alleviate insomnia, anxiety, headaches, and other symptoms commonly seen in patients with PTSD and trauma spectrum response.

As summarized in the 2010 white paper published by the Society of Acupuncture Research (SAR), "Paradoxes in Acupuncture Research, a Strategy for Moving Forward," future research should incorporate a translational approach with a lens which views acupuncture treatments as:

> (1) "top down" as multi-component "whole-system" interventions and (2) "bottom up" as mechanistic studies that focus on understanding how individual treatment components interact and translate into clinical and physiological outcomes. Such a strategy, incorporating considerations of efficacy, effectiveness and qualitative measures, will strengthen the evidence base for such complex interventions as acupuncture. [9]

As such, our improved understanding of the neurobiology of acupuncture together with emerging understanding of point specific effects on the brain and recent evidence from RCTs of acupuncture for PTSD referenced herein, support more extensive availability, use and study of this ancient therapy for the wounds of war which are often inadequately addressed by conventional approaches. Additionally, case reports such as those above, although viewed through the lens of modern science as a low form of evidence, are valuable in that they incorporate the profound response and essential narrative of the human being, the significance and meaning of which might otherwise be lost in the sorting of statistics and numbers.

References

1. Capra F. The web of life: a new scientific understanding of living systems. New York: Anchor Books; 1996.
2. Wang H, Qi H, Wang B, Cui Y, Zhu L, Rong Z, Chen H. Is acupuncture beneficial in depression: a meta-analysis of 8 randomized controlled trials? J Affect Disord. 2008;111:125–34.
3. Williamson JB, Porges EC, Lamb DG, Porges SW. Maladaptive autonomic regulation in PTSD accelerates physiological aging. Front Psychol. 2015;5(1571):12.

4. Fisher JP, Young CN, Fadel PJ. Central sympathetic overactivity: maladies and mechanisms. Auton Neurosci. 2009;148(1/2):5–15.
5. Otis JD, Gregor K, Hardway C, Morrison J, Scioli E, Sanderson K. An examination of the co-morbidity between chronic pain and posttraumatic stress disorder on U. W. Veterans. Psychol Serv. 2010;7(3):12–135.
6. Committee on the assessment of ongoing effects in the treatment of posttraumatic stress disorder, Institute of Medicine. Treatment for posttraumatic stress disorder in military and veteran populations: initial assessment. Washington, DC: National Academies Press; 2012.
7. Smith T, Ryan M, Smith B, et al. Complementary and alternative medicine use among US Navy and Marine Corps personnel. BMC Complement Altern Med. 2007;7:16.
8. Goertz C, Marriott BP, Finch MD, Bray RM, Williams TV, Hourani LL, Hadden LS, Colleran HL, Jonas WB. Military report more complementary and alternative medicine use than civilians. J Altern Complement Med. 2013;19(6):509–17.
9. Langevin HM, Wayne PM, MacPherson H, Schnyer R, Milley RM, Napadow V, Lao L, Park J, Harris RE, Cohen M, Sherman KJ, Haramati A, Hammerschlag R. Paradoxes in acupuncture research: strategies for moving forward. Evid-Based Complement Altern Med. 2011;2011, Article ID 180905, 11 pp.
10. Lee C, Crawford C, Wallerstedt D, York A, Duncan A, Smith J, Sprengel M, Welton R, Jonas W. The effectiveness of acupuncture across components of the trauma spectrum response (tsr): a systematic review of reviews. Syst Rev. 2012; 1:46.
11. Kim Y, Heo I, Shin B, Crawford C, Kang H, Lim J. Acupuncture for posttraumatic stress disorder: a systematic review of randomized controlled trials and prospective clinical trials. Evid-Based Complement Altern Med. 2013;2013 Article ID 615857, 12 pp.
12. Koffman RL, Helms JM. Acupuncture for PTSD: getting soldiers through the door. Healio Psychiatric Annals. 2013. http://www.healio.com/psychiatry/ptsd/news/online/%7B1a233a04-73be-42a8-8b4c-f89319359d4a%7D/acupuncture-for-ptsd-getting-soldiers-through-the-door. Accessed 18 March 2015.
13. Trivedi MH. The link between depression and physical symptoms. the primary car companion. J Clin Psychiatry. 2004;6(suppl 1):12–16.
14. Hui KA, Liu J, Makris N, Gollub RL, Chen AJW, Moore CL, Kennedy DN, Rosen BR, Kwong KK. Acupuncture modulates the limbic system and subcortical gray structures of the human brain: evidence from fMRI studies in normal subjects. Human Brain Mapp. 2000;9:13–25.
15. American Psychiatric Association. Diagnostic and Statistical Manual of Mental Disorders. 5th ed. DSM–5. Washington; 2013.
16. Sherin JE. Posttraumatic stress disorder: the neurobiological impact of psychological trauma. Dialogues Clin Neurosci. 2011;13(3):263–78.
17. Sang Hwan K, Schneider SM, Kravitz L, Mermier C, Burge MR. Mind-body practices for posttraumatic stress disorder. J Investig Med. 2013;61(5):827–34.
18. Tanielian T, Jaycox L, editors. Invisible wounds of war: psychological and cognitive injuries, their consequences, and services to assist recovery. Santa Monica: RAND Corporation; 2008.
19. Engle CC, Cordova EH, Benedek DM, Liu X, Gore KL, Goertz C, Freed MC, Crawford C, Jonas WB, Ursano RJ. Randomized effectiveness trial of a brief course of acupuncture for posttraumatic stress disorder. Med Car. 2014;52(12 Suppl 5):S57–64.
20. Cavalieri S, Rotoli M. Huangdi Neijing: a classic book of traditional Chinese medicine. Recenti Prog Med. 1997;88(11):541–6.
21. Capra F. The Tao of physics: an exploration of the parallels between modern physics and eastern mysticism. Boston: Shambhala Publications, Inc; 2010.
22. Milburn MP. The future of healing: exploring the parallels of eastern and western medicine. New York: Ten Speed Press (Division of Crown Publishing Group); 2001.
23. Zukov G. The dancing Wu Li masters: an overview of the new physics. New York: HarperCollins Publishers; 2001.
24. Scrimgeour A. What is the relationship between the Yi Jing (the classic of change) and Chinese medicine? Acupuncture dissertation for the College of Integrated Chinese Medicine 2011. http://www.academia.edu/4247873/YIJING_Dissertation_A_Scrimgeour. Accessed 29 April 2015.

25. Moss CA. Power of the five elements: the Chinese medicine path to healthy aging and stress resistance. Berkeley: North Atlantic Books; 2009.
26. Dharmandanda S. Acupuncture and herbs for mind and brain disorders. Institute for Traditional Medicine. http://www.itmonline.org/articles/acubrain.htm. 2000. Accessed 29 April 2015.
27. Yang J, Li Q, Li F, Fu Q, Zeng X, Liu C. The holistic effects of acupuncture treatment. Evid-Based Complement Alternat Med. 2014;2014, Article ID 73978, 10 pp.
28. Manni L, Albanesi M, Guaragna M, Garbaro Paparo S, Aloe L. Neurotrophins and acupuncture. Auton Neurosci. 2010;157(1/2):9–17.
29. Pillington K. Acupuncture therapy for psychiatric illness. Int Rev Neurobiol. 2013;111:197–216.
30. He T, Zhu W, Du S-Q, Yang J-W, Li F, Yang B-F, Shi G-X, Liu C-Z. Neural mechanisms of acupuncture as revealed by fMRI studies. Auton Neurosci. 2015;190:1–9.
31. MRI Reveals Acupuncture Modulates Brain Activity. Healthcare Medicine Web site. 2015. http://www.healthcmi.com/Acupuncture-Continuing-Education-News/1449-mri-reveals-acupuncture-modulates-brain-activity. Accessed 29 April 2015.

The Use of Stellate Ganglion Block in the Treatment of Panic/Anxiety Symptoms (Including Suicidal Ideation), with Combat-Related Posttraumatic Stress Disorder

13

Eugene Lipov

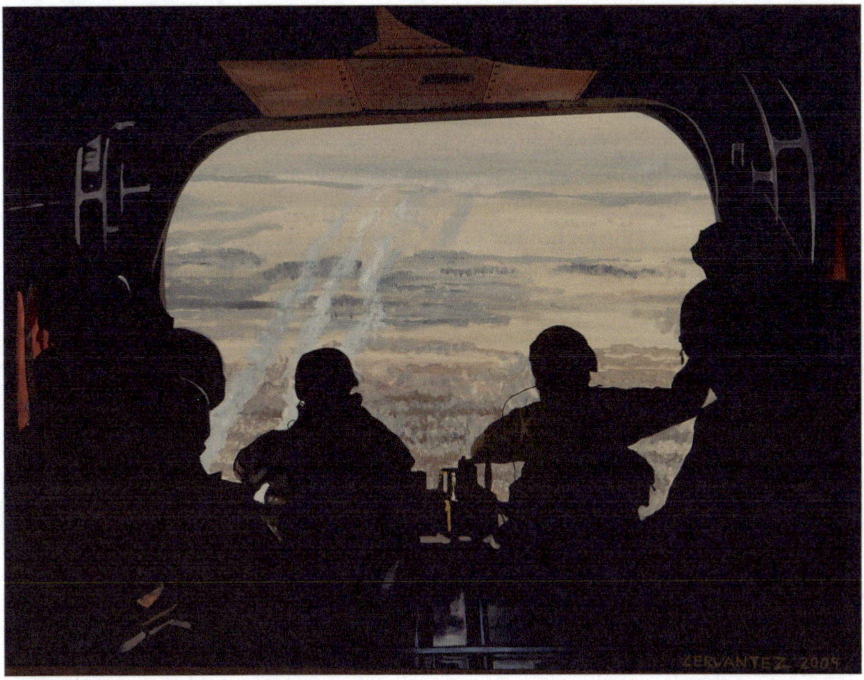

Tailgating Over the Valley, by MSG Martin J. Cervantez, courtesy of the Army Art Collection, US Army Center of Military History.

E. Lipov (✉)
Advanced Pain Centers, Hoffman Estates, 2260 W Higgins Rd, IL 60169, USA
e-mail: elipovmd@aol.com

E. C. Ritchie (ed.), *Posttraumatic Stress Disorder and Related Diseases in Combat Veterans,* DOI 10.1007/978-3-319-22985-0_13

Posttraumatic stress disorder (PTSD) is a chronic or pathological anxiety that is brought on by witnessing or experiencing severe trauma. In 1980, the American Psychiatric Association (APA) added PTSD to the third edition of its Diagnostic and Statistical Manual of Mental Disorders (DSM-III) [1]. However, multiple terms describing what is currently known as PTSD preceded its use. The first modern description of PTSD emerged during the US Civil War. Dr. Mendez DaCosta described war veterans as having irritable heart or "soldiers' heart" [2]. In his 1876 research paper, Dr. DaCosta described startle responses, hypervigilance, and heart arrhythmias.

The wisdom of this report is a biological description of the nervous system over activity. If PTSD can be recognized as biological trauma, it may respond to an approach that reverses or treats biological alteration of the nervous system. The division of the nervous system, which is likely to play a dominant role in the development and maintenance of PTSD, is the sympathetic system. If biological causes of PTSD are accepted, the utilization of a blockade of the sympathetic system supplying the brain is conceivable as opposed to a "FREAKY-PTSD-TREATMENT" as portrayed via an article in the Wired Magazine [3].

The focus of this chapter is to summarize clinical evidence available for the effectiveness of cervical sympathetic ganglion injection called stellate ganglion block (SGB), as well as demonstrate possible clinical applications of its use. The patient who is the subject of the case report, failed conservative treatments for over 40 years and presented to the author for an urgent SGB. What led the patient to present, including his follow-up, offers a glimpse into the understanding of SGB as a vital treatment option for PTSD treatment.

13.1 Methods

13.1.1 Right-Sided C6 Cervical Sympathetic Chain Blockade

Once written consent was administered, a right-sided SGB was performed. An intravenous line was started with a 22G IV in the right hand. The patient was positioned comfortably in the supine position, prepped and draped in the sterile fashion. After radiographic confirmation of the right C6 vertebral body, the skin was anesthetized with 1 cc of 2 % lidocaine. Using an anterior paratracheal approach, a 22-gauge Quincke needle was passed under fluoroscopic guidance until it contacted the anterior lateral aspect of the C6 vertebral body, and then it was pulled back 1 mm. Appropriate needle position was then confirmed by the injection of 2 cc of iohexol (180 mg/mL) radiopaque dye, and fluoroscopy was used to monitor its spread. After negative aspiration, 7 cc of 0.5 % bupivicaine was injected slowly in order to produce a sympathetic ganglion block. We observed the patient for facial anhidrosis (inability to sweat normally) and Horner's syndrome (i.e., enophthalmos-posterior displacement of the eye), ptosis (drooping of the upper eyelid), and miosis (constriction of the pupil) that was noted within 10 min. Horner's syndrome is considered demonstrative of a successful sympathetic block of the cervical sympathetic chain.

13.1.2 Psychometric Testing

The PTSD Checklist (PCL) is a 17-item psychometric test commonly used to screen for PTSD. It was developed based on PTSD criteria from the Diagnostic and Statistical Manual of Mental Disorders (DSM-IV). The PCL's initial validation [4] found that it was an effective brief screen for identifying PTSD, although the sample population did not include patients who experienced combat-related PTSD.

The PCL has since been validated for screening troops returning from combat to identify those with PTSD [5] as well as assessing symptom improvement as a result of treatment [6]. Different cutoff scores have been recommended for identifying PTSD, with ranges spanning from 30 to 50 PCL scores. Forbes et al. [6] concluded that the optimal cutoff score for identifying combat-related PTSD is a score of 50, with maximal score being 85.

13.2 Case Report 1

The patient is a 67-year-old male veteran of the Vietnam War. His military service began at age 19, where he served as a Medic for 19 months during the Vietnam War. Although the patient reported not seeing direct war combat, he witnessed horrific injuries and incidents of fellow military personnel. He experienced a very difficult transition as he attempted to settle back into a civilian lifestyle. His family and friends informed him how he was no longer the same person he was before he left for war. He also knew that what he experienced had fundamentally changed him.

Following his return home, the patient reported struggling with depression, insomnia, nightmares, flashbacks, alcoholism, and suicidal ideation for years. He dealt with fatigue, frequent headaches, and problems with concentrating, thinking, and recalling. His VA doctors prescribed him various medications to help alleviate his depression and sleeping problems. However, he was fired from 13 different jobs within his first year back home.

For 40 years, the patient lived with these symptoms. All the while, he was receiving individual counseling and was treated with many different medications. The veteran grew frustrated with the lack of relief these treatment modalities were providing. When the patient presented himself for treatment, he was noted to be severely anxious and agoraphobic. Although he denied being suicidal during the first evaluation, he informed the author after the treatment, "If I could not have the injection done I would have killed myself that night."

When the patient received his first SGB treatment, that night was the first time he slept without having nightmares. The day after the procedure, his PCL score dropped from 74 to 54. A few days after his first injection, he had noticed nightmares returning, and another SGB was performed 16 days later. Two weeks after the second SGB, the patient reported sleep improvements and he had been able to decrease his daily dose of Trazadone from 600 mg down to 350 mg. He was feeling calmer during the day and was finding himself better able to socialize. His flashbacks decreased and he found himself much less tense.

Two weeks after SGB #2, he was able to sleep through the night, increasingly more social than he had been prior to the injections, significantly less tense, less prone to flashbacks, and he was no longer experiencing suicidal thoughts. He also informed our staff members that he had been able to discontinue all PTSD-related medications. The patient no longer felt the need to attend therapy secessions. He stated, "SGB literally saved my life. I had nightmares which pretty much led to destruction of my house every night since 1968. I can honestly say that after the first night of receiving SGB #1 that was the first time I slept all the way through the night without a nightmare. I felt like I was at the end of my rope. I was unfortunately ready to commit suicide. The procedure is so simple and the results are so great."

The patient still has memories of the war, but he states the memories no longer cause him anxiety. He no longer takes any medications for PTSD nor does he require any counseling. During a recent follow-up, nearly 4 years following the original SGB, the patient's PCL was 29.

13.3 Case Report 2

13.3.1 Chronologic PCL-C Report for the Patient

The focus of this chapter is strictly related to military-associated PTSD; however, PTSD can occur in the civilian population as well. A brief example of SGB application for nonmilitary PTSD is also presented below.

The patient is a 23-year-old Caucasian female, nonmilitary, and first seen 1-year posttrauma. A formal diagnosis of PTSD was made by her psychiatrist. The patient was a rape victim. She was subsequently placed on multiple selective serotonin reuptake inhibitor (SSRI), which she felt provided about 20 % relief reduction in symptoms. The patient also attempted cognitive-behavioral therapy (CBT) but felt that it caused an increase in anxiety. The patient had a SGB at the C6 level and had a repeat block 4 months later. The procedure was unremarkable and no side effects were reported. The patient self-reported a reduction of symptoms by 90 %, soon after SGB. She also self-reported an 80 % reduction in anxiety 1 year after the last SGB and has returned to therapy; which is noted to be considerably more effective following SGB.

13.4 Discussion

13.4.1 PTSD Overview

The incidence of military-related PTSD is on the rise, partly due to increased awareness and better detection. The biggest driver, however, is the continued large-scale military mobilization in response to the sociopolitical violence of the past decade. The prevalence and profound impact on quality of life urgently demands effective PTSD treatments [7].

Although PTSD is the most commonly diagnosed service-related mental disorder among the US military personnel returning from Iraq and Afghanistan, an expert panel convened by the Institute of Medicine found little evidence for the efficacy of most currently employed PTSD treatment modalities [8]. As noted by Dr. Hoge in a JAMA 2011 editorial, current therapeutics has limited effect. He stated that veterans remain reluctant to seek care, with half of those in need not utilizing mental health services. Among veterans who begin PTSD treatment with psychotherapy or medication, there is a high percentage dropout which is commonly 20–40 % in randomized clinical trials (RCTs). "With only 50 % of veterans seeking care and a 40 % recovery rate, current strategies will effectively reach no more than 20 % of all veterans needing PTSD treatment" [9].

13.4.2 Conventional PTSD Treatment: Pharmaceuticals Plus Psychotherapy

13.4.2.1 Pharmaceuticals

Primarily used to address mood disorders, the SSRIs increase the amount of serotonin circulating in the synapse, but they have been shown to be helpful in mediating PTSD symptoms. The side effects, however, include sexual dysfunction [10], somnolence [11] and an increased risk for suicide [11]. Four SSRIs have undergone clinical trials for efficacy in treating PTSD; these include: citalopram (Celexa), fluoxetine (Prozac), paroxetine (Paxil), and sertraline (Zoloft). Of these SSRIs, only sertraline and paroxetine currently have a FDA indication for PTSD. The dual nighttime symptoms of PTSD—that is, nightmares and sleep disruption—are often unresponsive to medication [12].

While SSRIs are marginally effective for these symptoms among civilian populations [13], combat PTSD has been relatively impervious to pharmacological treatment [14]. Other drugs are beginning to take position on the front lines in the battle against PTSD, mainly atypical antipsychotics such as Seroquel.

Following the blood-thinner Plavix, Seroquel (quetiapine fumarate) is the VA's second most largest prescription drug expenditure each year since 2007; where in fiscal year 2010, the agency spent $ 125.4 million on Seroquel, up from $ 14.4 million in 2001 [15]. Similarly, the Department of Defense's spending on Seroquel has increased nearly 700 % since 2001, to $ 8.6 million in 2004, according to purchase records [16].

While the FDA approved Seroquel only for schizophrenia, it is often used off-label for PTSD. However, the potential side effects include diabetes, weight gain, and uncontrollable muscle spasms. In the past few years, Seroquel has been the subject of more than 25,000 product liability lawsuits, including one brought by federal prosecutors. In April 2010, AstraZeneca paid $ 520 million to settle the federal government lawsuit, although thousands of other civil lawsuits are still pending [17]. Researchers at Vanderbilt University published a study in the New England Journal of Medicine suggesting a new risk: sudden heart failure. The investigators found three cardiac deaths per year for every 1000 patients taking antipsychotic drugs like Seroquel [18].

Similar risks were reported by Dr. Kuehn who observed that, "taking atypical antipsychotics doubles the risk of sudden cardiac death" [19]. Furthermore, clinical consideration for the use of atypical antipsychotics to treat patients presenting with PTSD may be problematic, since this class of medications can increase the risk of suicidal attempts, as demonstrated by Dr. Hering. His findings suggest that a noncompliant patient using atypical antipsychotics has a 3.6 times increased risk of suicide attempts as compared to compliant patient using atypical antipsychotic [20].

13.4.2.2 Cognitive-Behavioral Therapy (CBT) and Other Psychotherapy

CBT involves a therapist who helps the client change how he or she thinks about the traumatic event and the client's response to that event. Exposure therapy is one component of CBT and is likely the most effective [21]. The main objective is to help the patient identify feelings associated with PTSD and then develop methods to cope with these feelings. The CBT component of treatment helps the patient change how he or she thinks about the traumatic event and the response to that event. Using exposure therapy, the client is reintroduced to portions of the traumatic event in a controlled, safe environment. The typical CBT course is of 3 months with one to two visits per week. Alternatives to CBT, with potentially similar efficacy, include eye movement desensitization and reprocessing (EMDR).

13.4.2.3 Eye Movement Desensitization and Reprocessing (EMDR)

Francine Shapiro first developed the EMDR therapy upon noticing that certain eye movements reduced the intensity of disturbing thought. She proceeded to conduct a scientific study, sampling trauma victims in 1988 and the research was later published in the Journal of Traumatic Stress in 1989 [22]. In a 2007 review of 33 randomized controlled trials of various psychological treatments for PTSD, EMDR was rated as an effective method, not significantly different in effect from Trauma-Focused CBT or stress management (SM) treatments [23]. EMDR did significantly better than other therapies, according to patient self-reports [23]. Dr. Salkovskis reported that the eye movement is irrelevant, and the effectiveness of EMDR was solely due to having properties similar to CBT, such as desensitization and exposure [24]. Most recent meta-analyses conducted in 2013, including the Cochrane review, have indicated that CBT and EMDR therapies are well-supported by research and superior to all other psychotherapies [25].

13.4.3 New, Cutting Edge Treatments for PTSD, Complementary Alternative Medicine (CAM)

13.4.3.1 Methylenedioxymethamphetamine (MDMA)

One of the newest PTSD treatments is the use of the drug MDMA, a street drug called ecstasy. In the early 1900s, this compound was developed in Germany as a parent compound to be used to synthesize other pharmaceuticals. The drug gained a small following among psychiatrists in the late 1970s and early 1980s. During which time, some psychiatrists even called it "penicillin for the soul" because MDMA was perceived to enhance communication in patient sessions and reportedly allowed users to achieve insights about their problems. Medical reviews have noted that MDMA has some limited therapeutic benefits in certain mental health disorders; however, it is unsafe due to the persistent adverse cognitive and neural effects associated with its use [26,27]. More research is needed in order to determine if the benefits of using MDMA in PTSD treatment outweighs the patients risk of persistent adverse neuropsychological harm [26,27].

13.4.3.2 Yoga

Patients experiencing PTSD which is exacerbated by stress and who have low heart rate variability (HRV) have been shown to improve in response to yoga-based interventions [28]. Dr. Streeter proposed a theory explaining the benefits of practicing yoga. It is hypothesized that stress induces (1) imbalance of the autonomic nervous system (ANS) with decreased parasympathetic nervous system (PNS) and increased sympathetic nervous system (SNS) activity, (2) increased allostatic load (allostatic load being defined as "the wear and tear on the body" which grows over time when the individual is exposed to repeated or chronic stress). It is further hypothesized that yoga-based practices (1) correct underactivity of the PNS in part through stimulation of the vagus nerves, the main peripheral pathway of the PNS, and (2) reduce allostatic load. According to the proposed theory, the decreased PNS underlying stress-related disorders can be corrected by yoga practices resulting in amelioration symptoms [27]. Interestingly, this theory is consistent with the SGB intervention because its effects are presumed to act via modulation of the SNS.

13.4.3.3 Mindfulness-Based Stress Reduction (MBSR)

Mindfulness-based stress reduction (MBSR) has shown promise as an intervention for PTSD [29]. Dr. Kearney reported significant improvements in PTSD symptoms; depression and behavioral activation, where 47.7 % ofveterans had clinically significant improvements in PTSD symptoms [29]. Dr. Hölzel reported that reductions in perceived stress correlated positively with decreases in right basolateral amygdala gray matter density. Stressed but otherwise healthy individuals ($N=26$) participated in an 8-week mindfulness-based stress reduction intervention. Following the intervention, participants reported significantly reduced perceived stress. Reductions in perceived stress correlated positively with decreases in right basolateral amygdala gray matter density, as measured by functional MRI. The more the participants' stress levels decreased, the greater the decrease of gray matter density in the right amygdala [30].

Dr. Hölzel went on to say that evidence suggests that mindfulness practice is associated with neuroplastic changes in the anterior cingulate cortex, insula, temporo-parietal junction, fronto-limbic network, and default mode network structures. The authors suggested that the mechanisms described work synergistically by establishing a process of enhanced self-regulation [30]. As with Yoga, the above theory is consistent with the effect of SGB intervention, since the effects of MBSR and SGB are theorized to be due to the effects modulated by the amygdala [31].

This summary provides an abridged overview of current interventions for treatments of PTSD. By no means does this review offer an exhaustive treatise on the aforementioned approaches discussed. Each treatment modality has its advocates as well as detractors. The remaining part of this chapter focuses on a relatively new treatment to the field of psychiatry, SGB.

Essentially, SGB is an injection of a local anesthetic in the cervical spine that modulates the SNS and has marked impact on PTSD symptoms that are apparent in 30 min following the procedure and may be long lasting. In evaluating SGB, as well as other methods, as a viable treatment option of PTSD, it is important to recall Dr. Hoge statement, "Interventions that will have the greatest potential for improving care on a population level are those focused on enhancing the reach of treatment (e.g., engagement, adherence, and acceptability [9])."

13.5 Treatment of PTSD by Modulation of the Sympathetic Nervous System

13.5.1 Overview Sympathetic Nervous System as Related to PTSD

The focus of this section is on the manipulation of the SNS, which the author believes is one of the new frontiers for treating PTSD. The SNS is part of the ANS. Its main role is to mobilize the body's resources under stress and to induce the fight-or-flight response. It is also constantly active at a basal level in order to maintain homeostasis.

In large part, the activation of the SNS is accomplished by the increase of catecholamines, mainly epinephrine and norepinephrine (NE). The role of NE in the brain is that of a neurotransmitter leading to arousal, selective attention, and vigilance which has been demonstrated in preclinical studies [32]. Specifically, elevated urinary NE has been identified among patients with PTSD [33]. Similarly, NE concentrations in cerebrospinal fluid (CSF) are significantly higher in subjects with PTSD than among healthy controls, and have been correlated with the severity of PTSD symptoms [34]. Such notable increase in noradrenergic activity among subjects with PTSD suggest that reducing CNS noradrenergic activity could be effective, especially for arousal symptoms such as nightmares and startle reactions [35].

13.5.2 Orally Active Noradrenergic Blocking Agents in Treatment of PTSD

Orally active noradrenergic blocking agents have been used to moderate an overactive SNS with previously reported psychiatric effects on PTSD, which include clonidine and prazosin.

13.5.2.1 Prazosin

A sympatholytic drug typically used to treat hypertension, prazosin, is in the class of alpha-adrenergic blockers which lower the blood pressure by blocking the effects of NE. In doing so, this process relaxes the vessel walls. Interestingly, significant psychiatric effect was noted in double-blind placebo-controlled trials of prazosin, which demonstrated a dramatic 70–80 % reduction in combat-related PTSD nightmares [12]. Although the evidence was less compelling, prazosin also reduced PTSD-related anxiety during the day, comparable to that observed with the SSRIs [12].

13.5.2.2 Clonidine

Clonidine is an alpha-2 adrenergic receptor agonist that suppresses the SNS outflow throughout the brain. Because clonidine activates the post-synaptic alpha-2 receptors in the central nervous system (CNS), it inhibits sympathetic activity [36]. Contrary to the effects of prazosin, clonidine does not block the effects of NE directly, but reduces the sympathetic activation of CNS. Clonidine has been shown to reduce hyperarousal symptoms of PTSD [37].

In addition to these oral agents, it is now possible to directly affect the SNS transmission to the brain. The neuroanatomy presented below provides a neuroanatomical explanation for brain sympathetic system manipulation outside the cerebrum. The stellate ganglion and upper thoracic ganglion (T-2) is the upper sympathetic ganglion that innervates the upper chest, the head, and the brain. Many of the efferent sympathetic fibers from the thoracic ganglia (T-2) pass through the stellate ganglion [38]. A connection from the stellate ganglion and the brain has been shown by the use of the pseudorabies virus injections [39]. Pseudorabies virus allows identification of neural pathway connections two to three synaptic connections from the injection site.

13.5.3 Minimally Invasive Modulation of SNS in Treatment of PTSD

13.5.3.1 Endoscopic Sympathetic Block (ESB) at the Second Thoracic Vertebra (T2)

Successful treatment of anxiety by the use of clipping the sympathetic ganglia via an endoscopic sympathetic block (ESB) at the second thoracic vertebra (T2) was first reported in 1998 [40]. In a follow-up publication to his 1998 paper, Dr. Telaranta noted the similarity in features between social phobias and PTSD—especially those caused by an overactive SNS, such as heart racing, hypervigilance, and avoidance of painful psychic situations [41].

13.5.3.2 Stellate Ganglion Block (SGB), a Cervical Sympathetic Injection

The SGB is an anesthetic injection in a group of nerves in the neck that are called the stellate ganglion. This procedure has been used to treat chronic pain since 1925, and recent studies have demonstrated great promise as a successful intervention for PTSD.

This author reported the first successful treatment of PTSD through the use of SGB in 2008 [42]. The subject of that report was a civilian robbery victim who presented for SGB treatment due to severe anxiety related to PTSD, 2 months post being robbed at gunpoint. The patient experienced excellent response to SGB and reported significant resolution of hyper vigilance and anxiety.

13.5.3.3 Potential Complications of SGB

SGB carry a very small risk of infection. Using prophylactic antibiotics can reduce the slight risk of infection. Although rare, severe complications following SGB do include bleeding, seizures, pneumothorax, and spinal cord trauma. A study of the incidence of severe complications was last undertaken in 1992 by German researchers Wulf and Maier; they reported 1.7 complications per 1000 blockades based on surveys completed by patients receiving a combined total of 45,000 blocks. No fatalities or persistent complications were reported [43]. This survey was conducted prior to the use of fluoroscopic guidance where the SGBs were performed at the C7 level rather than C6. The current improvements in guidance technology and changing the needle location to C6 are likely to reduce the chance of complications.

13.5.3.4 SGB and the Treatment of PTSD, Current Evidence

SGB has been used to treat PTSD since 2008. Dr. Navaie summarized available literature published between 2008 and 2013 on the use of SGB to treat PTSD [44]. She indicates that patients were predominantly male ($n = 21$, 88 %) and active duty military ($n = 14$, 58 %) or veterans ($n = 8$, 33 %) with combat-related PTSD. The average age was 40.5 years. All patients received more than 1 year of psychotherapy and pharmacotherapy before SGB. Seventeen patients (71 %) received one SGB, seven (29 %) received multiple SGBs. Clinically, meaningful improvements were observed in 75 % ($n = 18$) of patients after SGB, with significant differences in mean PTSD scores, pre and post treatment.

In clinical case reports reviewed above, two have specific merit.

Dr. Alino reported on a patient with a 2 year history of suicidal ideation had become free of suicidal thought two days after SGB [45]. Dr. Mulvaney reported on two patients with severe PTSD who were able to completely stop taking psychiatric medications after SGB [46]. Recently, further validation of SGB efficacy has been published.

Dr. Mulvaney, in a follow-up to a 2010 publication [46] observed that 166 service members with symptoms of PTSD that received SGB had clinically significant reductions in PCL scores. Specifically, 70 % of those treated with SGB reported significant reductions in PCL scores and the effects were sustained 3–6 months post procedure [47].

Further validation of SGB efficacy in 2014 came from Dr. Alkire. He presented an abstract titled: “Prolonged Relief of Chronic Extreme PTSD and Depression Symptoms in Veterans Following a Stellate Ganglion Block.” In this report, Dr. Alkire selected the most extreme PTSD cases in the veteran population and observed that SGB was greatly effective in helping 75 % (9/12) of the subjects [48].

13.5.3.5 Proposed Mechanisms for the Clinical Effect of SGB

The hypothesis for potential mechanism of action for SGB (or cervical sympathetic chain blockade) has been described in multiple peer-reviewed publications [31, 46–49]. The hypothesis rests on previously demonstrated evidence and was originally proposed by the author.

The first line of evidence in supporting the theory demonstrates a polysynaptic neurological connection from stellate ganglion to the part of the brain associated with PTSD, the amygdala [39] (Fig. 13.1). Specifically, Dr. Liberzon demonstrated increased activation of the amygdala in PTSD patients when compared to controls [50].

The second line of evidence relies on the nerve growth factor (NGF) increase observed as a physiological response to acute and chronic stress [51,52]. NGF increase is known to increase perivascular NE. This has been demonstrated by direct intracerebroventricular brain infusion of NGF into adult rats [53]. Stress-induced release of NE in amygdala and related structures has been shown to facilitate a number of anxiety-like behavioral responses that are mediated in these regions [54].

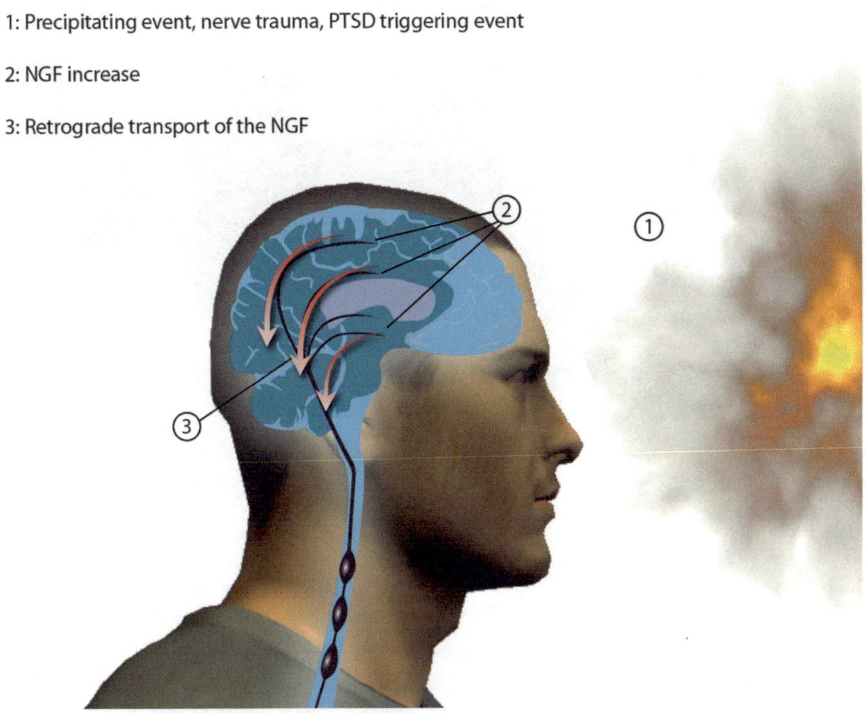

Fig. 13.1 The possible biologic mechanism exists for how sympathetic blockade may produce long-lasting systemic effects. There is a poly-synaptic neurological connection from stellate ganglion to the part of the brain associated with PTSD, the amygdala. (From Vlessides M, Anesthesia method suggests possible cure for post-trauma stress. Anesthesiology News 2012; 38:9, with permission)

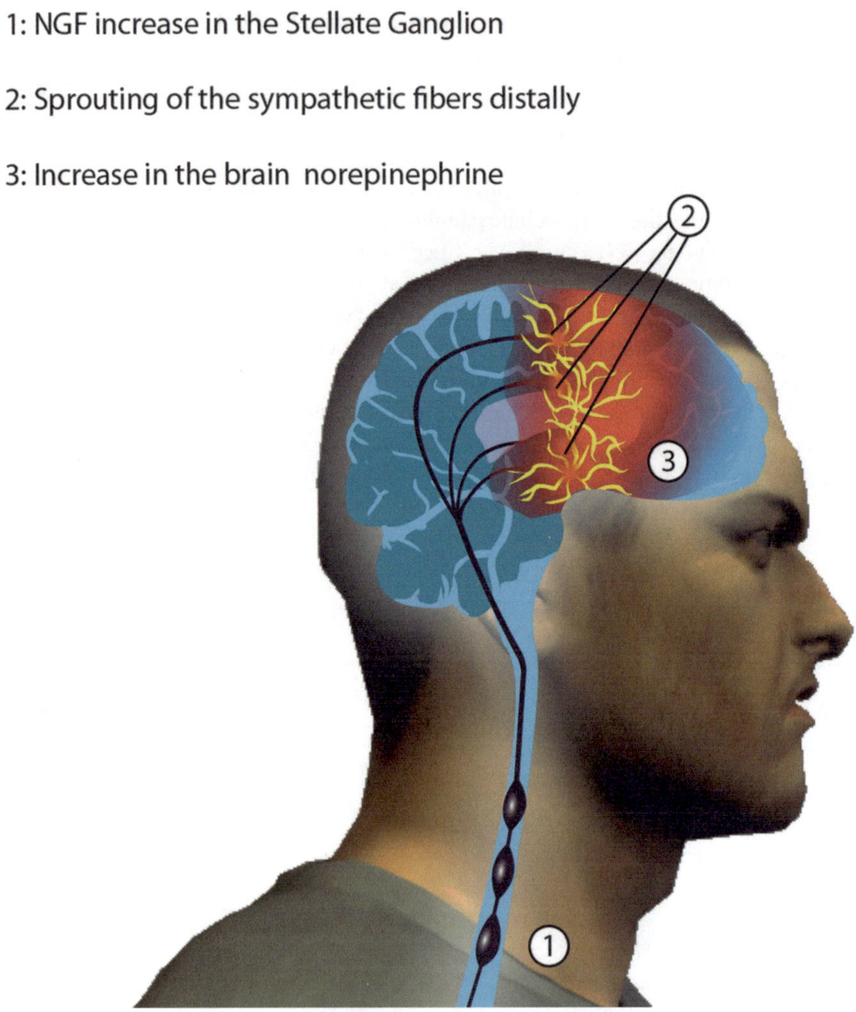

Fig. 13.2 The neurite outgrowth has been associated with NE increase. (From Vlessides M, Anesthesia method suggests possible cure for post-trauma stress. Anesthesiology News 2012; 38:9, with permission)

The NE increase has been shown to be associated with PTSD in urine [33] and cerebrospinal fluid [34] as discussed previously. The NE increase is likely due to NGF increase in the stellate ganglion which in turn is caused by retrograde NGF transport from the intracerebral site to the stellate ganglion [55]. NGF increase is also known to promote neurite outgrowth (sprouting) at the end terminals [56]. The neurite outgrowth has been associated with NE increase [57] (Fig. 13.2).

Finally, local anesthetic injections are known to suppress NGF [58], leading to dying of new nerve outgrowth since maintenance of sprouting is dependent on the

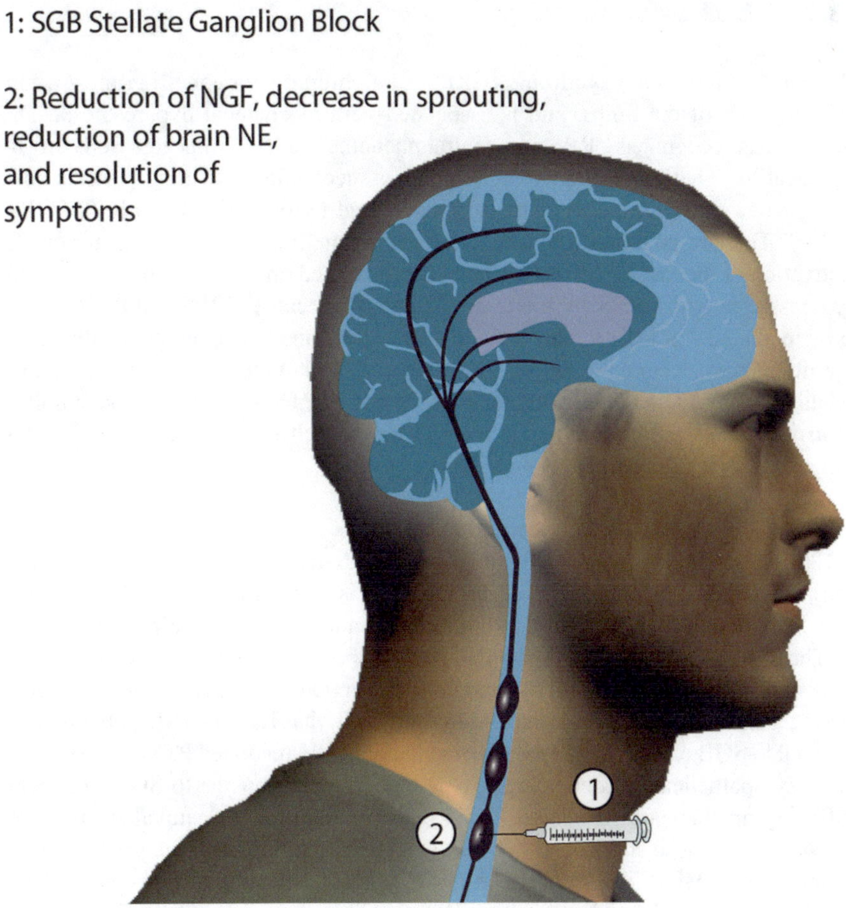

Fig. 13.3 It is hypothesized that the suppression of NGF would reduce NE levels and reverse the cascade of PTSD. (From Vlessides M, Anesthesia method suggests possible cure for post-trauma stress. Anesthesiology News 2012;38:9, with permission)

presence of NGF [59]. As a result, it is hypothesized that the suppression of NGF would reduce NE levels and reverse the cascade of PTSD [31] (Fig. 13.3).

The third and final line of evidence in support of the theory is based on EEG evaluation of rats following SGB. Dr. Jeong found that SGB with bupivacaine resulted in significantly decreased EEG activities in rats. These results suggest that SGB can induce a sedative effect in rats. The proposed mechanism of the effect described above was reduction in brain NE [60].

A possible new nomenclature for organization of PTSD etiology and treatment is based on the sympathetic system involvement. Complex regional pain syndrome (CRPS) and PTSD correlates.

13.5.4 Background

Complex regional pain syndrome (CRPS) is a chronic pain condition most often affecting one of the limbs, and is associated with mechanical hyperesthesia. Dr. Bogdak has recognized CRPS as a central phenomenon [61]. Repeated SGB utilizing local anesthetic are documented as being successful in treating patients suffering from upper limb CRPS, in prospective and retrospective trials [62]. CRPS and PTSD share common brain structure activation, mainly in the insular cortex. Activation of the insular cortex has been demonstrated on fMRI during mechanical hyperesthesia with CRPS [63], and in PTSD [64]. Because CRPS and PTSD seem to be mediated—at least in part—via insular cortex, one would anticipate that both conditions may occur simultaneously or one may lead to the other. One such report exists, where a Vietnam veteran had a recurrence of PTSD symptoms and simultaneous onset of CRPS in the leg, where the authors felt both the conditions have a common supraspinal mechanism [65].

13.5.4.1 A Possible New Nomenclature

CRPS is classified as being, sympathetically mediated pain (SMP) or sympathetically independent pain (SIP). By definition, SMP is responsive to SGB. Thus, CRPS with SMP diagnosis is made following a significant reduction in pain after SGB.

The SIP is defined as CRPS pain that is not responsive to SGB. The distinction of SMP and SIP is made to direct therapeutic intervention. Similarly, the author is proposing a similar diagnostic organization for PTSD, that is, the PTSD patients who respond to SGB can be diagnosed with sympathetically mediated PTSD (SMP), and those sympathetically independent PTSD who are irresponsive to SGB treatment (SIP). Sympathetically mediated PTSD (SMP) would be the equivalent of SMP, the way to diagnose and treat SMP; PTSD is by doing the SGB. The percentage of patients with SMP PTSD seems to be 70 % of PTSD patients based on current data. Sympathetically independent PTSD (SIP) would be equivalent of SIP. This diagnosis would be made following inadequate effect of SGB on PTSD symptoms, and no further SGB would be done.

The advantage of this nomenclature is a way to organize PTSD patients that have reversible sympathetic system activation and will respond to SGB.

The integration, of seemingly unrelated medical fields of study, has been predicted by Dr. Schore in 2002. He stated that neuropsychiatry and psychiatry would integrate for the treatment of PTSD [66]. He went on to report that data exists documenting episodes of trauma expressed in episodes of hyperarousal and dissociation; which are imprinted into the limbic and ANS of the right brain. These enduring structural changes lead to the inefficient stress-coping mechanisms that lie at the core of PTSDs [66]. SGB has been described as having therapeutic effect by affecting limbic and ANS, amygdala, and SNS, respectively [31].

13.6 Conclusion

Using the sympathetic system modulation as a new target for the treatment of psychiatric symptoms seems to have promise in the battle to resolve PTSD scourge. SGB has already changed a number of lives and has been used to help "save" four patients from suicide (unpublished data). It seems difficult to believe that an injection in the neck may lead to psychiatric effect at first glance; however, if one considers the persuasiveness of the sympathetic system and the well described SNS activation in PTSD, this effect becomes increasingly more plausible.

At the time of writing this chapter, over 2,000 military personal have been treated with SGB for PTSD in four military hospitals, with an over 70% success rate. The advantages of the SGB as a PTSD therapy lie in the fact that it offers virtually immediate relief, increases compliance with the therapy, consistently maintains a high efficacy rate, reduces the use of psychiatric medications, and significantly improves the psychotherapy efficacy. As such, this innovation may not only improve the quality of life for millions of patients but may also reduce the overall socioeconomic burden of treating PTSD on the health-care system. If SGB indeed lives up to its early potential, and is validated by formal studies, it may have substantial short-term and long-term benefits by alleviating suffering and hardships for PTSD patients and their loved ones.

References

1. PTSD VA. http://www.ptsd.va.gov/professional/PTSD-overview/ptsd-overview.asp. Accessed 16 Nov 2014.
2. Da Costa JM. On irritable heart; a clinical study of a form of functional cardiac disorder and its consequences. Am J Med Sci. 1871;121(1):2–52.
3. http://www.wired.com/2010/07/obama-loves-this-freaky-ptsd-treatment-the-pentagon-not-so-much/. Accessed 15 May 2012.
4. Blanchard EB, Jones-Alexander J, Buckley TC, Forneris CA. Psychometric properties of the PTSD checklist (PCL). Behav Res Ther. 1996;34:669–73.
5. Bliese PD, Wright KM, Adler AB, et al. Validating the primary care posttraumatic stress disorder screen and the posttraumatic stress disorder checklist with soldiers returning from combat. J Consult Clin Psychol. 2008;76:272–81.
6. Forbes D, Creamer M, Biddle D. The validity of the PTSD checklist as a measure of symptomatic change in combat-related PTSD. Behav Res Ther. 2001;39:977–86.
7. Gore AT, Richards-Reid GM. Posttraumatic stress disorder. 2006. eMedicine [serial online]. http://www.emedicine.com/med/topic1900.htm. Accessed 21 Oct 2007.
8. Institute of Medicine. Treatment of posttraumatic stress disorder: an assessment of the evidence. Washington, DC: National Academies; 2007.
9. Hoge CW. Interventions for war-related posttraumatic stress disorder: meeting veterans where they are. JAMA. 2011;306:549–51.
10. Balon R. SSRI-associated sexual dysfunction. Am J Psychiatr 2006;163:1504–163.
11. Giner L, Nichols CM, Zalsman G, et al. Selective serotonin reuptake inhibitors and the risk for suicidality in adolescents: an update. Int J Adolesc Med Health. 2005;17:211–7.
12. Raskind MA, Peskind ER, Hoff DJ, et al. A parallel group placebo controlled study of prazosin for trauma nightmares and sleep disturbance in combat veterans with Posttraumatic stress disorder. Biol Psychiatr. 2007;61(8):928–34.

13. Brady K, Pearlstein T, Asnis GM, et al. Efficacy and safety of sertraline treatment of posttraumatic stress disorder: a randomized controlled trial. JAMA. 2000;283:1837–283.
14. Zohar J, Amital D, Miodownik C, et al. Double-blind placebo controlled pilot study of sertraline in military veterans with posttraumatic stress disorder. J Clin Psychopharmacol. 2002;22:190.
15. Scott L. http://www.vawatchdog.org/10/nf10/nfaug10/nf083110-1.htm at VA Watchdog dot Org 08-31-2010. Accessed 22 Feb 2014.
16. Jones E, Wessely S. Shell shock to PTSD: military psychiatry from 1900 to the Gulf War 2005. Hove: Taylor & Francis. 2006; ISSN 0076–5465.
17. http://www.nolo.com/legal-encyclopedia/seroquel-product-liability-claims-32525.html. Accessed 23 Jan 2015.
18. Schneeweiss S, Avorn J. Antipsychotic agents and sudden cardiac death—how should we manage the risk? N Engl J Med. 2009;360:294–6.
19. Kuehn BM. FDA panel issues mixed decision on quetiapine in depression and anxiety. JAMA. 2009;301(20):2081–2.
20. Herings RM, Erkens JA, Increased suicide attempt rate among patients interrupting use of atypical antipsychotics. Pharmacoepidem Drug Safe. 2003; 12: 423–4.
21. Paunovic N, Öst LG. Cognitive-behavior therapy vs exposure therapy in the treatment of PTSD in refugees. Behav Res Ther. 2001;39(10):1183–97.
22. Shapiro F. Efficacy of the eye movement desensitization procedure in the treatment of traumatic memories. J Trauma Stress. 1989;2:199–223.
23. Bisson J, Andrew M. Psychological treatment of Posttraumatic stress disorder (PTSD). Cochrane Database Syst Rev. 2007.
24. Salkovskis P. Review: eye movement desensitization and reprocessing is not better than exposure therapies for anxiety or trauma. Evid-Based Ment Health. 2002;5(1):13.
25. Watts BV, Schnurr PP, Mayo L, et al. Meta-analysis of the efficacy of treatments for posttraumatic stress disorder. J Clin Psychiatr. 2013;74:e541–50.
26. Meyer JS. 3,4-methylenedioxymethamphetamine (MDMA): current perspectives. Subst Abuse Rehabil,2013;4:83–99.
27. Parrott AC. The potential dangers of using MDMA for psychotherapy. J Psychoact Drugs. 2014;46(1):37–43.
28. Streeter CC, Gerbarg RB, Saper DA, et al. Effects of yoga on the autonomic nervous system, gamma-aminobutyric-acid, and allostasis in epilepsy, depression, and Posttraumatic stress disorder. Med Hypotheses. 2012;78(5):571–9.
29. Kearney DJ, McDermott K, Malte C, et al. Association of participation in a mindfulness program with measures of PTSD, depression and quality of life in a veteran sample. J Clin Psychol. 2012;68(1):101–16.
30. Hölzel BK, Carmody J, Evans KC, et al. Stress reduction correlates with structural changes in the amygdala. Soc Cogn Affect Neurosci. 2009;5:11–7.
31. Lipov EG, Joshi JR, et al. A unifying theory linking the prolonged efficacy of the stellate ganglion block for the treatment of chronic regional pain syndrome (CRPS), hot flashes, and posttraumatic stress disorder (PTSD). Med Hypotheses. 2009;72(6):657–61.
32. Southwick SM, Bremner JD, Rasmusson A, et al. Role of norepinephrine in the pathophysiology and treatment of posttraumatic stress disorder. Biol Psychiatr. 1999;46:1192–204.
33. Mason JW, Giller EL, Kosten TR, et al. Elevation of urinary norepinephrine/cortisol ratio in posttraumatic stress disorder. J Nerv Ment Dis. 1988;176:498–502.
34. Geracioti TD, Baker DG, Ekhator NN, et al. CSF norepinephrine concentrations in posttraumatic stress disorder. Am J Psychiatr. 2001;158:1227–158.
35. Taylor FB, Lowe K, Thompson C, et al. Daytime Prazosin reduces psychological distress-to trauma specific cuesin civilian trauma post traumatic stress disorder . Biol Psychiatr. 2006;59:577–81.
36. Ma D, Rajakumaraswamy N, Maze M. Alpha2-adrenoceptor agonists: shedding light on neuroprotection? Br Med Bull. 2004;71:77–92.

37. Sutherland SM, Davidson JR. Pharmacotherapy for Posttraumatic stress disorder. Psychiatr Clin North Am. 1994;17:409–23.
38. Uchida K, Tateda T, et al. Novel mechanism of action hypothesized for stellate ganglion block related to melatonin. Med Hypotheses. 2002;59:446–9.
39. Westerhaus MJ, Loewy AD. Central representation of the sympathetic nervous system in the cerebral cortex. Brain Res. 2001;903:117–27.
40. Telaranta T. Treatment of social phobia by endoscopic thoracic sympathicotomy. Eur J Surg Suppl. 1998;580:27–32.
41. Telaranta T. Psychoneurological applications of endoscopic sympathetic blocks (ESB) [invited lecture]. Clin Auton Res. 2003;13(Suppl. 1):I120–1.
42. Lipov EG, Joshi JR, Lipov SG, Sanders SE, Siroko MK. Cervical sympathetic blockade in a patient with posttraumatic stress disorder: a case report. Ann Clin Psychiatry. 2008;20:227–8.
43. Wulf H, Maier CH. Complications of stellate ganglion blockade: results of a survey. Anaesthetist. 1992;41:146–51.
44. Navaie M, Keefe MS, Hickey AH, et al. Use of stellate ganglion block for refractory Posttraumatic stress disorder: a review of published cases. J Anesth Clin Res. 2014 5(403):2.
45. Alino J, Kosatka D, McLean B, et al. Efficacy of stellate ganglion block in the treatment of anxiety symptoms from combat-related Posttraumatic stress disorder: a case series. Mil Med, 2013;178:473–7.
46. Mulvaney SW, McLean B, De Leeuw J. The use of stellate ganglion block in the treatment of panic/anxiety symptoms with combat-related Posttraumatic stress disorder; preliminary results of long-term follow- up: a case series. Pain Pract. 2010;10:349–65.
47. Mulvaney SW, Lynch JH, Hickey MJ, et al. Stellate ganglion block used to treat symptoms associated with combat-related Posttraumatic stress disorder: a case series of 166 patients. Mil Med. 2014;179(10):1133–40.
48. Alkire MT, Hollifield M, Khoshsar R, et al. Prolonged relief of chronic extreme PTSD and depression symptoms in veterans following a stellate ganglion block. Presented at American Society of Anesthesiology. 11 Oct 2014.
49. Hickey AH, Hanling S, Pevney E, et al. Stellate ganglion block for PTSD. Am J Psychiatry. 2012;169:760.
50. Liberzon I, Martis B. Neuroimaging studies of emotional responses in PTSD. Ann N Y Acad Sci. 2006;1071:87–109.
51. Alleva E, Petruzzi S, Cirulli F, et al. NGF regulatory role in stress and coping of rodents and humans. Pharmacol Biochem Behav. 1996;54:65–72.
52. Smith MA. Hippocampal vulnerability to stress and aging: possible role of neurotrophic factors. Behav Brain Res. 1996;78:25–36.
53. Isaacson LG, Billieu SC. Increased perivascular norepinephrine following intracerebroventricular infusion of NGF into adult rats. Exp Neurol. 1996;139(1):54–60.
54. Morilak DA, Barrera G, Echevarria D J, et al. Role of brain norepinephrine in the behavioral response to stress. Prog Neuropsychopharmacol Biol Psychiatr. 2005;29(8):1214–24.
55. Johnson EM Jr, Taniuchi M, Clark HB, et al. Demonstration of the retrograde transport of nerve growth factor receptor in the peripheral and central nervous system. J Neurosci. 1987;7:923–5.
56. Chen PS, Chen LS, Cao JM, Sharifi B, Karagueuzian HS, Fishbein MC. Sympathetic nerve sprouting, electrical remodeling and the mechanisms of sudden cardiac death. Cardiovasc Res. 2001;50(2):409–16.
57. Madison R, Davis JN. Sprouting of noradrenergic fibers in hippocampus after medial septal lesions: contributions of the central and peripheral nervous systems. Exp Neurol. 1983;80(1):167–77.
58. Takatori T, Kuroda Y, Hirose M. Local anesthetics suppress nerve growth factor-mediated neurite outgrowth by inhibition of tyrosine kinase activity of TrkA. Anesth Analg. 2006;102:462–7.
59. Gatzinsky KP, Thrasivoulou C, Campioni-Noack M, Underwood C, Cowen T. The role of NGF uptake in selective vulnerability to cell death in ageing sympathetic neurons. Eur J Neurosci. 2004;20(11):2848–56.

60. Jeong S, Jeon Y, Yeo J, Baek W. The effects of stellate ganglion block on the electroencephalogram in rats. J Anesth. 2014:28(4):601–5.
61. Bogduk N. Complex regional pain syndrome. Curr Opin Anaesth. 2001;14:541–6.
62. Van Eijs F, Stanton-Hicks M, Van Zundert J, et al. Complex regional pain syndrome. Pain Pract. 2011;11(1):70–87.
63. Maihöfner C, Forster C, Birklein F, et al. Brain processing during mechanical hyperalgesia in complex regional pain syndrome: a functional MRI study. Pain. 2005;114(1–2):93–103.
64. Liberzon I, Martis B. Neuroimaging studies of emotional responses in PTSD. Ann N Y Acad Sci. 2006;1071(1):87–109.
65. Grande LA, Loeser JD, Ozuna J, et al. Complex regional pain syndrome as a stress response. Pain 2004;110(1–2):495–8.
66. Schore AN. Dysregulation of the right brain: a fundamental mechanism of traumatic attachment and the psychopathogenesis of posttraumatic stress disorder. Aust N Z J Psychiatr. 2002;36(1):9–30.

Canine Connection Therapy: Finding Purpose and Healing Through the Training of Service Dogs

14

Meg Daley Olmert, Michelle Nordstrom, Marshall Peters, Matthew St Laurent and Rick Yount

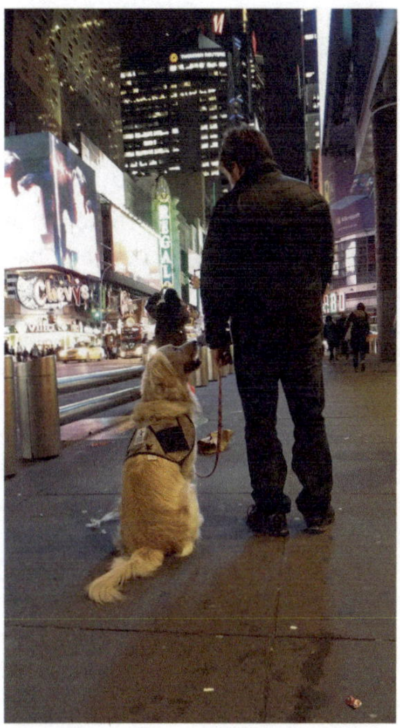

John navigating Times Square with Lundy, November 2014 (courtesy of Marshall Peters, SDI).

M. St Laurent (✉)
Department of Rehabilitation, Walter Reed National Military Medical Center, Bethesda, MD 20889, USA
e-mail: Matthew.G.StLaurent.mil@mail.mil

M. D. Olmert · R. Yount
Warrior Canine Connection, Brookeville, MD 23222, USA
e-mail: megolmert@gmail.com

E. C. Ritchie (ed.), *Posttraumatic Stress Disorder and Related Diseases in Combat Veterans,* DOI 10.1007/978-3-319-22985-0_14

14.1 History and Overview of the Therapeutic Service Dog Training Program Offered at Walter Reed National Military Medical Center

A pilot of the service dog training therapy program (SDTTP) model was launched in July 2008 at The Men's and Women's Trauma Recovery Program at the Veterans Administration (VA) Hospital in Menlo Park, CA. The SDTTP was conceived as a safe and effective complementary treatment to reduce the symptoms of posttraumatic stress disorder (PTSD). The perception of this program as an opportunity to reengage in a meaningful mission had a strong appeal to the powerful warrior ethos of this patient population. Over the next 2 years, this volunteer SDTTP proved to be highly popular and demonstrated a low dropout rate. In 2009, patient reports of reductions in their PTSD symptoms and clinical observations of the program's success were presented at the Veterans Administration National Mental Health Conference and the annual meeting of International Society for Traumatic Stress Studies. Approximately 200 service members participated in the pilot SDTTP program, five service dogs were placed with veterans in need, and two warrior trainers (WT) have become accredited service dog trainers currently pursuing careers in this field.

In 2009, the SDTTP was integrated into the Walter Reed's occupational therapy (OT) and recreational therapy (RT) programs. Clinicians at Walter Reed continued to observe reduction in patients' PTSD symptoms and patients reported improved wellness and high satisfaction with the program. The SDTTP, which is staffed by professional service dog trainers with clinical experience, is now also offered as an adjunct therapy for PTSD at the National Intrepid Center of Excellence (NICoE), WRNMMC, Ft Belvoir Community Hospital, the VA hospital in Menlo Park, CA, and NeuroRestorative's residential treatment program in Germantown, MD. Approximately 3000 active-duty service members and veterans have participated in the SDTTP since February 2009 [1].

The golden and labrador retrievers used in the program are bred for the health and temperament necessary for mobility service dogs. It takes approximately 2 years to mature and train a service dog. From day one, these purpose-bred dogs are gently handled and exposed to increasing social and sensory experiences bolstering their devotion and confidence in humans. Patients and their families participate in this fun and essential early socialization training. Around 3 months of age, the young dogs are ready to start the training program. Participants begin to teach the dogs

M. Nordstrom
Occupational Therapy Mental Health Services, Walter Reed National Military Medical Center, Bethesda, MD 20889, USA

M. Peters
Walter Reed National Military Medical Center, Bethesda, MD 20889, USA
e-mail: marshall.ptrs@gmail.com

basic commands and eventually work toward completing the list of 90 commands which each dog must be competent in to become qualified as skilled, certified, service dogs. The patients' participation in the SDTTP depends on their needs as well as the length and flexibility of their treatment program. Some WTs may work with the dogs for 2 weeks, while others are in the program for a year or more. This means that over 50 WTs can experience the psychological, physiological, and behavioral therapeutic value of the program during the course of training one service dog.

14.2 Case History/Presentation (John)

ID: 40-year-old male, married, white, AD/USN/E7 Chief Navy SEAL

John joined the Navy in 1992 (21 years service)

Current Military Status: Active Duty

Family History: John was married to his current wife in 2005 and together, they have five children.

John completed 11 deployments including Operation Iraqi Freedom (OIF) and Operation Enduring Freedom (OEF). He was exposed to multiple blasts during the deployments, including one in November 2010 when he sustained shrapnel wounds to his head. John began experiencing memory loss, loss of balance, and severe headaches. He did not seek medical attention until February 2012, after returning to the USA. John also experienced numerous significant emotional loss throughout his career, including but not limited to, losing 40+ friends who were killed in combat.

May 2011, John returned from deployment in Afghanistan to his home in Virginia Beach, VA. He had an extremely difficult time readjusting to normal family life. John continued experiencing constant headaches, loss of balance, increased irritability, speech difficulty, and episodes of memory loss. Combat-related dreams and daydreams, avoidance of social situations, hypervigilance, isolating himself from people, and increasing marital and family conflicts were a few of the challenges he was facing at that time.

14.2.1 Diagnosis and Treatment

May 2012, John was diagnosed and treated for traumatic brain injury (TBI) at NICoE located on the WRNMMC campus, where he received 6 weeks of intensive evidence-based and complementary, alternative medicine (CAM) treatments. His treatment continued over the next 15 months with therapies provided by both Portsmouth Naval Hospital Brain Trauma Outpatient Clinic and also the Richmond VA Inpatient Transitional Rehab Program. However, John's symptoms continued to worsen.

September 2013, John was transferred to WRNMMC's inpatient TBI ward (7E). Neurological examinations were normal and behavioral observations ruled out TBI as the cause of John symptoms. PTSD became the working diagnosis.

John began a 7-month comprehensive, intensive psychological and behavioral rehabilitation program consisting of: OT , RT, and speech-language pathology (SLP). John's medications were evaluated and adjusted to increase efficacy and decrease pharmacological burden. At this time, John and his wife also started intensive marital counseling. The counseling resulted in a significant decrease in marital discord and subsequently correlated with improvement in some of John's symptoms.

14.2.2 SDTTP Clinical Notes from Service Dog Trainer and Recreational Therapist

14.2.2.1 September 25, 2013: First Encounter with SDTTP

Shortly after his arrival on 7E, John was invited to participate in a volunteer SDTTP as part of OT/RT services. The intent was for this program to help improve his verbal fluency, increase independence in recreation/leisure participation, and increase community functioning. John liked the idea that these dogs would be partnered with veterans in need. He agreed to work with the therapist and the service dog instructor (SDI) even though he was skeptical that training the dogs would help his recovery. As part of his inpatient treatment he attended hour-long service dog training sessions 2–3 times per week for approximately 5 weeks.

John: I felt like, sure I'll play with your dog for a little bit, but what I really need to be doing is working on brain games or getting help for my speech and math issues.

SDI: In our first session, John's presentation was one of quiet and reserve. Speech and sequencing was a noticeable issue. A verbal greeting that would normally take seconds was challenging and proved to be a point of frustration.

RT: John was attentive and demonstrated bright affect as evidenced by smiling and laughing intermittently when directly interacting with the service dog. He responded appropriately to constructive feedback from the SDI and agreed to continue participation in the program.

14.2.2.2 Weeks 2 and 3 of the SDTTP

SDI: John seemed to be somewhat disinterested in our appointments initially, but would dutifully attend them anyway. Within the first few sessions working with Lundy (9 month-old male Golden Retriever) there was a noticeable and distinct bond forming between the two of them. Although John was having trouble initially remembering commands or even our names, his affect was noticeably more positive and he appeared more resilient to the challenges of remembering/verbalizing commands.

John: On the third visit I couldn't remember Lundy's name, even though, just days before, I had said it a hundred times. I couldn't remember the commands or say them because of my speech issues. I thought it was a waste. On the fourth session, it suddenly dawned on me that the dog training demanded the same brain skills as the computer games—except in real life/time. This training was helping me, I was helping Lundy become a service dog, and we were both working toward helping a Veteran in need. That's when I started to take program seriously.

SDI: At first we were conducting training sessions on the ward. As our sessions progressed and John formed an even closer bond with Lundy, we ventured to the first floor of the hospital—a crowded, noisy environment that would begin to challenge his arousal and avoidance issues. Lundy is routinely mistaken for a hospital therapy dog and was often abruptly approached and engaged by random people. These situations allowed John to practice and become more comfortable with healthy confrontation and setting boundaries with people.

John: As part of OT, I'd have to navigate the Metro or go shopping. These were stressful experiences, but I could manage to do them without talking to any strangers. Going out in public with Lundy meant that many people would approach and I would have to talk to them. I could talk to Lundy and I could talk to guys I knew, but memorizing, 'I'm sorry Ma'am he's a service dog in training,' and articulating that to a stranger made me very apprehensive. The first couple of outings were pretty stressful. I just focused on Lundy and said, okay, let's get through this. But Lundy was excited to be around me and just having him at my side gave me a sense of confidence and pride. My speech really improved as I worked with Lundy and I found it was getting easier to talk to strangers. That was a real confidence builder for me.

RT: John demonstrated active listening and learned training skills with verbal feedback requiring minimal demonstrations by the SDI. The dogs are rewarded with verbal praise, treats, and petting. He successfully ambulated through crowded hallways with a dog using verbal cues and adjusting his pace for proper training technique. John was initially distracted with passers-by, however his attention increased until he was able to focus on the task independently. John engaged in a conversational task while sitting in a public eating area with minimal difficulties noted. 10 Oct 2013.

14.2.2.3 18 October 2013: Week 4 of SDTTP: Public Training Outing (Bethesda Lunch with Metro)

SDI: Because John's attention was focused greatly on Lundy and the success of his training, we were able to successfully introduce increasingly stimulating environments for John and Lundy. Four weeks into the training program he agreed to an outing that involved taking the underground Metro train from WRNMMC to downtown Bethesda. Upon arrival at the metro station John was noticeably agitated at the task of riding the 230-foot escalator, down the dark tunnel, to the train. He gathered himself and was ready to step towards the downward escalator: Lundy however, was not. Lundy, being a puppy, had not yet been exposed to escalators and he stopped in his tracks. Since John's "white-knuckle, grit-your-teeth and bear it" coping strategy was not going to work for Lundy, in this situation, John was now confronted with slowing down and encouraging Lundy onto the escalator. As he focused on helping Lundy to feel more comfortable with the new experience, John effectively convinced himself to become comfortable with it as well.

John: My stuttering and stammering made me very self-conscious in public and I had very low confidence. I knew that I had to display confidence so that Lundy would feel confident. I tried to just focus on Lundy and move directly to the task, but Lundy stopped short when he saw the moving steps. With the SDI's help I slowed down the process by walking back and forth so that Lundy could get used to the idea of this strange machine. I had to keep praising him and encouraging him. Finally, we were able to get on the escalator and both Lundy and I became more and more confident as we rode it up and down.

RT: Overall, John maintained exceptional emotional regulation when training the service dog while in the community. He required minimal cueing to offer verbal commands to the dog when appropriate.

14.2.2.4 21 October 2013: Week 5 of SDTTP. Public Training Outing - Walter Reed Navy Exchange (NEX)

RT: John attended a therapeutic SDTTP session with RT and SDI on an outing to the NEX. He demonstrated appropriate affect and required intermittent cueing to praise the dog when necessary. John ambulated throughout the session with independence. John demonstrated good emotional regulation skills when teaching simple commands to "stay" and "heel" when near dog food aisles. John was noted to require distant supervision as he and Lundy approached the escalator. John was also required to practice providing verbal commands when in the electronics area due to the increased distractions such as visual and auditory stimulation. He was noted to demonstrate fluid speech in 95 % of session and independently participated in conversational tasks.

John: Working with this young puppy was very challenging. Remembering the commands and being able to find and produce the words was very frustrating. Timing is incredibly important in dog training and my timing was not there. My depression and anxiety made it hard to express the happiness Lundy needed for encouragement, but the sense of purpose punched through. I didn't want to mess this dog up, get him off-track, and keep him from helping a Vet. I was determined to display the confidence and support Lundy needed so that we could help somebody else.

14.2.3 Additional Service Dog Training Program Effects Reported by John

14.2.3.1 Reading Out Loud

John: "I was also having a lot of trouble reading. My doctor suggested I try reading aloud. I would do this in my room, but it was a struggle. I mentioned it the SDTTP Director and he suggested I try reading to Lundy. I thought it was a funny idea, but I quickly found that I could read much more smoothly while reading to Lundy."

14.2.3.2 Sleep

April 15, 2014: John received permission from 7E medical director to have the service dog spend the night in his room to see if his sleep might improve with the dog present.

Medical Notes: John slept through night. Patient denies having any dreams or nightmares.

John: With Lundy at my side, I slept through the night for the first time in a year. I did not wake up even once during the nurses' hourly 'fall-checks.' The four nights Lundy spent with me I slept great and woke up feeling alert and like a different person.

14.2.3.3 Headache, Pain, and Depression

John: Working with Lundy also helped me with my migraines. On many occasions I thought I was in too much pain to work with Lundy. Still, I did not want to quit this mission, so I'd try. I'd start out in pain and unable to focus. When we came back an hour later the nurses would ask about my pain levels and I'd realize I had none. If I started out depressed, I came back laughing.

14.2.3.4 December 2013–March 2014

John was enrolled in a 10-week PTSD program at Oasis (San Diego, CA). John progressed well. Zoloft was discontinued. Lamictal 100 mg PO Qam was begun. John's depression resolved. John's conversion type symptoms resolved. Some anxiety symptoms have improved.

14.2.4 Outcomes and Case Resolution

March 12, 2014: John readmitted to 7E of WRNMMC for reevaluation and final disposition planning. SDTTP sessions recommenced.

14.2.4.1 24 March 2014: SDTTP Public Training Session (Naval Bowling Alley)

RT: John attended an on-base community reintegration outing to Naval Base Bowling Alley with therapist, wife, service dog in training and SDI. John demonstrated bright affect as evidenced by smiling and laughing throughout. He practiced heeling with dog while ambulating in the outdoor environment; required minimal cueing from SDI. John initiated bowling activity with independence. John did not demonstrate overt signs and symptoms (s/s) of distress when being exposed to loud noises from bowling pins, balls, and children laughing/yelling. John and wife were observed encouraging each other throughout session as evidenced by intermittently cheering, clapping and giving "high-fives." John's wife was noted to put her arm around him when sitting beside him. Both John and wife participated in conversational tasks with others. At the end, John reported that he enjoyed the session.

14.2.4.2 14 April 2014: Service Dog Note—Recreational Therapy

RT: John demonstrated bright affect and smiled while talking about his weekend–in particular the time spent at the collaborative nonprofit SDTTP organization's Puppy Center. John reported he is seriously considering training service dogs as a future employment. John and therapist discussed options for him to pursue service dog training opportunities post discharge, either through internship, employment, or both.

14.2.4.3 November 3–7, 2014 PT Accompanied SDI to a Concert Event in Times Square, NYC.

SDI: John independently navigated Times Square NYC, comfortably interacted with strangers, all while successfully handling Lundy. John demonstrated a significant improvement in symptoms and ability to reintegrate (see Figure on opening page).

14.2.4.4 18 April 2014—Discharge Summary

Psychiatric notes: John reports that he is better at conversing with people, and this only causes him minor anxiety now. John reports that he still has the tendency to isolate from people, but he is actively trying to overcome this habit. Currently, John reports that he is "hopeful and optimistic". He reports 0/10 for depression.

Neurological notes: John no longer has any complaints regarding his spoken communication (this is an improvement from previously). John's headache markedly improved.

Hospital Notes: John gained significant benefit from helping to train service dogs and worked well with the animal.

14.2.5 Concluding Remarks Excerpted from Patient Interview (12 December, 2014)

"My TBI rocked our family, but the lessons learned from teaching Lundy translated back to my home and personal life. I am able to talk and laugh. My kids have their Dad back and my wife and I are doing much better. When my teenage daughter challenges me, I am able to think it through more logically and not just lose it.

The brain games were good. They were challenging and I could see and track my progress, but they weren't real life applications. The OT, Speech, and other therapies were also good, but in the end, it was the dog training that helped me.

This program is special and it worked for me. I know there are so many other Wounded Warriors it can help. I saw that when Lundy came to spend the night with me on the ward. The guys on the ward liked having Lundy up there as much as I did. One guy really liked talking to him. The nurses later told me that this patient never talked.

I am about to retire from 20 years of military service and will be entering an internship to become a Service Dog Training Instructor."

14.3 Case History/Presentation (Bob)

ID: 34 y/o male, white, coast guard, lieutenant

Length of service: 15 Years

Military status: Active duty

Family Status: Married: 2000. Four sons ages: 12, 9, 8, and 6

Bob completed a number of stateside disaster missions with the coast guard including rescue and evacuation of victims during Hurricane Katrina. These missions required him to gain and maintain order while conducting dangerous rescue and retrieval operations. Bob reported having always thrived "off adrenaline." This fact was demonstrated by his desire to perform incredibly dangerous missions, take on increasingly challenging home front assignments, and risk his life while performing many high-risk leisure activities.

Alcohol became a social lubricant turning into a daily habit starting at a very young age. After sustaining knee and back injuries he also had easy access to narcotics. Bob recognized that he was on a very dangerous path but felt that he was in control and was still functioning at work so there was not really a problem. During this time he was hospitalized multiple times for Rhabdomyolysis or "Rhabdo": a life-threatening syndrome due to muscle injury. "Rhabdo" results from the death of muscle fibers and release of the contents into the bloodstream requiring immediate medical attention. His home front mission also changed from the adrenalin-producing ship duties to working in an office and going home to his wife and four young children every night. He was getting away with alcohol and drug dependence and no longer routinely risking his life onboard the ship. He started an extramarital affair, which was the final point of contention for his wife.

14.3.1 Diagnosis and Treatment

14.3.1.1 December, 2013

Voluntary admission to Walter Reed Psychiatric Inpatient for treatment/evaluation for depression, risky behavior, suicidal ideation, and alcohol and drug addiction. Bob has a history of deployment-related PTSD and marital discord.

14.3.1.2 January, 2014

Patient transferred to 6-week, Intensive Outpatient Program for Addiction Treatment Services. Begins participating in SDTTP.

14.3.1.3 May 8, 2014

Begins a course of OT for behavioral health—specifically to continue participation in SDTTP.

Bob is currently undergoing genetic testing to understand why he has frequent bouts of Rhabdomyolysis, excessive pitting edema in bilateral lower extremities, chronic fatigue, and reduced strength. Bob is currently participating in outpatient OT at WRNMMC.

14.3.1.4 SDTTP Clinical Notes from Service Dog Training Instructor and Occupational Therapist

14.3.1.5 December, 2013

Bob had been in WRNMMC inpatient psychiatric ward (7 W) for 2 weeks when he was invited to volunteer for a program to help train service dogs for wounded warriors as part of the SDTTP.

Bob: I have always loved and owned dogs and so was very happy to 'get a dog fix.' I like the idea of helping to train dogs for amputees and guys who need them. I felt the benefit of working with the dogs immediately. The positive energy generated during that first hour, left me feeling much better.

14.3.1.6 January, 2014

Bob transferred to intensive outpatient program for addiction treatment services and continued to partake in the training of Lundy (12-month-old golden retriever) during weekly group SDTTP sessions.

Bob: The SDI showed the group how to use positive and nurturing encouragement and praise to teach the dogs. It was not easy for me since I was depressed, but the SDI instructed us to fake the high-pitched, happy voice for the dog's sake. I had used harsher, heavy-handed training methods on my own dogs. However, seeing how well these young dogs responded to our supportive friendly efforts and enthusiastic praise was very impressive. So this has been a very refreshing and new way to learn how to train dogs. I called my wife and told her how great it was working with the dogs and how much I was looking forward to each session.

SDI: Bob participated in one-hour per week group service-dog training session for four weeks while in Addiction Treatment Services. He was very attentive and receptive to SDI instructions and worked appropriately with the dogs in training. Positive affect/high emotion praise was challenging for Bob but with coaching and demonstration, he was ultimately successful in feigning positive emotion to praise the dog in training.

14.3.1.7 June 2014

Patient enters outpatient OT program including one-on-one therapeutic service dog training sessions (Total of 5 h of SDTTP instructions).

OT: Bob was socially withdrawn and had a hard time making eye contact. Functional limitations from fatigue. Behavioral therapies had limited effect on his ability to cope with pressures on the home front. He is very concerned about his mental and physical wellbeing as well as the implications for his future and the future of his family. Bob reports sobriety × 150 days.

Bob: By the time I began my one-on-one training sessions, as part of out-patient OT, I was no longer faking my positive feelings when encouraging the dog's efforts. I had begun to get through my weeks, just looking forward to these sessions. The 'dog time' was carrying me through my weekend too.

For so long I had isolated myself. I dreaded the public and going anywhere near crowds. The first time I took Lundy on a public training session, I felt a sense of calm and empowerment with him at my side. By focusing on Lundy, I was able to see a path through crowds. It was as if Lundy parted it for me. That was when I first considered applying for a service dog for myself.

Alcohol was always a social lubricant that helped me talk to people and get to know them. The dog is now that social lubricant. It also takes the attention off me and directs it to the dog.

Training these young dogs is very challenging. I was easily frustrated. The SDI really helped me shift my attitude and use positive reinforcement methods to succeed with the dogs. Working with the dogs taught me patience and understanding of the dog's needs. I only wish I could have used these training methods while I was working with those under my command.

14.3.1.8 June 30, 2014

OT: Bob's wife said she was thrilled with the change in Bob she was seeing at home. She came to one of the training sessions so she could, "see how a dog could be creating so much change." She quietly joined SDI and Bob during their session. When they returned to my office after the session she was smiling from ear to ear. Later, when I spoke to her separately she commented on how amazing it was to see her husband so calm and collected, focusing on Lundy instead of everything else. This is the change she had been noticing around the house but did not understand what we were doing to make it happen.

Bob: In 2012, my wife and I were seeing a marriage counselor. My alcoholism, drug abuse, depression, risky behavior and infidelity had brought us to the brink of divorce.

Learning the skills of positive affect and praise in service dog training has helped me to experience empathy for my wife, my sons, others, and myself. Family members comment on how much more affectionate and present I am now.

The way that I used to parent was harsh—focusing on the negative consequences of behavior–'life is hard and you learn hard lessons.' That's how I was raised. Now, I engage my children in conversation and try to identify with their issues; helping them visualize what they can work towards. It's motivating– just like with the dogs. I am more connected with my family than I've ever been. My boys see the change and they are forgiving me for not being there for them in the past.

14.3.1.9 July 2014

Bob: Of the programs offered to me, some were good and others were a waste of time. The service dog training program was the best. Training a service dog for a Veteran is a huge service to provide. It gives me a tremendous sense of purpose and accomplishment. When you're working through an injury, finding a sense of purpose is really, really key to feeling successful. I know there are so many out there just like me—who can't ask for help, but could benefit from working with these dogs.

14.3.2 Outcomes

14.3.2.1 January 7, 2015

OT: Over the course of treatment in the OT program, Bob began to slowly make progress in his ability maintain a positive outlook, continued to maintain his sobriety and continues to make progress with his family. He has accepted that the physical challenges which once invigorated him are now debilitating and is accepting his more limited physical capacity. His relationship with his wife and children significantly improved when he started using the positive, encouraging, focused, behavior-shaping strategies of the SDTTP when relating to them. Bob benefited significantly from his involvement in the SDTTP.

Bob: "I have just completed my first year of sobriety. My depression has lifted and I feel connected to my family. I still struggle with pain and fatigue, but I feel much more positive. I am able to pace myself better and allow myself to take the time to rest and regain my emotional and physical strength. I am much more aware of what will trigger my arousal response and find that I can cope better when unexpected stressors occur. My frustration tolerance has significantly improved. My empathy and patience levels have also improved. I am better at setting healthy social boundaries and prioritizing time for my family. I'm really enjoying and committed to sharing my story and the healing lessons I've learned from the SDTTP with other Wounded Warriors. I am looking into pursuing a career as a Service Dog Instructor.

14.4 Concluding Remarks

Research has shown that the presence of animals in a psychological therapy setting can increase the willingness to enter into therapy, facilitate therapeutic alliance, reduce the rate of attrition, and reduce the symptoms of trauma [2–4]. Most recently, Hunt and Chizkov (2014) [5] showed that adults who recalled and wrote about trauma in the presence of dogs found the essay exercise less distressing and had significantly reduced symptoms of depression at follow-up than those who completed the writing exercise without a dog.

Over the last 20 years, there has been an increasing scientific awareness of the similarities between the neural, neurohormonal, and genetic mechanisms that regulate stress and social behaviors in all mammals. A growing body of evidence shows that the nurturing training methods, similar to those used in the SDTTP program provides positive sensory stimulation that can activate the antistress/pro-social brain network in both humans and dogs [6–10]. These findings illuminate how and why this service dog training program can be so emotionally and therapeutically powerful and emphasizes why therapy based on clinical theory and positive dog training skills can be effective at reducing the full range of symptoms in a condition as complex as PTSD [11–15].

Over the next several years, the collaborative nonprofit SDTTP organization—in partnership with researchers from the Uniformed Services University of Health Science, NICoE, WRNMMC, and the University of Maryland—will be testing this hypothesis in order to establish therapeutic service dog training as an evidence-based therapy for the reduction of symptoms of combat-related PTSD.

References

1. Yount RA, Lee MR, Olmert MD. Service dog training program for treatment of posttraumatic stress in service members, AMEDD, April-June, 2012; 63–9.
2. Beck AM, Seraydarian L, Hunter F. Use of animals in the rehabilitation of psychiatric patients. Psychol Rep. 1986;58:63–6.
3. Wilkes JK. The role of companion animals in counseling and psychology: discovering their use in the therapeutic process. Springfield: Charles C. Thomas; 2009.
4. Wesley MC, Minatrea NB, Watson JC. Animal-assisted therapy in the treatment of substance dependence. Anthrozoos. 2009;22(2):137–48.
5. Dietz TJ, Davis D, Pennings J. J Child Sex Abus. 2012;21(6):665–83. doi:10.1080/10538712.2012.726700.
6. Hunt MG, Chizkov RR. Are therapy dogs like Xanax? Does animal-assisted threapy impact processes relevant to cognitive behavioral psychotherapy? Anthrozoos, 2014;27(3):457–69.
7. Olmert MD. Made for each other, the biology of the human-animal bond. Cambridge: DaCapo Press; 2009.
8. Nuemann ID, Landgraf R. Balance of brain oxytocin and vasopressin: implications for anxiety, depression, and social behaviors. Trends in Neurosciences. 2012;(35)11:649–59.
9. Beetz A, Uvnas-Moberg K, Julius H, et al. Psychological and psychophysiological effects of human-animal interactions: the possible role of oxytocin. Front Psychol. 2012;3:234. doi:10.3389/fpsyg.2012.00234.
10. Olff M. Bonding after trauma: on the role of social support and the oxytocin system intraumatic stress. Eur J of Psycho-Traumatolog 2012;3:18597. doi:10.3402/ejpt.v3i0.18597.
11. Pitman RK, Orr SP, Lasko NB. Effects of intranasal vasopressin and oxytocin on physiologic responding during personal combat imagery in Vietnam veterans with posttraumatic stress disorder. Psychiatry Res. 1993;48(2):107–17.
12. Olff M, Langeland W, et al. A psychobiological rationale for oxytocin in the treatment of posttraumatic stress disorder. CNS Spctr. 2010;15(8):436–44.
13. Meyer-Lindenberg A, Domes G, et al. Oxytocin and vasopressin in the human brain: social neuropeptides for translational medicine. Nat Rev Neurosci. 2011;12:524–38. doi:10.1038/nrn3044.
14. Ayers LW, Missig G, et al. Oxytocin reduces background anxiety in a fear-potentiated startle-paradigm: peripheral vs central administration. Neuropsychopharmacolog. 2011;36:2488–97.
15. Eckstein M, Becker B, Scheele D, et al. Oxytocin facilitates the extinction of conditioned fear in humans. Soc Biol Psychiatr. 2014; doi:10.1016/j.biopsych.2014.10.015.

Part IV
Comorbidities

Trauma and Pain: Linking Emotional and Physical Symptoms

15

Genelle Weits

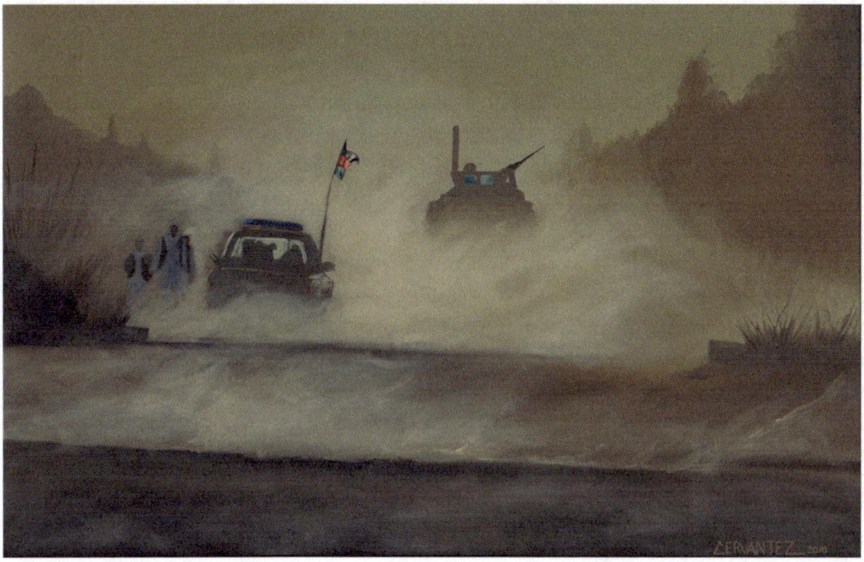

Dust Devils, by MSG Martin J. Cervantez, courtesy of the Army Art Collection, US Army Center of Military History.

Chronic pain is a common complaint in the retired military settings with veterans administration (VA) patients rating significantly worse pain than those in the general public [1]. The higher incidence of pain may be due to the heightened exposure to trauma and psychological stress [2]. The combination of pain and posttraumatic stress disorder (PTSD) creates greater self-reported pain and affective distress when

G. Weits (✉)
Behavioral Health Psychology Department, Navy Medical Center, San Diego, CA, USA
e-mail: Genelle.I.Weits.civ@mail.mil

E. C. Ritchie (ed.), *Posttraumatic Stress Disorder and Related Diseases in Combat Veterans*, DOI 10.1007/978-3-319-22985-0_15

compared to pain in patients without PTSD symptoms [3]. Indeed, childhood abuse has been associated with greater chronic pain in adulthood [4] with emotional neglect predicting lifetime trauma exposure over and above physical or sexual abuse [5]. Abuse is also positively correlated with anxiety, depression, somatic symptoms, and PTSD. Childhood emotional neglect may also predict later emergence of an inability to identify or express emotions (alexithymia) and somatization [6], with alexithymia a known risk factor for psychiatric and psychosomatic disorders.

Theories addressing the relationship of PTSD and pain have been proposed but not well researched. The mutual maintenance model [7] highlights various factors that may occur, including attentional biases with patients attending more to threatening or painful stimuli, pain as a reminder of the trauma events, and avoidance to minimize pain and disturbing thoughts.

The triple vulnerability model for PTSD [8] can also be applied to chronic pain. It asserts that life events and one's emotional reactions to the events are perceived as unpredictable and uncontrollable, leading to impairment. Additionally, development and attachment theories describe the effects of abuse and neglect on self-efficacy and trust.

It is imperative that both the physical and emotional conditions are addressed simultaneously. One such way is to educate patients on the ways that they maintain and exacerbate one another and to use strategies to minimize both the cognitive and behavioral avoidance that is observed so frequently in both conditions [9]. As patients begin to decrease avoidance and increase their participation in appropriate activities, their level of distress and disability may decrease, leading to an improved quality of life. However, the lack of healthy role models for emoting and the use of poor coping skills, such as the overuse of avoidance, are pivotal in maintaining impairments.

In this case study, the interplay between pain and trauma experiences will be exemplified, as well as the investigative process that is required to understand the connection.

15.1 Biopsychosocial Assessment

Cole is a 22-year-old, married, Caucasian, male corporal with approximately 3 years of continuous active duty in the US Marine Corp. He initially was on limited duty status for his pain and disability after fracturing his thoracic vertebral body (T12) and was eventually started on a Medical Evaluation Board for possible medical separation from the military. He worked in communication as a radio operator until his injury prevented him from performing his work tasks. He was referred to health psychology, a mental health specialty clinic, to aid with pain management and anxiety related to feelings of vulnerability due to his physical limitations.

Pearl Beginning the assessment with a focus on the pain symptoms and treatment experience portrays the belief that his pain is real. Validation is paramount to rapport building and successful therapy.

Cole was participating in CrossFit training at a public gym and was lifting 165 lbs. of weights when his hands slipped and the dumbbell fell on his right shoulder and neck. He tried to bring the weight above his head again, but he could not feel his extremities and subsequently fell to the floor. At that point, he blacked out for approximately 15 seconds and next recalled being in the hands of a trainer stabilizing his neck. He admitted that he did not want to go to the hospital, not wanting to "frighten my wife…and because of my pride." While applying ice, he lay on the gym floor for an hour. He then stood and drove home on his own, took a shower, and proceeded to bed. However, he soon felt as if he could not breathe and was gasping for air. He had his wife take him to the emergency department for immediate attention.

He received X-rays and a computed tomography (CT) scan, which confirmed he had fractured his T12 vertebra, and was given a torso brace and pain medications. Surgery was discussed and was not recommended. He received a prognosis that he would begin to feel better after 12 weeks. He was placed on convalescent leave and was required only to phone his command daily for accountability as he was unable to drive.

He initially wore a back brace that spanned from his pelvis to neck, creating difficulties with movements. He progressed to a smaller torso brace and over time used no support. However, his pain continued. He complained of constant throbbing in his mid-back and episodes of shooting pain down his left leg to the mid-shin, mainly felt when moving (such as walking). Sitting or standing for more than a few minutes would increase the pain. He was unable to complete many activities of daily living independently, including bathing and dressing his lower half, as he could not bend over.

His wife would aid him with these tasks; although when she was unavailable, he would struggle unsuccessfully. Due to his discomfort, he could not cook or clean as he could prior to the injury. Eventually, he avoided such tasks. The limitations brought on intense frustration, sometimes leading to anger or sadness and other times leading to anxiety about his future and ability to protect his wife.

He admitted sleeping with a knife next to his bed as he felt vulnerable and less able to protect himself and others without the aid of weapons. He agreed that although he did not fear for intruders prior to his injury, his physical limitations brought up feelings of vulnerability. Further, he felt worthless. Continuing to only have contact with his battalion via phone calls, he gained no sense of accomplishment from work. Rather, he felt he had no skills to offer.

He spent his days at his apartment complex, attempting to walk daily (100 yards) and otherwise staying indoors playing video games, watching movies, or reading. The latter activities caused little pain as his symptoms were lessened when lying flat on his back. These activities became monotonous and no longer offered him distraction. He did not emerge from his home unless required for appointments and socialization ceased. The only consistent contact with others included his wife, who was only home 1 day per week, and a peer from his battalion who he would see inconsistently; sometimes meeting every day and other times not speaking for months.

He presented to sessions with a slow and labored gait, getting up cautiously from his seat in the waiting room.

Pearl Gaining an understanding of the experience throughout the evolution of pain symptoms and dysfunction creates a holistic view of the person.

During sessions, he sat stiffly in the seat leaning to one side and changing positions throughout in attempts to ease his pain. He often did not show outward expressions of pain; however, with movements he would show subtle signs of discomfort.

Cole often felt down and hopeless about his future as he did not see significant improvements in his physical functioning. He had a sense of feeling disconnected to others and an overall numbness of emotions. He used to be quite social and outgoing but justified to the therapist that he was content with not having friends.

Cole reported an inability to relax due to the constant pain. He often reacted to his depressed and anxious feelings with self-blame and deprecation, feeling he had let himself and others down. He thought he was not fulfilling his role as a husband since it was likely he could not maintain a military career.

While he was hopeless, he denied any suicidal thoughts, plan, or intent, stating he lived for his wife and best friend. He reported significant fatigue, which he attributed to pain interfering with his sleep. He showed insight into the effect of worrisome thoughts on his sleep; however, he stated the concerns were only about his lessened ability to protect his wife at night. There was significant overlap in his symptoms between pain, depression, and anxiety, with fatigue, sleep difficulties, and poor concentration being symptoms of all three conditions.

Cole further mentioned a difficult incident during his first field operation training 3 years prior. He said that he and two peers were awoken with kicks and yelling and made to do manual labor as punishment for something they did not do. Post-trauma symptoms were denied, and thus that diagnosis was initially ruled out.

Pearl Chronic adjustment disorder can be a diagnostic consideration since the lifestyle changes and effects on military career evolve over time.

He endorsed symptoms consistent with depression and anxiety and was diagnosed with major depressive disorder, moderate, single episode.

15.2 Interventions

15.2.1 Initial Treatments and Responses

With a diagnosis of moderate clinical depression, the overarching treatment goals were to improve Cole's self-esteem and identity when faced with his current physical limitations. His depressive symptoms were understood to be in response to his changed physical status and limiting pain. He readily noted his frustration with his limitations. He focused on getting better quickly, pushing himself to walk a little further every day.

However, this resulted in flares of intense pain that would keep him from reaching his goal the following day, thus bringing on more frustration and hopelessness.

Efforts to improve his daily functioning and pain management were initiated. He was challenged to pace himself to his current ability level, adjusting his expectations for physical tasks. Pacing required acknowledging his limits and honoring them. Practicing self-awareness and listening to the body's signals were the skills he needed to learn. This process can take time, especially when one's identity is often tied to physical fitness [10].

Cole was focused on what he was no longer able to do, such as running, lifting weights, and getting out on his own. The new limitations to his physical functioning were explained in terms of grief and loss, with loss including his identity as an active, strong person. This identity was threatened since he was dependent on others for necessities, such as bathing, dressing, and driving. He loathed relying on his military command—not wanting others to see him in his "broken" state.

Taking time to grieve these losses validated his emotional reactions, such as sadness, anger, and jealousy of others' unchanged physical status. It was reframed that although some aspects of his identity had changed, there were still many parts of his identity that were the same. Defining in clear terms what he believed were important aspects of a husband, son, employee, and friend enabled him to see how he still fulfilled these roles. However, until he more fully accepted the reality of his situation, he could not progress in adjusting his identity to incorporate these changes in a healthy manner.

He often blamed himself for his shortcomings, and he needed constant reminding that he did not choose to have the injury and the subsequent difficulties. Adjusting Cole's expectations was one way to prevent feelings of worthlessness and failure. He said that he and his wife used to spend time together walking at the mall, and he predicted that his need for frequent breaks to sit down would frustrate his wife. He felt it would not be fun for her, so he stopped going altogether.

Pearl Including a loved one in the treatment plan offers support and accountability.

His wife was present at a session, and she said she would be happy to take breaks with him if it meant going out again. Further, she was comfortable going to a store without him while he rested. It appeared that his avoidance of past-enjoyed activities was due to concurrent poor communication and self-esteem. Once Cole discussed his concerns with his wife and modifications were problem-solved, he was more likely to follow through with the plan.

He was introduced to the idea of having a limited amount of resources per day now, and once that resource was used up, he would either be "borrowing" from the next day's resources or faced with the increased level of pain. He learned to make conscious decisions about what activities would be worthy of his precious resources for that day. In this way, he had choices, even if they were not ideal.

Cole had some insight into the mind–body connection, noticing he was more agitated and irritable when in pain. However, he did not yet show an understanding of the opposite relationship: negative emotions leading to increased pain symptoms.

Pearl The mind–body connection is best understood by eliciting examples from the patient, rather than the provider proving it to the patient.

Meditative practices were introduced as a way to elicit the relaxation response [11] to calm the physical reaction to emotional strain. Mindfulness meditation was specified as a way to increase awareness of the interconnections of body sensations, thoughts, and emotions [12]. This enabled Cole to observe his experiences and gain insight into his pain and mood. Further, this was modeled in sessions, asking Cole to focus on his bodily sensations whenever he discussed a troubling situation. In this way, he started to see how his thoughts and emotions could affect his physical symptoms.

After a substantial amount of time honoring his losses and exploring the effects of relaxation, he was asked to focus on his abilities more than the disabilities. Adjusting his expectations to meet his current functional level helped him have more realistic goals. He began to set attainable goals, such as increasing his exercise only once he maintained a certain level for a week without major flares. He also learned that comparing his current level of fitness to levels prior to his injury was unfair and led to disappointment and hopelessness. Over our time working together, he added water walking in his community pool as well as daily walks. Knowing he was actively doing something for his health every day, and adding more activities to his schedule, his self-esteem and mood improved—but only slightly.

Cole's motivation wavered as he noted few outward signs of progress. For a provider, slow progress can bring into question the usefulness of therapy. However, grief and loss issues and identity shifts take a considerable amount of time. Repetition of the aforementioned concepts and consistent trial and error practice to determine physical limitations for each day are required. This also necessitates an extreme amount of patience on the part of the patient and provider. Often, significant mood improvements are not seen for several months, especially if the patient is in denial of his or her changed abilities. While there may be improvements in physical functioning in the future, the treatment should be aimed at honoring current limits.

While it was understood that physical limitations inherently bring on feelings of vulnerability, the intensity of his anxiety regarding trust and safety appeared disproportionate to what he had discussed thus far.

Pearl A person with an abusive past is constantly, albeit mainly unconsciously, testing the provider to determine whether there is sufficient trust, understanding, and a genuine willingness to help.

After 2 months of weekly sessions, it was theorized that perhaps the impact of the military abuse was minimized.

He was asked to discuss the traumatic incident in more detail. He divulged vague information at first, but over time and with increasing trust, he detailed the incident more thoroughly.

In summary, the events played out as follows. Cole was suddenly awoken from his sleep with kicks to his face and chest from outside of his tent and shouts of insults and vulgarity. He and two peers were demanded to dress in full attire and proceed to their communications locker within minutes. They were reprimanded by two superiors for the poor organization of the locker; however, it was quickly clarified by the awakened that this was in fact not their locker. One superior apologized, asked them to go back to sleep, and began to leave. The other superior stated he was not yet done with them and embarked on hours of shouting insults and ordered them to repetitively reorganize and pack the locker of equipment. He created parameters for failure while they repeated these tasks throughout the night.

When the ordeal was apparently over, the superior made the remark "This isn't over," which proved to be true, according to Cole. The abusive superior remained in Cole's immediate chain of command for the next 3 years, and Cole described especially menial tasks being asked of them, even as they promoted. He was the target of ridicule and emotional abuse, leading Cole to "feel as if they were treating me like a 5 year old" and continuing to fear further punishments. The initial event was perceived as traumatic and he claimed intense fear, which did not decrease while being in close contact with that superior for the following 3 years.

A trauma treatment, cognitive processing therapy (CPT) [13], was begun with the belief that by addressing the trauma incident the symptoms would lessen or dissipate. Cole reported intense anxiety whenever he discussed the event, but with few outward signs of such distress. He would make little to no eye contact while recounting, became sweaty and flushed, and had some word production issues.

However, his mental dysfunction was significant. He described heightened anxiety reactions being in public, especially in close proximity to others, such as walking toward another person on a sidewalk. He would avoid stores or only attend late at night or early in the morning, to avoid being around others. He rarely slept at night, fearing intruders and hearing all noises as such. He kept a knife next to his bed and investigated sounds in his house throughout the night with great fear. He felt completely vulnerable with his physical limitations and feared he would be unable to fight off anyone with violent intentions.

CPT was continued with much resistance to sharing the details of the incident and often was vague with what was actually said or done. He further needed direct prompting to include his emotional reactions.

Cole strongly held the beliefs that others could not be trusted and he was always in danger. The treatment challenged these beliefs and increased awareness of his cognitive distortions, including all-or-nothing thinking extremes, overgeneralizing, catastrophizing, and personalizing. While Cole was learning to question his automatic thoughts and use reasoning and logic to aid in viewing the situations in a more balanced manner, he admitted that he still fully prescribed to these negative beliefs.

Pearl Trust your clinical intuition when events disclosed do not seem to match up with the emotional experience or level of impairment—there may be more to uncover.

When Cole would describe the trauma, he was asked to pay attention to any physical sensations. Along with increased heart rate and becoming sweaty, his back pain increased. Connecting the trauma to his physical status was enlightening for Cole.

He was able to see how his current status of physical vulnerability triggered memories of when he felt similarly vulnerable during the nighttime trauma and subsequent interactions with that superior. He was quoted saying, "If it was just [back] pain, I could handle it. It's all the other stuff that's making it worse."

He now understood the relationship of the mind and body, noticing increased pain when he discussed his upsetting military experiences. CPT brought to light the connections between his thoughts, emotions, and behaviors, highlighting his tendency to predict the situation as unsafe before looking at all the information. He could state logical challenges to his faulty beliefs; however, emotionally the strength of the distorted thoughts did not lessen. His unyielding beliefs were not budging with this therapy. While he met criteria for PTSD, it was not clearly understood why he was having such a subjectively intense reaction. Thus, the CPT protocol was discontinued after nine sessions for further exploration of his past.

15.2.2 Exploration of the Past

Over multiple sessions, childhood experiences were explored with curiosity, rather than with an attitude of trying to find something to account for his symptoms. Relationships with his parents, school events, and childhood and adolescence experiences were discussed. Bits and pieces were offered throughout sessions and over time the following discoveries were made that aided in understanding the events that led to his current symptom cluster.

Pearl When recent events do not seem to account for the current impairments, delve into the remote past.

Cole grew up in poverty in a factory town. His parents worked overlapping shifts and often took on additional shifts for income. Cole described living in a house with meager standards, including a kitchen lacking an interior ceiling as it had been overcome by mold. Cole described the neighbors as "immature" since children were poorly supervised by parents, who would drink excessively amidst nightly loud and raucous parties (breaking bottles, yelling, cursing, and fights breaking out).

Cole's father drank excessively as well and his parents' marriage faltered with the home feeling "tense." He was sent to live at his maternal grandparents' home in the country from 1st to 4th grade while his parents "figured things out." After his father's third offense of driving under the influence, his license was revoked, and he was sent to jail for a period of time, during which his mother came to live with Cole too. Although his grandparents were older and there were not many activities planned, he felt safe and included in their lives. They would watch the Grand 'Ol Opry on television nightly and eat supper as a family. He fondly recalled the comfort he felt knowing these activities were a consistent occurrence.

When he returned to his previous home, he yearned for time together with his parents, yet they only spent time with Cole if he joined them for grocery shopping or other errands. The structure he enjoyed at his grandparents' home was also absent since his parents would sleep during the days and they rarely ate meals together. Since his father's license was revoked, Cole often was awakened late in the night to accompany them for the drive to his father's work, so as not to stay home alone.

When Cole turned 15 and earned a driver's permit, he was placed in charge of driving his father to work at night. He described nights when there was a snow or ice storm and he would voice his discomfort in driving in such conditions; however, his father scoffed at his fears and demanded he drive him to work. Cole recalled feeling resentful and angry at this role he was required to fill. Although this was the only time Cole spent with his father, they rarely spoke.

Cole spent the majority of his time outside of school at a friend's home, where the parents "were involved" by being present in the evenings and "eating supper together." He often ran home around dinnertime in hopes that his parents may be awake to eat with him, but he found them asleep or away and would disappointedly return back to his friend's home.

Themes of desiring parental attention and disappointment in not receiving it were found throughout his development. He earned high grades and his parents would not remark on them. He was on the football team, and although they would attend some games, they showed no outward emotions when he looked at them in the stands after a good play. He responded by going to extremes to gain attention or praise. After football games, he would remain alone at the field for hours continuing to train, often resulting in exhaustion and vomiting due to the physical strain.

He felt a strong need to be "better," believing he was not good enough; otherwise, he would have earned some recognition. This transformed his self-view to one of personal deficiency that he strived to improve. He believed that he needed strength and skills to avoid living in poverty. This became a major theme in sessions since he now found himself less physically strong, bringing up concerns that he would be unable to provide for or protect his family.

Cole used to interpret his parents' lack of interaction with him as proof they did not care. As an adult, he viewed their dogged focus on work as a means to provide him with shelter, food, and clothing. In turn, he felt these were the essentials for living and little more was required. He relied on himself and trusted few others, learning that even parents would not be available for his needs. However, it was palpable in sessions that he felt great disappointment that he had not been cared for in other ways. This was interpreted as emotional neglect, and Cole stated he felt abandoned. Emotionally distant parents and unstable environments can have a strong impact on the development of self.

Abandonment was felt in many of his life experiences, including being taken to live at his grandparents' home for years and the lack of consistent contact with his parents. Additionally, his extended family ceased contact with him after his mother and her siblings had a falling out. He then expected the military to care for him, believing in the brotherhood and how they would not hurt their own. After being abused by a leader, he felt abandoned by the military as a whole.

Since Cole did not have examples of positive regard by others, he would assume neutrality if nothing blatantly negative was stated. Without clear positive or negative feedback, he extrapolated how others felt. While miniscule expressions offered him a feeling of positive regard, similarly minute details led to negative appraisals, triggering low self-worth and mistrust of others.

Cole voiced his desire for more open communication and expression of emotions with his parents, wife, and friend. Yet he feared negative reactions, risking further abandonment. Identity issues resurfaced as he strived to preserve how his wife historically viewed him. He was ashamed of his emotions and believed that she would rebuke this "weaker" man.

In sessions, although he reported feeling anxious, angry, or sad, he presented flat. Even with humor, he showed a partial smile and faintly let out one whispered laugh, although sharing how it was "very funny." Besides having no role models or practice in expressing emotions, he admitted purposely hiding his emotional reactions. He did not want to offer others insight into his internal experience, leaving him vulnerable to rejection. With therapy, he challenged the utility of keeping his emotions to himself and set goals of more honest communication with trusted others.

Cole's past exemplified the chaotic and unpredictable events in his life, which harken to the more recent unexpected events in the military. The lack of control felt in the childhood and military events was triggered once his physical abilities were drastically changed. It was this combination that threatened his sense of independence and control.

Since he could not physically defend himself as he used to, he tried to prevent catastrophes from occurring. This proved to be an overwhelming responsibility in public settings; thus, he avoided leaving his home. He continued to have severe anxiety that negative deeds could befall him at any moment, internalizing the words of his superior: "This isn't over." He often had nightmares of home intruders killing his friend and threatening the lives of others, leaving him panicked and hypervigilant. His fear of violence was unwavering. He projected his need for protection throughout his own life onto his wife, needing to keep her safe.

Pearl It can be frustrating when progress seems to have ceased. Remember that outward change can be slow and the therapist may not witness the positive effects of therapy.

15.3 Future Treatment: To Be Continued

Unfortunately, therapy with Cole terminated before relief from his PTSD symptoms was attained. He medically retired from the military and subsequently moved out of the area to be near family. His continued guardedness regarding emoting and disclosing inner experiences to others maintained his fears and low self-esteem. He expressed frustration with the slow progress and often did not see the relevance of the improvements highlighted. He wanted to trust the process, but admitted that he felt "awkward" attempting the assignments. He was praised for trying, noting he would not improve without acting outside of his comfort zone.

The exploration of the past and linking it to his current beliefs offered him a greater understanding of the origins and past utility of his behaviors. He more fully believed in the importance of opening up to others with genuine emotional expression, even if he was not consistently practicing it. He saw the value in supportive others and realized that communication was a necessary step to create trusting relationships. His wife's pregnancy motivated him to change, rather than only providing the basics for survival, as he was raised.

Cole looked forward to teaching his child about praise and disappointment, communicating both clearly, rather than his child relying on interpretations, which he now knew could be harmful. He was able to express his own disappointment at the lack of comfort offered by his parents and connect these experiences with his current inability to allow others to care for him. He began showing more outward emotions in sessions. His willingness to make these changes was a testament to his trust in the therapist. This supportive relationship boosted his confidence, enabling him to make more extreme changes, such as remaining in the moment instead of impulsively reacting to his anxious thoughts.

With chronic pain, he will continually be adjusting his expectations and modifying activities to meet his needs. Cole no longer expressed desperation to find a fix for his pain. He accepted his physical status and attempted to move forward despite it. He left therapy with an enhanced sense of control over his future. His self-confidence soared as he felt supported and encouraged by his wife's parents. He tried not to let physical status and fears of failure limit his dreams.

15.4 Final Remarks

Treatment of persons with complicated and lengthy trauma histories in combination with pain issues will not likely show great improvements in short-term outpatient mental health military settings. The rapport and stability required for such work often is not available; thus, the patient may never feel secure enough to disclose pertinent information. As a consequence, the façade remains and symptoms continue or worsen over time. By offering a safe environment for honest expression, the foundation for positive therapeutic interactions is laid, leading to greater potential for future disclosure.

As shown in this case, several months of intensive work did not show gains appreciable to the patient. However, to the skilled eye of a therapist, many gains were made. The healthy shifts in beliefs about himself and others and the importance of human emotions were important foundational goals to foster positive relations. Cole's journey to improved health will continue via self-exploration. CPT, an evidence-based therapy, was not apparently helpful at the time it was introduced. The necessary step of challenging his beliefs and then taking action are predicted to be more successful now that Cole has internalized the therapist's positive regard and support, helping him trust in himself again.

References

1. Kazis L, Ren X, Lee A, Skinner K, Rogers W, Clark J, Miller DR. Health status in VA patients: results from the Veterans health study. Am J Med Qual. 1999;14(1):28–38.
2. Arnstein P, Cadill M, Mandle C, Norris A, Beasley R. Self-efficacy as a mediator of the relationship between pain intensity, disability and depression in chronic pain patients. Pain. 1999;80:483–91.
3. Geisser ME, Roth RS, Bachman JE, Eckert TA. The relationship between symptoms of Posttraumatic stress disorder and pain, affective disturbance and disability among patients with accident and non-accident related pain. Pain. 1996;66:207–14.
4. Davis DA, Luecken LJ, Zautra AJ. Are reports of childhood abuse related to the experience of chronic pain in adulthood? A meta-analytic review of the literature. Clin J Pain. 2005;21(5):398–405.
5. Spertus IL, Yehuda R, Wong CM, Halligan S, Seremetis SV. Childhood emotional abuse and neglect as predictors of psychological and physical symptoms in women presenting to a primary care practice. Child Abuse Negl. 2003;27:1247–58.
6. Güleç MY, Altinaş M, İnanç L, Bezgin ÇH, Koca EK, Güleç H. Effects of childhood trauma on somatization in major depressive disorder: the role of alexithymia. J Affect Disord. 2013;146:137–41.
7. Sharp TJ, Harvey AG. Chronic pain and posttraumatic stress disorder: mutual maintenance? Clin Psychol Rev. 2001;21:857–77.
8. Keane TM, Barlow DH. Posttraumatic stress disorder. In: Barlow DH, editor. Anxiety and its disorders. New York: Guilford; 2002. pp. 418–53.
9. Otis JD, Keane TM, Kerns RD. An examination of the relationship between chronic pain and Posttraumatic stress disorder. J Rehabil Res Dev. 2003;40(5):397–406.
10. Harris S, Morley S, Barton SB. Role loss and emotional adjustment in chronic pain. Pain. 2003;105(1–2):363–70.
11. Benson H. The relaxation response. In: Goleman D, Gurin J, editors. Mind/Body medicine. Yonkers: Consumer Reports Books; 1993. pp. 233–57.
12. Kabat-Zinn J, Lipworth L, Burney R. The clinical use of mindfulness meditation for the self-regulation of chronic pain. J Behav Med. 1985;8(2):163–90.
13. Monson CM, Schnurr PP, Resick PA, Friedman MJ, Young-Xu Y, Stevens SP. Cognitive processing therapy for veterans with military-related posttraumatic stress disorder. J Consult Clin Psychol. 2006;74:898–907.

The Multifactorial Approach to PTSD in the Active Duty Military Population

16

Rita Richardson, William D. Rumbaugh and Hanna Zembrzuska

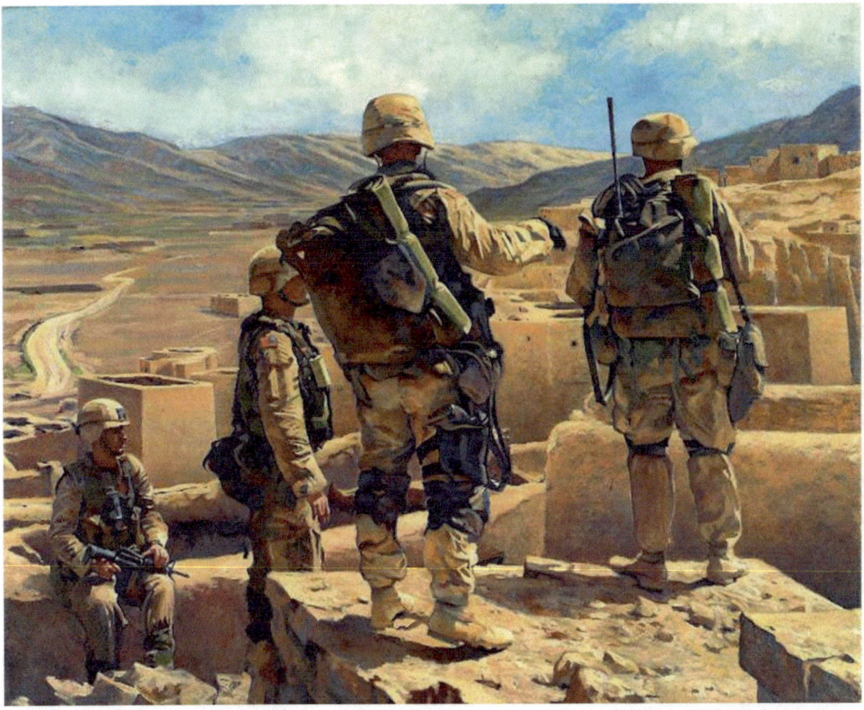

Hizara Province, by SFC Elzie Golden, courtesy of the Army Art Collection, US Army Center of Military History

W. D. Rumbaugh (✉) · R. Richardson · H. Zembrzuska
National Capital Consortium, Walter Reed National Military Medical Center Bethesda, Bethesda, MD, USA
e-mail: william.d.rumbaugh.mil@mail.mil

E. C. Ritchie (ed.), *Posttraumatic Stress Disorder and Related Diseases in Combat Veterans,* DOI 10.1007/978-3-319-22985-0_16

16.1 Case Presentation

A biopsychosocial approach is required when treating the active duty service member or veteran with posttraumatic stress disorder (PTSD) due to the complex integration of medical and psychological elements with ever-evolving social dynamics. Additionally, there are military-specific issues (administrative, cultural, etc.) that must be considered for comprehensive treatment for the active duty military population.

A 35-year-old female, active duty enlisted soldier, with history significant for alcohol use disorder, PTSD, and chronic low back pain, presents to outpatient adult behavioral health clinic complaining of depressed mood, chronic nightmares, with worsening hyperarousal and avoidance behaviors. Her military service is significant for a history of two deployments as a mechanic during Operation Iraqi Freedom and Operation Enduring Freedom (OIF/OEF) which were noted for involvement in three separate improvised explosive device (IED) blasts, one during a convoy movement resulting in vehicle rollover and death of all other service members in her vehicle. The patient was diagnosed with PTSD after her second deployment and experienced a significant escalation in symptoms over the 2 years following the deployment including hyperarousal and nightmares. The patient reported heavy alcohol consumption to assist with insomnia secondary to nightmares and hyperarousal as well as her chronic back pain. Additionally, escalation in symptoms in conjunction with increased alcohol use led to marital discord which culminated in divorce. A few weeks after the divorce was finalized, she became increasingly depressed with new onset suicidal ideation resulting in inpatient psychiatric admission at a civilian hospital. While hospitalized she was started on sertraline for mood and PTSD symptoms in addition to quetiapine for insomnia resulting in significant weight gain. Two weeks following initiation, sertraline was discontinued secondary to significant nausea and patient was transitioned to escitalopram. During admission, providers continued her outpatient opiate regimen for chronic low back pain. The patient was discharged from the hospital after 2 months with plan to continue quetiapine and escitalopram and scheduled for follow-up with a civilian outpatient psychiatrist; however, the patient self-discontinued all medications except for opiates and did not attend the follow-up appointment. Approximately 1 month after discharge, she presented to her military primary care physician for continued PTSD symptoms and low back pain. After evaluation, her primary care provider recommended initiation of Medical Evaluation Board (MEB) for the purpose of medical retirement from the military.

16.2 Assessment and Diagnosis

This patient represents a common, multifactorial presentation of service members with combat-related PTSD with comorbid physical conditions, such as chronic pain. Psychologically, she is experiencing extreme survivor's guilt regarding the IED blast during her second deployment. Biologically, she continues to struggle with opiate dependency for management of chronic pain as well as heavy alcohol use. Socially, her marriage ended in divorce, resulting in a limited support network. The problem list is lengthy and could include anxiety, depression, alcohol use disorder, opiate use disorder vs. physiological dependence for the purpose of pain control; however, the unifying diagnosis is PTSD.

Notable changes to the diagnostic criteria for PTSD were made for the DSM-5 as compared to the DSM-IV-TR. Per DSM-IV-TR, the individual needs to react with horror to the traumatic event; however, the military population is trained to maintain composure when faced with a potentially traumatic event (Table 16.1). The DSM-5 removes the requirement of reacting with horror. The symptom triad of reexperiencing, avoidance, and hyperarousal has been expanded to include an additional requirement of negative alteration of mood, such as depression, anger, or irritability [1, 2].

Table 16.1 Comparison of DSM-IV-TR and DSM-5 criteria for PTSD

DSM-IV-TR	DSM-5
Criterion A: exposure	Criterion A: exposure
First-hand exposure to trauma	First- *OR* repeated/extreme second-hand exposure
Reacting with horror, fear, helplessness	*NO* requirement of reacting with horror
Criterion B: reexperiencing	Criterion B: *intrusion* symptoms
Recollections, intrusive thoughts	Intrusive memories
Dreams	Dreams
Flashbacks	Dissociative reactions
Criterion C: avoidance	Criterion C: avoidance
Avoiding thoughts, activities reminding of trauma	Avoiding emotions/thoughts
Diminished interest/participation in significant activities	Avoiding external reminders of trauma
Inability to recall aspects of trauma	
Criterion D: hyperarousal	Criterion D: *negative alteration of cognition and mood*
Sleep difficulty	Inability to recall aspects of trauma
Irritability	Negative beliefs about oneself, others, or the world
Hypervigilance	Negative emotional state
	Diminished interest/participation in significant activities
	Inability to experience positive emotions
	Criterion E: hyperarousal
	Sleep disturbance
	Irritability
	Hypervigilance

PTSD remains a clinical diagnosis, though multiple assessment tools may be helpful in screening and tracking progression of treatment. The PTSD checklist (PCL) has a military-specific version (PCL-M) for combat-associated PTSD that consists of 17 questions answered by patient self-report [3]. The Department of Veterans Affairs (VA) and Department of Defense (DoD) have now adopted the PCL-5 for screening purposes. Given the push for more objective measures of patient progress in clinical practice, these tools can be helpful in tracking a patient's response to treatment.

Initial psychiatric evaluations must include a safety assessment which is of noted importance in the military population, where the rate of suicide is higher than the general population [4]. Many service members and veterans own firearms, a known risk factor for suicide [5]. Counter to popular belief, a recent publication noted no association between deployment and suicide rate. Increased suicide risk was associated with early separation from the military (<4 years) and other-than-honorable discharge from military service [6].

There are inherent challenges in developing rapport between the civilian provider and a military patient due to perceived cultural differences and possible language barriers with regard to military jargon. Examples include the numerous acronyms used in the various services and military slang to refer to individuals, weapons, etc. Identifying these barriers and differences early in the treatment process can aid in developing rapport, potentially leading to improved outcomes [7]. Possible strategies include providers familiarizing themselves with acronyms and military slang specific for their patient's branch of service as well as open dialogue acknowledging the provider's deficits regarding military culture.

16.3 Treatment/Management

Significant advancements have been made in the understanding of PTSD pathology and treatment since the beginning of the Global War on Terror, including structured practice guidelines for both military and civilian mental health providers, such as the VA/DoD clinical practice guideline on management of posttraumatic stress published in 2010 [8]. The current first-line medications for PTSD include selective serotonin reuptake inhibitors (SSRIs) and serotonin-norepinephrine reuptake inhibitors (SNRIs) with specifically sertraline having evidence of best long-term efficacy [9, 10]. Sertraline and paroxetine have both received Food and Drug Administration (FDA) approval for treatment of PTSD. Fluoxetine has shown mixed evidence for efficacy in randomized trials and to date has not received FDA approval, specifically for PTSD. The patient in the above case was initially treated with sertraline; however, due to provider preference, the patient was transitioned to escitalopram after experiencing intolerable side effects. An alternative treatment method would be transition to paroxetine, another SSRI specifically FDA approved for PTSD, or transition to venlafaxine, an SNRI, all of which are considered to be first-line according to VA/DoD guidelines.

The case demonstrates a common practice of utilizing the sedation effect of quetiapine for treatment of insomnia. Quetiapine for insomnia is an off-label but commonly utilized regimen; current evidence, including VA/DoD guidelines, note second-generation antipsychotics such as quetiapine have unknown benefit in treatment of PTSD. Of note, mirtazapine has been shown to have some benefit in the treatment of PTSD and has a common side effect of sedation which can be utilized for management of insomnia with nightly dosing. Numerous studies have demonstrated that prazosin can benefit PTSD-associated insomnia and nightmares, leading many to consider it first-line treatment [11–13]. Additionally, recent evidence illustrates prazosin may help mitigate hyperarousal symptoms and improve global functioning, but this requires twice a day dosing due to its relatively short half-life [14].

Benzodiazepines are no longer considered to have a place in the treatment of PTSD [15]. Not only is there little evidence for their effectiveness, but mounting evidence demonstrates benzodiazepines are harmful to patients including the potential of interference with the extinction of fear [16]. Per current VA/DoD guidelines for PTSD treatment, benzodiazepines have no benefit at any phase of PTSD treatment and may cause harm. Another concern is the high abuse potential of benzodiazepines. Once started, benzodiazepines can be extremely difficult to discontinue [17]. Similar to the effects of alcohol, benzodiazepines can lead to disinhibition in an already volatile patient population. The rates of comorbid substance use disorders may be as high as 40–50% in veterans. In addition, non-benzodiazepine hypnotics, including zolpidem and eszopiclone, may induce more vivid nightmares and the dissociative effects may potentiate dissociative component of PTSD. For these reasons, benzodiazepines and non-benzodiazepine hypnotics should be avoided [8, 18].

The VA/DoD guidelines also mention multiple psychotherapy modalities useful in treatment of PTSD, including exposure-based therapies, cognitive-based therapies, stress inoculation therapy, and eye movement desensitization and reprocessing. Similar to treatment recommendations for depressive disorders, mild to moderate PTSD patients could be managed via monotherapy of either medication or psychotherapy; however, any complicated PTSD patient, such as those with comorbid psychiatric conditions and/or chronic pain syndromes, may require a dual treatment approach utilizing both medications and one or more psychotherapy modalities. In addition, complicated PTSD patients may benefit from referral to specialized care centers, such as dual-diagnosis mental health facilities [8]. These therapies are addressed in other chapters of this book.

16.4 Military-Specific Administrative Issues

Numerous administrative considerations must be accounted for when treating an active duty service member whose job is to defend our nation and, if necessary, go to war [7]. Medications can profoundly impact a service member's ability to serve in the military. For example, medications that may lead to significant impairment (e.g., benzodiazepines) can affect a service member's judgment and reaction time. Medications that lead to significant weight gain (e.g., second-generation antipsychotics) can create problems in maintaining height/weight and physical fitness standards. Other medications (e.g., lithium) can limit the service member's ability to deploy to an "austere environment," and if a service member becomes non-deployable, his or her continued military service may be put in jeopardy. For the civilian provider who is unfamiliar with military regulations and policies, it may be helpful to discuss treatment planning with a military health-care provider. Another resource available to providers is the Defense Health Agency Pharmacy Operations Division, which is responsible for the policies covering medications available in theater (the CENTCOM pharmacy) and medications limiting deployment or other active duty engagements (MOD-12) [19].

Acting as a liaison between the service member and their command is another important consideration when initiating a treatment. If the condition itself is severe enough to impact the service member's ability to perform their duties, the command has a right to know for the safety of the service member and unit. Certain patients will require a restriction of access to firearms, and others operating complex machinery may become impaired when given certain medications. This can lead to the loss of expensive equipment, but more importantly, the unnecessary loss of human lives. If the service member is to deploy in the future, their illness must be stable and they must be without medication changes for 90 days prior to deployment or transfer to another military installation [19].

Finally, a service member struggling with addiction issues may require a mandatory referral to an addiction treatment program, such as the Army Substance Abuse Program (ASAP). If referred to ASAP, the service member will undergo an addiction-specific evaluation, followed by determination of appropriate level of further care, if any, required. ASAP can be especially helpful for service members with comorbid pain and addiction issues as the service member's treatment plan will include a dialogue between the pain management team and the addiction management team in order to provide the service member with a patient-centered approach to recovery. While programs such as ASAP are helpful tools for the patient and provider, patients with comorbid PTSD and substance use disorders may require higher level of care, such as admission to a dual-diagnosis unit which specializes in a holistic approach including comprehensive management of all comorbid conditions [8, 18].

16.5 Conclusion: Pearls and Pitfalls

- Service members with combat-related PTSD commonly present with multiple comorbidities such as chronic pain and substance use disorders.
- First-line treatment includes SSRIs and SNRIs with sertraline showing best evidence for long-term efficacy.
- Prazosin has demonstrated efficacy for treatment of PTSD-associated sleep disturbances and nightmares and treatment of severe hyperarousal symptoms when given twice a day.
- Benzodiazepines and other hypnotics should be avoided as they have been shown to cause harm.
- Antipsychotics have implications for height/weight and fitness standards and have unknown benefit for treatment of PTSD.

- Administrative policies unique to the military may impact the service members to continue on active duty status, thus providers must maintain open communication with service member's command.
- VA/DoD guidelines recommend utilization of dual-diagnosis programs for service members with comorbid PTSD and substance use disorders.

References

1. American Psychiatric Association. Diagnostic and statistical manual of mental disorders. 4th ed., text rev. Washington, DC: American Psychiatric Association; 2000
2. American Psychiatric Association. Diagnostic and statistical manual of mental disorders. 5th ed. Washington, DC: American Psychiatric Association; 2014
3. Wilkins KC, Lang AJ, Norman SB. Synthesis of the psychometric properties of the PTSD checklist (PCL) military, civilian, and specific versions. Depress Anxiety. 2011;28:596–606.
4. Martin J, Ghahramanlou-Holloway M, Lou K, Tucciarone P. A comparative review of U.S. Military and civilian suicide behavior: implications for OEF/OIF suicide prevention efforts. J Ment Health Couns. 2009;31(2):101–18.
5. Kellermann AL, Rivara FP, Somes G, et al. Suicide in the home in relation to gun ownership. N Engl J Med. 1992;327(7):467–72.
6. Reger MA, et al. Risk of suicide among US military service members following operation enduring freedom or operation Iraqi freedom deployment and separation from the US military. JAMA Psychiatry. 2015. doi:10.1001/jamapsychiatry.2014.3195.
7. Rice TR, Sher L. Suicidal behavior in war veterans. Expert Rev Neurother. 2012;12:611–24.
8. Department of Veterans Affairs, Department of Defense. VA/DoD clinical practice guideline for the management of Posttraumatic stress. Washington, DC: VA/DoD; 2010.
9. Rapaport MH, Endicott J, Clary CM. Posttraumatic stress disorder and quality of life: results across 64 weeks of sertraline treatment. J Clin Psychiatry. 2002;63:59–65.
10. Londborg PD, Hegel MT, Goldstein S, et al. Sertraline treatment of posttraumatic stress disorder: results of 24 weeks of open-label continuation treatment. J Clin Psychiatry. 2001;62:325–31.
11. Kung S, Espinel Z, Lapid MI. Treatment of nightmares with prazosin: a systematic review. Mayo Clinic Proc. 2012;87:890–900.
12. Raskind MA, Peskind ER, Kanter ED, et al. Reduction of nightmares and other PTSD symptoms in combat veterans by prazosin: a placebo-controlled study. Am J Psychiatry. 2003;160:371–3.
13. Raskind MA, Peskind ER, Hoff DJ, et al. A parallel group placebo controlled study of prazosin for trauma nightmares and sleep disturbance in combat veterans with Posttraumatic stress disorder. Biol Psychiatry. 2007;61:928–34.
14. Raskind MA, Peterson K, Williams T, et al. A trial of prazosin for combat trauma PTSD with nightmares in active-duty soldiers returned from Iraq and Afghanistan. Am J Psychiatry. 2013;170(9):1003–10.
15. Viola J, Ditzler T, Batzer W, et al. Pharmacological management of Posttraumatic stress disorder: clinical summary of a five-year retrospective study, 1990–1995. Mil Med. 1997;162:616–9.
16. Hart G, Panayi MC, Harris JA, Westbrook RF. Benzodiazepine treatment can impair or spare extinction, depending on when it is given. Behav Res Ther. 2014;56:22–9.
17. Kosten TR, Fontana A, Sernyak MJ, Rosenheck R. Benzodiazepine use in posttraumatic stress disorder among veterans with substance abuse. J Nerv Ment Dis. 2000;188:454–9.
18. Department of Veterans Affairs, Department of Defense. VA/DoD clinical practice guideline for the management of substance use disorders. Washington, DC: VA/DoD; 2009.
19. Defense Health Agency Pharmacy Operations Division. Pharmacy operations division. http://www.health.mil/About-MHS/Defense-Health-Agency/Healthcare-Operations/Pharmacy-Division. 2015. Accessed: 20. Dec. 2014.

17 Comorbid PTSD, Bipolar I, and Substance Use Disorder

Rachel Sullivan

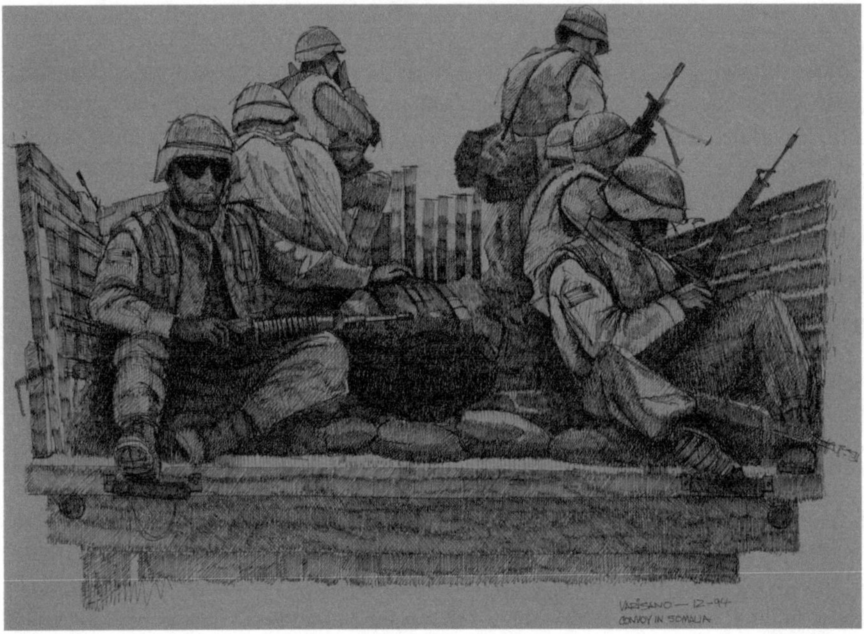

Convoy in Somalia, by Peter Varisano, courtesy of the Army Art Collection, US Army Center of Military History.

On its own, posttraumatic stress disorder (PTSD) is a devastating disorder. However, it is not always seen as the sole diagnosis: the most challenging PTSD patients are often the ones whose symptoms do not fit neatly into one diagnosis, but in-

R. Sullivan (✉)
Child and Family Behavioral Health System, Department of Behavioral Health, Madigan Army Medical Center, 9040 Jackson Ave., Tacoma, WA, 98431, USA
e-mail: rmr.sullivan@us.army.mil

E. C. Ritchie (ed.), *Posttraumatic Stress Disorder and Related Diseases in Combat Veterans,* DOI 10.1007/978-3-319-22985-0_17

stead present with symptoms that span multiple diagnostic categories. In particular, the constellation of PTSD, bipolar I disorder, and substance use disorder creates a daunting challenge, as each diagnosis brings with it a set of symptoms that interfere with treatment of the others, and the synergies between co-occurring disorders yield a result far more complex than just a sum of the component disorders' symptoms.

For example, PTSD is typified by avoidance, which reinforces the desire to use substances for escape. The same avoidance can lead to the patient's noncompliance with their treatment plan for bipolar I disorder. Also, bipolar I disorder can take the paranoia and reexperiencing seen in PTSD and bring it to the level of true psychosis, making these symptoms more real and terrifying to the person reexperiencing his trauma. In addition, substance use in PTSD can blunt the ability to participate in psychotherapies requiring higher-level cognition, such as exposure therapy, and may even reinforce the disordered brain chemistry that medications prescribed for bipolar I disorder attempt to correct [1]. Finally, all three can interfere with sleep, which is often one of the most important symptoms to manage in the pursuit of recovery.

The following two examples will explore these issues in case format, and were created with compiled details from multiple active duty patients treated by the author. It will discuss the risks of polypharmacy, additional areas of caution for medication management, and the consideration of somatic and complementary treatments. It will also discuss the goals of an appropriate treatment plan and the prognostic indicators for the patient suffering from all three disorders.

17.1 Case 1

17.1.1 Case Presentation/History

17.1.1.1 Identifying Information

SPC Jones is a 43-year-old married Caucasian male diagnosed with PTSD, bipolar I disorder, and alcohol use disorder, severe. He is an activated US Army National Guard reservist, and completed a 9-month deployment to Operation Iraqi Freedom 6 months ago. As will be described below, he had significant exposure to death and combat during this deployment. He is a combat support specialist (31B) with 4 years' time in service. When not activated, he works as a commercial building inspector for his home state.

He was referred to the clinic for medical management after having been stabilized in the inpatient unit for a manic episode with psychosis. He has gone back and forth between hospitalizations and the partial hospitalization program over the past 6 months, with sometimes less than 24 h between admissions.

A chart review reveals that he also showed hypomanic and depressive symptoms during his deployment, though the deployed behavioral health assets were able to help him remain in theater and avoid early return. Psychiatric testing done by the partial hospitalization team confirmed these diagnoses.

17.1.1.2 History of Present Illness

SPC Jones arrived on time for his initial appointment, but took 20 min longer than average to fill out the clinic paperwork. When he finally finished, it was incomplete and confusingly written, with arrows and extrapolations filling the blank sides of the form for some questions, while others were left blank. He appeared hypomanic with pressured, barely interruptible speech, flights of ideas, psychomotor agitation, and frequent tangents.

He had some insight into his current state however, saying, "This is nothing Doc, usually I'm at a 10/10, but today I'm just a 7!" When asked to explain what that means he reported that he always feels "keyed up" and cannot relax. He was entertaining in his long-winded and tangential stories, but very difficult to interview. He also interrupted to mention that his main agenda today is to convince the provider to increase his lithium in the hopes that this might help him "chill out." After reviewing his recent lithium blood level of 1.1 and providing education on therapeutic range and toxicity risks, he agreed to not take more than prescribed. He denied recent depressive symptoms, though he has gone through severe depressive episodes in the past.

When asked, he reported that he sleeps "okay." However, when pressed for more detail he admitted that his roommates in the barracks have complained that he screams, yells, cries, and kicks the walls at night. He does not remember these episodes now that he is taking risperidone and quetiapine fumarate every evening, but he sometimes wakes up feeling sore.

He first began drinking at age 15, and told the provider that he does not remember most of his 20s or 30s due to his heavy drug and alcohol use. While he admitted to using multiple drugs, alcohol was always his drug of choice. Despite that history, his last drink was 7.5 years ago due to extensive involvement in Alcoholics Anonymous (AA).

During the periods of heavy alcohol and drug use he had numerous encounters with law enforcement. The reasons for arrest were always related to his substance use, to include several Driving Under the Influence (DUIs). When asked how he was able to enlist with that background, he reported that it was during the height of the Iraq and Afghanistan conflicts when recruiters were unable to meet their minimum quotas, especially in the National Guard. His recruiter had minimal difficulty helping him obtain waivers, especially since none of his convictions were felony charges.

In regard to his PTSD diagnosis, he reports that during his deployment, "We were in a complete industrial wasteland… People just hobbling down the street… kids begging for water and food…." He had to dispose of body parts regularly; the worst was when he was ordered to transport a killed civilian Iraqi's head in a bag and then pry open an eye in order for the receiving personnel to perform biometric iris scanning. He was also regularly exposed to mortar attacks and the occasional chaotic combat mission where his unit took active fire and casualties.

He described intrusive, vivid memories/flashbacks/hallucinations of these incidents, and used to experience nightmares prior to his current med regimen. At his worst he "sees severed heads everywhere," and this combined with his increasing mania led to his most recent hospital admission. He avoids everything that might remind him of these events, and this has begun to include all public transportation and crowded locations. He has not left the base that houses the hospital and his barracks since arriving, and has refused to go on therapeutic outings sponsored by the hospital or warrior transition unit.

He has started to generalize this fear to the base as well, and sometimes believes he is seeing snipers hidden in various places when he walks from building to building. He showed the provider the knife that he wears on his belt to protect himself when he has to leave his barracks room, and does not respond well to the request that he should not bring weapons to the clinic, though he put the knife away without making any threats.

He has no interest in any of his old pre-deployment activities outside of AA, and while he is still married he feels very disconnected from his wife, friends, and family. His wife has chosen to stay in their home state instead of joining him while he goes through the medical board process. He speculates that she must be having an affair and probably intends to leave him, but feels too removed to care.

17.1.2 Diagnosis/Assessment

This is a patient who meets the criteria for PTSD, bipolar I disorder, and alcohol use disorder, severe. The diagnoses for this patient are clear, and have been verified by multiple providers across various medical settings as well as with psychological testing. The challenge here is not diagnosis, but coming up with a treatment regimen able to control his symptoms and get him well enough to return to post-deployment life.

Contributing to his current presentation are his history of substance use, military deployment with repeated traumatic exposure, and long-standing mood symptoms. These symptoms have led to decades of dysfunction starting in his teen years, though he was able to hold a steady job and maintain his marriage for a few years prior to the deployment. While he has a wife and extended family, his support system is tenuous at best. His long history of sobriety might be considered a positive prognostic indicator, though the severity of his previous substance use history puts him at high risk for relapse during this time of significant stress.

17.1.3 Treatment/Management

There are two important considerations to keep in mind for medication management in such cases. The first is the risks versus benefits of polypharmacy. The medications tried for this patient include aripiprazole, olanzapine, lithium, gabapentin, fluoxetine, trazodone, propranolol, buspirone, quetiapine fumarate, hydroxyzine, clonazepam, and ziprasidone, at various times over 1 year of treatment. Though he never suffered from extrapyramidal side effects, neuroleptic malignant syndrome, or serotonin syndrome, he was at high risk for all three, as well as p450 interactions.

This is of course in addition to the myriad other side effects that each medication could cause on its own.

In addition to interactions and side effects, polypharmacy for a patient like this can lead to poor medication compliance and accidental overdose. An unintentional overdose did occur when this patient accidentally took his evening medication twice, leading to mental status changes, QT prolongation, temporary renal injury, and a brief hospitalization, but luckily no long-term complications.

The second consideration is that medication used as first-line treatment for one diagnosis might be contraindicated for another. For example, clonazepam (for acute mania only) and second-generation antipsychotics are recommended treatments for bipolar I disorder, yet both carry D-level recommendations (harms outweigh benefits) in Veterans Affairs/Department of Defense (VA/DOD) guidelines for the treatment of PTSD [2]. As stated in these guidelines:

> There is theoretical, animal, and human evidence to suggest that benzodiazepines may actually interfere with the extinction of fear conditioning or potentiate the acquisition of fear responses and worsen recovery from trauma. Benzodiazepine should be used especially cautiously in combat veterans with PTSD because of the very high comorbidity of combat-related PTSD with alcohol misuse and substance use disorders (upwards of 50 percent of co-morbidity) and potential problems with tolerance and dependence. [3]

Of course, benzodiazepines are also contraindicated in someone with a substance use disorder, and their use would not be recommended in a patient like this unless he were in active withdrawal.

In regard to non-pharmacologic treatments, one difficulty with these three severe psychiatric comorbidities is that his response to standard treatment may be suboptimal. He is unlikely to resemble the standardized and highly screened populations studied in clinical trials for each diagnosis separately, and there have been no studies on evidence-based treatments for patients suffering from all three [4]. There is some evidence to suggest that patients with bipolar disorder will have more severe PTSD symptoms than a patient with PTSD alone [5], but otherwise there are very little data to help guide clinical treatment for a patient with all three diagnoses.

Another problem is that one diagnosis directly interferes with treatment for the other; his bipolar I symptoms made him unable to participate in standardized treatments for PTSD, such as eye movement desensitizing processing (EMDR) or prolonged exposure therapy, despite repeated attempts by his treatment team. They also interfered with his ability to meet acceptance criteria for dual diagnosis residential treatment programs.

His nightmares from PTSD caused his sleep to be poor, perpetuating his bipolar symptoms and preventing him from getting appropriate amount of sleep. His PTSD and bipolar disorder put him at much greater risk for substance use relapse, and the combination of all three made performing activities of daily living to include compliance with treatment very difficult. While on active duty his command could be relied upon to bring him to appointments, but this was no longer available once he left the service.

17.1.4 Outcomes/Case Resolution

This soldier went through the medical board process and was medically retired from the military with 100 % VA service connection. He was lost to follow-up for a period of 4 months when transitioning from military medical care to the VA system, and during that time he relapsed on alcohol. He was ultimately stabilized on olanzapine 15 mg PO QHS, prazosin 15 mg QHS [6], lithium 1500 mg PO QHS, gabapentin 900 mg QAM/1200 QHS, hydroxyzine pamoate 50 mg BID PRN severe anxiety, and naltrexone 50 mg. His only noted side effects were hyperlipidemia and a 20-lb weight gain. On average, he managed to attend one out of every three scheduled appointments, sometimes going months at a time without being seen by his provider.

His reasons for poor compliance were reportedly the reminder of military life that going to the VA triggers, the fear that he will be rehospitalized whenever a doctor evaluates him, and the lack of hope that he will ever get better. His alcohol relapses continued off and on for 2 years, but he ultimately managed to return to the AA community with the help of supportive family and the addition of naltrexone to his medication regimen. His wife chose to end their relationship because the patient's paranoia about her fidelity caused constant fighting, and due to the concern that his drinking and erratic behavior put her safety and financial security at risk. As per the last recorded report, he now lives with a supportive older sister and her family. He has yet to return to his work as a building inspector, and is instead only able to do occasional odd jobs while relying on disability to make ends meet.

17.1.5 Clinical Pearls

Be aware of polypharmacy and the risks associated with it.

Consider the impact comorbid disorders have on treatment if you are attempting to focus on one diagnosis for treatment.

Be aware of medications used to treat one disorder but that are contraindicated for another.

Sobriety is an important component of treatment, since substance use interferes with the treatment of PTSD and other comorbidities.

Continuity of care is paramount but difficult without a strong support network.

17.2 Case 2

17.2.1 Case Presentation/History

17.2.1.1 Identifying Information

SGT Garcia is a 23-year-old single Active Duty Army Hispanic male diagnosed with PTSD, bipolar I disorder, most recent depressive episode with mixed features, and alcohol use disorder, moderate. He was transferred to the inpatient psychiatric unit after a 3-month ICU/surgical hospitalization status post suicide attempt by self-inflicted gunshot wound. He had placed a pistol in his mouth with the intent to die, but the bullet veered to the left of vital structures, causing soft tissue and mandible wounds requiring multiple procedures for bone reconstruction, tongue and parotid gland reconstruction, as well as additional complications from infection.

Plastic surgery assisted and they were able to obtain good cosmetic results and restore full function of facial muscles and structures. The psychiatric consult liaison team followed him throughout his surgical hospitalization, and recommended a switch from their initial recommendation of aripiprazole and lamotrigine to lithium and olanzapine after adequate trial of the first regimen revealed no benefit. They also kept him under direct suicide watch at all times while on the surgical floor. He had been on active duty for 5 years at the time of admission, and he had no prior psychiatric hospitalizations or history of psychiatric treatment.

17.2.1.2 History of Present Illness

The patient was transferred to the inpatient psychiatric unit with unresolved major depressive symptoms as well as racing thoughts, feeling that he was fully rested after 2 h of sleep per 24-h period, pressured speech, disorganized thinking and increased sexual impulses to include masturbating multiple times a day and inappropriately touching staff and other patients, despite frequent redirection.

He was not cooperative with therapy, refused basic hygiene, and had difficulty participating in the milieu. His suicidal thoughts continued, and he expressed intent to reattempt suicide, but denied a plan while on the ward since he did not have access to a weapon. Despite treatment, his symptoms did not show any improvement over 3 weeks on the inpatient unit, and his sleep did not respond to various medication trials. His condition began to worsen, showing signs that he might progress to catatonia, so his treatment team decided to pursue electroconvulsive therapy (ECT). After four sessions, he began to show some improvement in cognition and mood, and his sexual acting out subsided.

As he regained mental clarity, he began to relate some experiences and additional symptoms. He explained that he had begun to have symptoms consistent with major depressive disorder starting around age 12, though he never sought treatment or let his parents know. His first manic episode was during the summer before junior year in high school and lasted for 2 weeks, culminating in a severe depressive episode that still did not garner medical attention due to his chaotic family environment, as his parents were divorcing and his mother was suffering from her own depression. He did not use substances during high school, and in general did well in school with decent grades and good athletic performance in varsity sports, despite his psychiatric symptoms.

He began drinking heavily at age 18 when he joined the military, and he described heavy binging, blackouts, and ever increasing amounts needed to achieve the same effect, but no withdrawal symptoms or legal consequences. After basic and advanced training, he worked as an infantryman (11B), and quickly progressed in rank due to excellent performance. He was accepted for training in an elite unit, and during the training did well overall, though he ultimately did not pass the course.

He related a traumatic event that happened during that training. He described an exercise that involved a water obstacle course where he was blindfolded and thrown into an indoor pool. He had been told that his objective was to make it to the other side of the pool, but was not told that the training cadre would be in the water making it more difficult to progress by dunking him, holding him under for brief periods, etc. He described himself as an insecure swimmer at best, and during the obstacle course he experienced his first and only panic attack. He recalled feeling certain he would die right before losing consciousness and failing the training task.

He soon developed PTSD symptoms to include violent nightmares, frequent intrusive thoughts of the event while awake, difficulty functioning at work because being around other soldiers reminded him of the event, avoidance of places that echo in ways that remind him of the indoor pool or smell like chlorine or bleach, fear of water to the point of being unable to shower, a sense that he had no value to others and no future, constant guilt and shame, inability to feel positive emotions, and a sense of complete alienation from others. He was unable to concentrate and was always hypervigilant around other men, with an exaggerated startle response if touched unexpectedly. These symptoms, as well as increasing alcohol use, worsened over the course of 9 months, and this exacerbation in symptoms ultimately culminated in his suicide attempt and hospitalization.

Collaborative history was collected from his unit. They corroborated that he did not graduate from the elite training program, but was failed and then assigned to another infantry unit similar to the one he had been in previously. His commander acknowledged some low-level concern about the soldier's performance, but had no idea that he was suffering from psychiatric symptoms or using alcohol to excess. He was by no means the worst performer in their unit, and had never required disciplinary action. He was regarded as a "quiet loner," who did not tend to socialize with others. They had never noticed anything that would lead them to consider referring him for substance use treatment or psychiatric assessment.

17.2.2 Diagnosis/Assessment

This is a patient who meets the criteria for PTSD, bipolar I disorder, and alcohol use disorder, moderate. He has a long-standing history of depressive, manic, and hypomanic symptoms prior to military service, though he had no trouble enlisting since he had never sought treatment. He developed a substance use disorder over the course of his active duty service as well. He performed remarkably well prior to the traumatic event described above, and was able to do well in school, sports, and the military, despite his ongoing mood symptoms and substance use.

It is unclear if his unit turned a blind eye to his symptoms during his decline, was just not psychologically minded as some infantry units may be, or if he really was able to perform well enough to avoid suspicion. The latter seems difficult to believe, but because he was such a high performer at baseline it remains within the realm of possibility.

17.2.3 Treatment/Management

After 12 sessions of ECT treatment, this patient was ultimately stabilized on olanzapine 20 mg QHS, lithium ER 900 mg PO BID, and trazodone 150 mg PO QHS. He had no significant side effects from the medication, but did have some short-term retrograde amnesia and mild memory loss from the ECT. Other medications tried during his hospitalization were prazosin, hydroxyzine, and buspirone, but all were discontinued due to inefficacy or side effects. After the ninth session of ECT his symptoms and suicidality improved enough to allow for discharge to the partial hospitalization program. At the time of discharge, he was able to shower but continued to be too fearful to take a bath or go on a therapeutic outing to the hospital indoor therapy pool.

He strongly desired to continue his military career, but a medical board was initiated due to the severity of his symptoms. He remained in the partial hospitalization program for 3 months, which is significantly longer than the program is designed to support, but he was too ill to transition to a lower level of care. He had one short rehospitalization secondary to alcohol use during that time. He dropped out of an exposure therapy clinical trial, but was ultimately able to complete a course of EMDR with some success.

He responded well to the provided classes on coping skills, and was able to put some of them into practice. He also benefitted from art therapy, and his artwork progressively showed a decrease in dark themes. Eventually, his mood symptoms were stabilized enough that he was able to attend a residential dual diagnosis treatment program to address his PTSD and substance use. He was able to participate in therapeutic outings sponsored by the medical facility, to include professional sports events in large, crowded stadiums and government buildings with large, echoing rooms. However, he continued to avoid taking baths, swimming, and bodies of water.

17.2.4 Outcomes/Case Resolution

The soldier was found unfit for duty by his medical board, and so chose to enroll in an unpaid internship program for veterans at a local government agency. Due to strong performance and a good work ethic, he was offered an entry-level government service job, which he accepted. He was assigned to an open position in his home state, though once there he very rarely saw his family.

His job performance was considered good and he was promoted twice. He continued to maintain sobriety per report, and he has remained in mental health treatment through the VA, with few missed appointments. He continued to have difficulty with close relationships, and still struggled with a strong sense of shame and guilt. His facial reconstruction surgeries left minimal visible damage, yet he continued to worry about his appearance. He continued to have occasional periods of depression or mild hypomania, but nothing like previous episodes and no further hospitalizations or reported suicidality.

This service member, while extremely ill initially, had several factors that led to a better prognosis than the first case presented in this chapter. He was younger, with less severe substance use, and only one trauma related to his PTSD, as opposed to multiple. He also never presented with significant psychotic symptoms. His intelligence can be estimated to be higher as evidenced by his ability to achieve during high school and military service even while suffering from severe mood symptoms. Overall, he was able to participate in and benefit from treatment in a way that the first patient was never able to do.

Clinical factors that benefitted this patient the most were his course of ECT, his ability and desire to get better and return to active duty, his ability to tolerate the disappointment of being medically retired, and the flexibility to find a reasonable and successful plan to transition into civilian life. He was also more open to treatment and found it much easier to be compliant with medical recommendations.

17.2.5 Clinical Pearls

Consider ECT or other non-pharmacological treatment in resistant cases of comorbid PTSD and mood disorders [7].

Consider all available treatment options, to include art therapy and nontraditional treatments.

Consider previous level of functioning when trying to assess the patient's prognosis.

Successful substance use treatment is a significant factor in returning to and maintaining recovery from all comorbid disorders.

17.3 Conclusion

Comorbid PTSD, bipolar I, and substance use disorders can lead to extremely severe and complicated presentations, as the above cases exemplify. The symptoms of each diagnosis are not merely seen alongside one another, but interact in complex and synergistic ways to create an extremely complex and difficult to treat clinical picture.

Such patients often require their prescriber's vigilance for inadequate response to standard medication regimens, the risks of polypharmacy, difficulty maintaining a strong support network, the challenges of med regimens recommended for one diagnosis conflicting with recommendations for another, and challenges to long-term sobriety.

Prognosis for these patients can vary widely, from ongoing disability to relative normalcy in the long term. This depends on many factors such as premorbid functioning, the ability to comply and participate in treatment, response to available treatments, the ability to remain connected to a support network, and other unique qualities such as adaptive or maladaptive personality traits and varying levels of resilience.

References

1. Chitty KM, Lagopoulos J, Kaur M, Hickie IB, Hermens DF. The N-Methyl-D-Aspartate receptor as a neurobiological intersection between bipolar disorder and alcohol use: a longitudinal mismatch negativity study. Int J Neuropsychopharmacol. 2015. doi:10.1093/ijnp/pyu113.
2. MEDCOM OTSG Policy. 14-094, 18 Dec 2014.
3. VA/DoD clinical practice guideline for management of Posttraumatic stress department of veterans affairs department of defense, page 112. http://www.healthquality.va.gov/guidelines/MH/ptsd/cpg_PTSD-FULL-201011612.pdf.
4. 2013 0010-3853 Community Mental Health Journal 49, 6, R 10.1007/s10597-013-9620-8 lifetime trauma, subjective distress, substance use, and PTSD symptoms in people with severe mental illness: comparisons among four diagnostic groups. http://dx.doi.org/10.1007/s10597-013-9620-8. Springer US, 2013-12-01.
5. Raskind MA, Peterson K, Williams T, et al. A trial of prazosin for combat trauma PTSD with nightmares in active-duty soldiers returned from Iraq and Afghanistan. Am J Psychiatry. 2013;170(9):1003–10.
6. Nakama H, Garcia A, O'Brien K, Ellis N. Case report of a 24-year-old man with resolution of treatment-resistant major depressive disorder and comorbid PTSD using rTMS. J ECT. 2014;30(1):e9–10. doi:10.1097/YCT.0b013e182a2705d.
7. Margoob MA, Ali Z, Andrade C. Efficacy of ECT in chronic, severe, antidepressant- and CBT-refractory PTSD: an open, prospective study. Brain Stimul. 2010;3(1):28–35. doi:10.1016/j.brs.2009.04.005.

Psychosis Masquerading as PTSD 18

Eric G. Meyer and Brian W. Writer

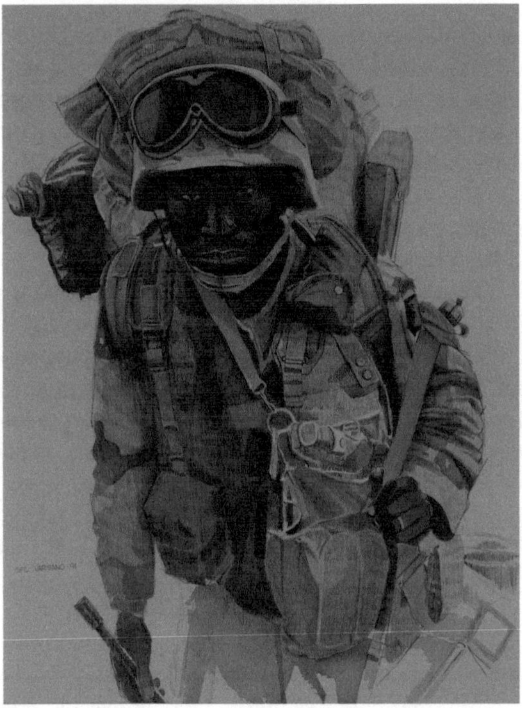

Don't Mess with the 101st, by Peter Varisano, courtesy of the Army Art Collection, US Army Center of Military History.

E. G. Meyer (✉)
Department of Psychiatry, Uniformed Services University of the Health Sciences, Bethesda, MD, USA
e-mail: eric.meyer@usuhs.edu

B. W. Writer
Department of Psychiatry, Adjunct Faculty, Audie L. Murphy VA Hospital, University of Texas Health Science Center San Antonio, San Antonio, TX, USA

E. C. Ritchie (ed.), *Posttraumatic Stress Disorder and Related Diseases in Combat Veterans*, DOI 10.1007/978-3-319-22985-0_18

The overlap between posttraumatic stress disorder and psychosis is marked and well documented [1]. Psychosis and psychotic disorders may be provoked by a traumatic event: patients with schizophrenia are four times more likely to have PTSD compared to the general US population [2]. The overlap also influences treatment, as patients with psychotic disorders have more difficultly processing trauma and are thus typically excluded from evidence-based therapies for PTSD [3]. Additionally, patients with PTSD and schizophrenia have high rates of substance abuse, a phenomenon that can complicate, and worsen, both conditions. A family history of a psychotic disorder confers both heritability risk for such disorders and vulnerability to traumatic childhood exposures with subsequent PTSD.

Differentiating the two diagnostically can also be a challenge, as several PTSD symptoms overlap with symptoms of psychosis:

- The experience of a flashback is described as the patient believing that they are not just remembering a trauma, but are reexperiencing it. Although patients are often able to reality test such experiences after the fact, during a flashback they are convinced that the event is actually reoccurring; making it challenging to differentiate a flashback from a perceptual disturbance. The overlap between PTSD and psychosis is so profound that previous studies defend the use of antipsychotics like quetiapine for the off-label treatment of nonpsychotic trauma-related nightmares and flashbacks [4].
- PTSD patients may avoid people and places out of fear that they will be re-traumatized. For military patients, this often includes avoiding large public areas or feeling panic when driving on the highway due to recollections of the combat environment. Depending on the level of their conviction, attempts to assure patients that these external reminders pose little threat to them may not reduce their concerns. Such vigilance may resemble delusional paranoia or represent transient delusional states.
- Feeling emotionally detached and engaging in interpersonal avoidant behaviors are common PTSD findings, which can look surprisingly similar to a variety of negative symptomatology found in schizophrenics.

Teasing out the difference between trauma-related symptoms including PTSD-related psychosis and primary psychotic disorder-related psychosis requires a thoughtful approach. Further complicating matters is that the presence of schizophrenia confers vulnerability to trauma exposure and hence concurrent PTSD. Differentiating a psychotic PTSD flashback from schizophrenic psychosis can be accomplished by assessing a patient's ability to return to reality after the flashback: did they realize the event was not real? A schizophrenic patient will likely maintain a prolonged disruption in reality testing relative to a PTSD flashback, especially early in course of their disease. However, patients with chronic perceptual disturbances of schizophrenia may eventually learn to recognize and maintain some degree of functionality despite their hallucinations. The content of the flashback can also be helpful—it is related to a specific trauma in the patient's history, or is it a novel experience for the patient? Distinguishing schizophrenic paranoid delusions from PTSD hypervigilance and avoidant behaviors requires a similar approach. A delusional schizophrenic patient may not have insight into where their fears are coming from, or their answers may not be entirely logical. A hypervigilant PTSD patient with avoidant symptoms should be able to account for how the stimuli they are avoiding reminds them of their traumatic event in some way. Additionally, the modality of the false sensory experience can aid in differentiation. PTSD flashback perceptual disturbances often involve several perceptual modalities and are much more likely to include nonauditory disruptions, such as olfactory disturbances, as compared to schizophrenic psychosis which are typically limited to auditory hallucinations. Lastly, and perhaps most importantly, the emergence of schizophrenic psychosis occurs in the absence of a putative potentially traumatic exposure (PTE), which is the defining characteristic of PTSD that is requisite for a determination of PTSD-related symptomatology.

Unfortunately, patients with PTSD related to military trauma can have several additional diagnostic challenges. Multiple military (and non-military) traumatic experiences across their lifespan can coalesce, leaving the patient's intrusion symptoms vague and difficult to connect to a specific event. Military patients who suffer from a traumatic brain injury (TBI) may have a difficult time recalling important events independent of potential PTSD-related memory avoidance. Such difficulties in recalling trauma exposures along with ongoing difficulties in processing can interfere with cognitive and exposure therapies—the standard of care treatments for PTSD. The very nature of their military service may bias a provider's interpretation of symptoms toward PTSD and away from other considerations. The following case demonstrates some of the complexities in presentation and treatment of a military patient who, despite appearing to have PTSD, was ultimately determined to be suffering from schizophrenia.

18.1 Case Presentation

A 43-year-old African American Major in the US Air Force presented to the mental health clinic due to difficulty sleeping and concerns regarding his "routines." He had been having difficulty maintaining asleep over the past few years, which he attributed to recurrent distressing dreams associated with previous deployments to Iraq and Afghanistan. He noted that somewhere during his seven deployments he started having nightmares of falling in a black void and waking up afraid of "something." He recently started checking the locks on his house every night and walking the perimeter of his property due to concerns related to being attacked. He believed that these behaviors were also due to traumatic events that had occurred during his deployments. These symptoms appeared to worsen after he and his family moved out into the country a few months ago. Specifically, he admitted that his wife was concerned about the fact that he had cleared a 10 ft swath around the perimeter of their property and routinely watched the small country road they lived on, noting cars that "should not be there."

On further exploration of the patient's trauma, it was determined that the most distressing event during his deployments was being woken in the middle of the night with a Red Cross message alerting him that his elderly father had become ill.

He felt helpless in that he could not return to his family during their time of need and, ultimately, felt guilty for not being present for his father's death or funeral. He perceived waking up in the middle of the night as "re-living that terrible night." He acknowledged that, although the event was traumatic for him, it did not seem to relate to his paranoia about being attacked in his home. He reflected that over his multiple deployments he had also been shot at, exposed to mortar attacks, had numerous friends die, and participated in convoys that were attacked. Although he denied that any of these events caused him distress, he felt that they might be the source of his safety concerns.

The Major also reported feeling uncomfortable in crowded places, to include his own office: "I'd rather work in my car, out in the parking lot." He confirmed feeling disconnected from his emotions and his wife. He recognized that he avoided thinking about his deployments and the death of his father. He had never visited his father's grave and was hesitant to attend extended family reunions due to fear people would talk about his father.

On psychiatric review of symptoms, the patient described some overlapping depressive symptoms with PTSD including anhedonia and reduced concentration. He associated his reduced energy to his sleep disturbances and his vigilant mind/behavior. Mania was not detected, given a lack of concurrent elevated/irritable mood with increased energy or goal-directed activity. He denied any other obsessions, compulsions, or anxiety symptoms. He denied perceptual disturbances and delusions.

Clinical Pearl Clinicians should make longitudinal inquiries beyond the initial evaluation regarding the possible presence of PTSD-related psychosis because many victims of trauma exposure are either too embarrassed or have not yet established the prerequisite level of trust to disclose such symptoms early on in the treatment relationship [1].

Regarding his fear of being attacked, his ability to reality test these thoughts was inconsistent with delusional paranoia. He reported occasional use of alcohol, denied evidence of misuse, and denied use of any other substances. He denied any history of loss of consciousness or confusion due to being exposed to an explosion or mechanical injury. He denied any thoughts of death or suicidal ideation. He also denied any homicidal intent, but qualified his answer with, "unless someone attacked me—then I'd have to defend myself."

On medical review of symptoms, he endorsed snoring at night and that his wife had told him that he often made gasping sounds. He also endorsed occasional morning headaches that required over the counter medication (ibuprofen), but otherwise denied any current signs or symptoms of a medical condition. Medically he was being treated for essential hypertension with hydrochlorothiazide and elevated cholesterol with simvastatin.

Clinical Pearl Consider screening for organic causes in any patient experiencing disrupted sleep. Following up with a sleep study can confirm the diagnosis and guide treatment. Resolution of organic contributions can enhance the treatment of any remaining symptoms [5].

He denied any previous personal or family psychiatric history. He grew up in a stable home, denied abuse, had a good relationship with parents, and reported doing well in school. He had completed a master's degree a few years ago and was doing well occupationally: He had been in the military for 16 years and was up for promotion to Lieutenant Colonel, he was getting along well with others at work and had recently been praised for performance by his commander. He described his job as section lead for operations where he helped plan missions. He had been married for 15 years and had four children. He denied any legal or financial issues.

Clinical Pearl Military patients often define themselves occupationally. A brief military history can provide insight into the patient's functional levels and put the remainder of their history in a contextual frame. For example, promoting to Lieutenant Colonel around 16 years of service infers that this military patient is "on track" [6].

In addition to routine screening tools, the patient completed a Beck Depression Inventory (BDI-II), which showed some symptoms of depression but was not positive for a depressive disorder. He also completed the Yale-Brown Obsessive Compulsive Scale (Y-BOCS), which did not reveal any additional obsessions or compulsions. The patient's posttraumatic stress disorder check list (PCL-5) supported a diagnosis of PTSD and demonstrated moderate clinical distress.

Clinical Pearl While routine screening tools are not diagnostic, they can help clarify and support your diagnosis. Repeat use can also assist with symptom monitoring to access for treatment response and/or success [7].

Based on the patient's initial assessment, he was diagnosed with PTSD. As noted above, there was evidence of PTSD-related unipolar depressive difficulties and potentially, an independent organic sleeping disorder. Treatment options were discussed, and the patient agreed to routine blood work and a sleep study to identify any comorbid organic contributions. He also agreed to a trial of a selective serotonin reuptake inhibitor (SSRI) for his anxiety and depressive symptoms along with prazosin at night to assist with nightmares. It was also agreed that after the patient's acute symptoms of distress were improved with medication that he would engage in an evidence-based psychotherapy for PTSD. After describing prolonged exposure (PE) therapy and cognitive processing therapy (CPT), the patient opted to start the latter.

Clinical Pearl CPT and PE are equally efficacious in the treatment of PTSD [8], but are also often difficult therapies to initiate for patients with a history of trauma. Minimizing patient distress prior to starting therapy can greatly improve their chances of starting and completing a protocol. Reducing trauma-related nightmares with off-label prazosin, has been found to be beneficial [9]. The sustained use of benzodiazepines and similar hypnotics are relatively contraindicated in the setting of PTSD [10], but short-term use, prior to therapy, can be helpful in reducing avoidance. Coordinating symptom focused medication management with therapy can serve to frame a patient's entire treatment: with successful completion of therapy such medications may no longer be necessary.

Clinical Pearl Some patients are more behavioral/experiential in their approach, while others are more cognitive. Describing the differences between PE and CPT can allow patients to take control of how they will be engaging their trauma. For some patients, core components of each therapy may be needed to "meet patients where they are" [11]. Fostering autonomy and thereby sense of control by allowing patients to choose their treatment has also been shown to improve adherence/outcomes [12]. Promotion of agency is especially important to this patient population given the core themes of disrupted control inherent to most trauma exposures.

Routine blood work was normal. The patient dutifully completed the sleep study and was diagnosed with obstructive sleep apnea. He was started on continuous positive airway pressure (CPAP) treatment with a noticeable improvement in his sleep quality and a decrease in his headaches.

At 3-month follow-up, he reported that he was tolerating the SSRI well, with no side effects. He felt that his depression had somewhat improved, but reported minimal reduction in his safety concerns or associated anxiety. He reported that the prazosin had been helpful in reducing the number of times he woke up from nightmares, which further improved his sleep. His BDI-II and PCL-M scores had both dropped slightly. The patient was provided a titration schedule for his SSRI and scheduled for an intake with psychology later that month to initiate CPT.

The psychologist reported that the patient appeared "off," echoing that the patient had a hard time relating his trauma to his current symptoms. The patient also seemed confused at times, perseverating on concerns about his safety and requiring extensive clarification on several simple questions when completing the clinician assessment of PTSD symptoms (CAPS). It was agreed that these behaviors were unexpected in a patient with such a high level of education and occupational functioning. The psychologist supported a diagnosis of PTSD, but was concerned that something was "just not right." Both providers agreed to maintain an open differential given these observations.

Several weeks later, the psychologist reported that the patient was having a difficult time with the CPT protocol. Specifically, the Major not only had difficulty identifying his affective experiences in his trauma account, but he also struggled to make sense of the account itself. The psychologist referenced specific examples where the patient's logic would jump from an event to another and then ultimately end with the patient reporting not feeling safe. The patient was scheduled for follow up with psychiatrist in 2 weeks, and it was agreed that the patient would be further assessed for an independent neurocognitive disorder at that time.

Clinical Pearl Evidence suggests that mild TBI is highly prevalent in veterans from recent conflicts and has a high concordance with PTSD [13]. Repetitive mild TBI can result in neuropsychological difficulties with functional impairment. Routinely screening for prior TBI events and/or cognitive testing of any patient that appears to have difficulty processing information can assist with management planning and improved health outcomes [14].

One week prior to that appointment, the patient was emergently hospitalized due to a self-inflicted gunshot wound. Psychiatric evaluation in the hospital revealed that it was not a suicide attempt. Rather, the patient had intentionally shot himself in the thigh to reduce, or distract, himself from a headache. He denied thinking that this plan was dangerous or that there might be a better method of treating such a headache.

After he was medically stabilized, he was transferred to the inpatient psychiatric unit. Magnetic resonance imaging (MRI), electroencephalography (EEG), and routine blood work did not reveal other organic contributions. Due to his ongoing disorganized thinking he was started on second-generation antipsychotic (SGA).

Clinical Pearl The age of initial onset of a psychotic disorder is bimodally distributed in males, peaking at the ages of 21.4 and 39.2 [15]. Regardless, all initial episodes of psychotic symptoms should be evaluated for general medical and/or substance-use related etiologies.

Collateral from his wife revealed that he had been adherent to his medications and CPAP, but that he had continued to be very concerned about the safety of his family. She shared that a few weeks ago he started to patrol the border of their property every night. She also clarified that he not only watched for unfamiliar cars, but also kept a log of vehicle types and colors. She confided that the whole reason they had moved to the country was to get away from "the crowds," which she initially thought was part of their lifelong dream, but had recently come to realize it was actually due to his paranoia.

After a brief inpatient hospitalization, the Major was discharged with improved insight regarding his recent behavior and decreased disorganized thinking. After a month of treatment with an SGA, the patient was better able to account for the events he had experienced. Reassessment clarified that his nightmares were solely related to the death of his father, while the remaining symptoms of paranoia were not related to a traumatic experience. The patient continued SGA treatment and discontinued the other medications as his anxiety, depression, and nightmares appeared to resolve with treatment of his delusional paranoia.

Due to requiring treatment with an antipsychotic and having a diagnosis of schizophrenia, the patient was no longer qualified for military service. A Medical Evaluation Board was conducted and the Major was medically separated from the military. The patient's care was transferred to the Veterans' Administration for continued treatment.

Clinical Pearl Several psychiatric diagnoses and treatments can result in separation from the military. Each branch of the military has different policies. When starting a new psychotropic or providing a new diagnosis for an active duty, guard, or reserve member it can be especially helpful to consult with a representative from the patients assigned "Military Treatment Facility" to determine the implications. In the Air Force, for example, even off-label use of an SGA can result in separation—prompting many providers to instead use trazodone or mirtazapine.

18.2 Discussion

This patient was suffering from a paranoia that was initially attributed to his cumulative trauma experiences and, as such, was conceptualized as a symptom of PTSD. Similarly, his nightmares, affective blunting, avoidance, and depression were also initially attributed to PTSD. However, given the divorced nature of his paranoia from any identifiable potentially traumatic exposure (PTE), it subsequently became apparent that his paranoia, emotional blunting, and interpersonal avoidance were representative of schizophrenia as opposed to PTSD-related psychosis. His nightmares also became more clearly related to the death of his father, which appeared consistent with a sustained loss response. Such a reaction may be representative of persistent complex bereavement disorder, which has been proposed as an area for further study in the DSM-5 [16]. Although he had always seemed confused, and the association of his trauma to his intrusive reexperiencing appeared discordant, it was not until he shot himself that it was apparent how disorganized his thinking was—ultimately meeting criteria for schizophrenia. In the end, the patient did not have PTSD at all.

How was there such discordance with the initial diagnostic impression and his actual pathology? The patient's disjointed initial presentation was confusing in many regards. The loss of his father did not correlate to the posttraumatic reaction being described. His exposure to combat and loss of life may have, but the patient framed it in a way that was divorced from any clinical distress. However, an unclear history is not an uncommon presentation for military PTSD and is rarely considered psychotic.

Although evidence-based therapies have been found to be efficacious for patients with TBI [17], such patients may require adjustment to their therapy based on their level of function (e.g., simplifying cognitive approaches and/or starting with more behavioral approaches) [18]. Additionally, patients with multiple combat deployments can have an almost unending list of trauma accounts—with an unclear understanding of which is the most troubling. Those who deploy multiple times are often skilled in compartmentalization and will report that none of their trauma experiences are terribly upsetting until much later in therapy.

The Major's symptoms of hyperarousal started several years ago, somewhere in the middle of all of his deployments. These symptoms may have been a transient combat operational stress reaction (COSR), subsyndromal PTSD that resolved on its own, or an acute stress reaction. Because this ambiguity often exists in the military, the mismatch between the patient's trauma exposure and his hyperarousal symptoms appeared justifiable, and was not further challenged.

Consistent with being paranoid, the patient also underreported the extent of his paranoid behavior. His wife's account was much more concerning and demonstrated a severe change in behavior that would have likely prompted a more aggressive assessment. The use of collateral information is often avoided in outpatient treatment due to concerns of privacy. This is certainly one scenario where asking the patient for permission to get his wife's perspective early on represented a missed opportunity that may have dramatically changed the course of his diagnosis and treatment.

The last, and potentially most troubling, contribution was the context of the patient's treatment and the expectations of his providers. The patient was a senior officer, serving for almost two decades in a grueling and often unforgiving occupation. The possibility of having a psychotic disorder was heavily deflated because of his rank and position, not just his age. Similarly, he was seeking care at a military mental health clinic, which are often given titles like "Warrior Clinic" to reduce stigma. Such clinics are streamlined for the conditions associated with combat: Consults for sleep disorders and TBI are prioritized, psychologist have entire templates built around completing CPT and PE protocols, and psychiatrists are well versed in recent research on the pharmacologic treatment of PTSD. As a consequence of this focus, when a member with seven deployments presented with nightmares and avoidance symptoms it seemed difficult to imagine the diagnosis as anything other than PTSD.

A key principle in psychodynamic therapy is to be cautious of assumptions made regarding patients. This is especially true of patients who are culturally similar to the provider, as the provider is more likely to believe assumptions to be fact [19]. In a military clinic designed for trauma-related conditions, filled with military providers, certain assumptions were made regarding this military patient. In this case, such assumptions led to concessions in diagnostic scrutiny, which contributed to a poor outcome.

18.3 Conclusions

Our understanding of PTSD has advanced dramatically in the past decade. Tools for assessing and diagnosing PTSD have progressed, while pharmacologic and therapeutic management of PTSD has advanced dramatically, along with acceptance of the importance in treating concurrent medical and psychiatric conditions. Despite these advances, PTSD remains a complicated reaction to trauma and is often not as linear as described.

In even the most straightforward of cases, a broad differential should be maintained, with consideration of the potential overlap and/or co-occurrence of psychosis with PTSD. Careful exploration for a potentially traumatic event is imperative: It is this event that anchors any intrusions, alterations in cognitions, reactivity, and avoidance in PTSD. Looking beyond an etiologic framework, individual symptoms should be carefully assessed. Whereas schizophrenic psychotic perceptual disturbances and paranoia are often persistent, flashbacks are more transient in nature and trauma-related paranoia is limited to the content of the trauma event. Lastly, poor or limited response to well-established pharmacologic or therapeutic-based treatments can be an indication that a patient's diagnosis may require further exploration.

The ability to differentiate symptoms can be especially difficult in military patients. Exposure to repeated and varied traumas over an extended period of time can make their awareness of what caused their posttraumatic stress difficult to ascertain. Exposure to TBI can result in difficulty in processing information that may cause patients to appear disorganized. Furthermore, while patients and the medical record will typically reflect awareness of historical moderate to severe

TBI events—repeatative mild TBI may be more difficult to detect without routine screening. Lastly, the temptation to have military patients fit into an archetype of PTSD can blind providers to the possibility of another process.

In these instances, ongoing assessment and consideration of other potential processes are critical. Seeking collateral can be paramount in understanding how a patient has deviated from their baseline. As the field of psychiatry continues to become more process oriented, with cavalcades of best practice guidelines, this case stands to underscore the complexity of diagnosis and the need for thoughtful examination.

References

1. Hamner MB. Psychotic symptoms in posttraumatic stress disorder. FOCUS Psychiatry. 2011;9(3):278–85.
2. Buckley PF, Miller BJ, Lehrer DS, Castle DJ. Psychiatric comorbidities and schizophrenia. Schizophr Bull. 2009;35(2):383–402.
3. Powers MB, Halpern JM, Ferenschak MP, Gillihan SJ, Foa EB. A meta-analytic review of prolonged exposure for posttraumatic stress disorder. Clin Psychol Rev. 2010;30(6):635–41.
4. Hamner MB, Deitsch SE, Brodrick PS, Ulmer HG, Lorberbaum JP. Quetiapine treatment in patients with posttraumatic stress disorder: an open trial of adjunctive therapy. J Clin Psychopharmacol. 2003;23(1):15–20.
5. Sharafkhaneh A, Giray N, Richardson P, Young T, Hirshkowitz M. Association of psychiatric disorders and sleep apnea in a larger cohort. Sleep. 2005;28(11):1405–11.
6. Meyer EG. The importance of understanding military culture. Acad Psychiatry. Available online. Feb 2015.
7. Ursano JU, et al. Practice guidelines: treatment of patients with acute stress disorder and posttraumatic stress disorder. Am J Psychiatr. 2004;161(11):3–31.
8. Resick PA, Williams LF, Suvak MK, Monson Cm, Gardus JL. Long-term outcomes of cognitive-behavioral treatments for posttraumatic stress disorder among female rape survivors. J Consult Clin Psychol. 2012;80(2):201–10
9. Writer BW, Meyer EG, Schillerstrom JE. Prazosin for military combat-related PTSD Nightmares: a critical review. J Neuropsychiatry Clin Neurosci. 2014;26(1):24–33.
10. Friedman M, Ruzek J, Lowry P. VA/DoD Practice Guidelines for Management of Posttraumatic Stress (v2.0). Department of Veterans Affairs/Department of Defense. 2010.
11. Hoge CW. Interventions for war-related posttraumatic stress disorder meeting veterans where they are. JAMA. 2011;306(5):549–51.
12. Le AQ, Doctor JN, Zoellner LA, Feeny NC. Cost-effectiveness of prolonged exposure therapy versus pharmacotherapy and treatment choice in posttraumatic stress disorder (the optimizing PTSD treatment trial): a doubly randomized preference trial. J Clin Psychiatry. 2014;75(3):222–30.
13. Hoge CW, McGurk D, Thomas JL, Cox AL, Engel CC, Castro CA. Mild traumatic brain injury in U.S. Soldiers returning from Iraq. N Engl J Med. 2008; 358(5): 453–463.
14. Bryan CJ. Repetitive traumatic brain injury (or concussion) increases severity of sleep disturbance among deployed military personnel. Sleep. 2013;36(6):941–6.
15. Castle D, Sham P, Murray R. Differences in distribution of ages of onset in males and females with schizophrenia. Schizophr Res. 1998;33:179–83.
16. American Psychiatric Association. Diagnostic and statistical manual of mental disorders: DSM-5. Washington, DC: American Psychiatric Association; 2013.

17. Sripada RK, Rauch SAM, Tuerk PW, Smith E, Defever AM, Mayer RA, Messina M, Venners M. Mild traumatic brain injury and treatment response in prolonged exposure for PTSD. J Trauma Stress. 2013;26:369–75.
18. Hsieh MY, Ponsford J, Wong D, McKay A. Exploring variables associated with change in cognitive behavior therapy (CBT) for anxiety following traumatic brain injury. Disabil Rehabil. 2012;34(5):408–15.
19. Rodriguez CI, Cabaniss DL, Arbuckle MR, Oquendo MA. The role of culture in psychodynamic psychotherapy: parallel process resulting from cultural similarities between patient and therapist. Am J Psychiatry. 2008;165(11):10.

19 The Mefloquine Intoxication Syndrome: A Significant Potential Confounder in the Diagnosis and Management of PTSD and Other Chronic Deployment-Related Neuropsychiatric Disorders

Remington Lee Nevin and Elspeth Cameron Ritchie

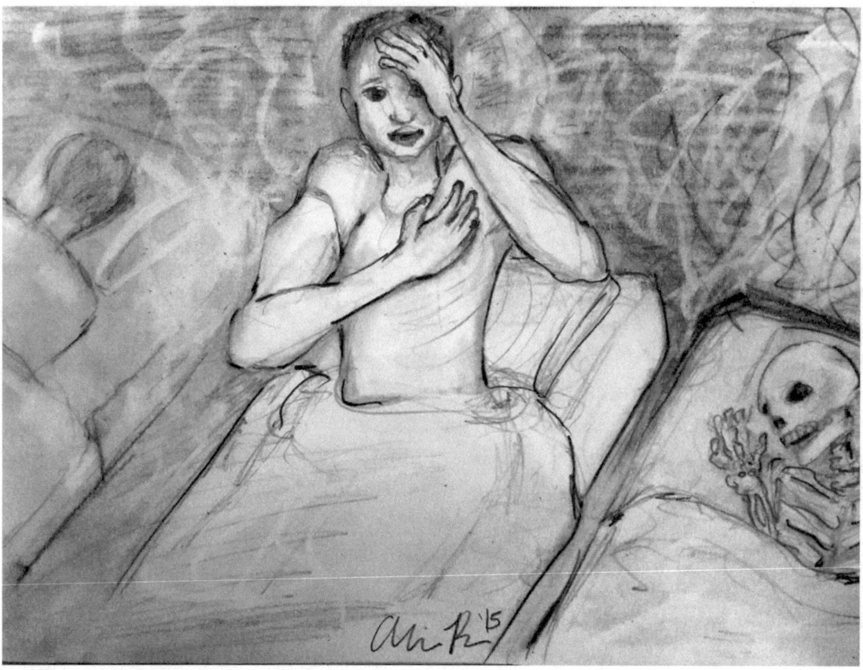

Acute mefloquine intoxication may produce vivid, hyper-realistic nightmares that may precede a manic, paranoid, dissociative or confusional psychosis, often marked by horrific auditory and visual hallucinations. Courtesy of Allison Stroh Rabin.

R. L. Nevin (✉)
Department of Mental Health, Johns Hopkins Bloomberg School of Public Health, 624 N. Broadway, Rm 782, Baltimore, MD 21205, USA
e-mail: rnevin@jhu.edu

E. C. Ritchie (ed.), *Posttraumatic Stress Disorder and Related Diseases in Combat Veterans*, DOI 10.1007/978-3-319-22985-0_19

Mefloquine intoxication has significant but previously overlooked relevance in military and veteran populations. Since the early 1990s, mefloquine has been widely used as an antimalarial prophylaxis during large-scale military operations, particularly in Somalia, Iraq, and Afghanistan [1]. However, only recently has intoxication with mefloquine been recognized as potentially confounding the diagnosis and management of certain deployment-related neuropsychiatric disorders, including posttraumatic stress disorder (PTSD) [2]. In this chapter, a well-publicized case of missed diagnosis of mefloquine intoxication is presented as background to frame a discussion of the symptomatology of acute mefloquine intoxication and its chronic sequelae.

The chapter discusses methods for the appropriate prevention, diagnosis, and management of this condition in military and veteran populations potentially exposed to this neurotoxic drug [3].

The chapter then discusses the relevance of recent insights [4] into the lasting and even permanent nature of many of the sequelae of mefloquine intoxication for the evaluation and care of exposed veterans, and concludes by considering the possibility that even mild subclinical intoxication may have similar chronic effects.

Given the prior widespread use of the drug in military and veteran populations, the chapter concludes with a recommendation that health-care providers screen for mefloquine exposure, particularly when assessing a patient who appears to have PTSD or other chronic neuropsychiatric disorders whose diagnosis may be plausibly confounded by prior intoxication.

19.1 Case Presentation[1]

In September 2003, a 33-year-old male soldier presented to a combat stress control unit in Iraq complaining of the acute onset 4 days earlier of symptoms of marked anxiety, paranoia, auditory and visual hallucinations, delusions of persecution, and confusion, with worsening physical complaints of photophobia and dizziness. The soldier was a newly arrived member of the US Army Special Forces unit based in a small team house in Samarra.

The night his symptoms began, he reported being awakened by a terrifying and "hyperrealistic" nightmare in which his room was exploding in a giant fireball as if under attack. Fearing the enemy was infiltrating his team house, the soldier quickly donned his combat gear and grabbed his weapon, and conducted a tactical room-to-room search. He was horrified to perceive the peacefully sleeping members of his unit as mangled corpses; eerily similar to the mangled corpse of an Iraqi insurgent

[1] It was adapted from my work published in reference [1]. This title is a US Government Work to which there should be no copyright or licensing requirements.

E. C. Ritchie
Uniformed Services University of the Health Sciences, 4301 Jones Bridge Road, Bethesda, MD 20314, USA
e-mail: elspethcameronritchie@gmail.com

he had seen the evening prior while on a mission. The soldier returned to his room experiencing visual and auditory hallucinations, unable to sleep, helpless, anxious, and paranoid.

The next day, his hallucinations continued. He perceived his team members as horrific "talking skeletal remains" and he heard nearby muffled voices plotting his death. He reluctantly informed his immediate supervisor of his hallucinations and anxiety and stated his fears that he was experiencing a "nervous breakdown." However, his concerns were initially attributed to cowardice and he was advised to return to duty.

His sense of helplessness and persecutory delusions worsened the following day. After finally insisting on medical care, and fearing for their safety, his unit members disarmed and confined him while they awaited his transport to a nearby combat stress control unit where he received an evaluation 2 days later.

On evaluation, his medical history was significant only for an episode of concussion in his mid-teens, for which he was briefly hospitalized and from which he had no residual symptoms. He had no family or personal history of mental illness. He was serving as an interrogator and human intelligence collector and had been granted a top secret security clearance after passing a full background investigation.

His only medication was mefloquine, which he had begun approximately 2 weeks prior to his departure to Iraq. He had taken his third 250-mg weekly dose 2 days prior to the onset of his symptoms. He had consumed a modest amount of alcohol with meals while awaiting air transport to Iraq, but none following his arrival. In the days prior to the acute onset of his psychosis, he recalls having experienced no vivid dreams, change in personality, anxiety, restlessness, depression, or confusion.

At the time of his initial evaluation at the combat stress control unit, his symptoms were attributed to a panic attack stemming from his initial encounter with the deceased Iraqi insurgent. The symptoms were deemed consistent with a combat stress reaction. Although combat stress control had recommended he should receive local treatment, his unit had elected to initiate legal proceedings for his earlier behavior. He was subsequently returned to the USA to be charged with cowardice by the Army under Article 99 of the Uniformed Code of Military Justice (UCMJ), a crime that carries a maximum penalty of death.

The possibility that the patient's symptoms could represent an adverse reaction to mefloquine was not initially suspected either by his command or medical personnel, nor the soldier himself. Although the soldier had been issued the drug some months after the US Food and Drug Administration (FDA) first required issuance of a medication guide "wallet card" [5], he neither received this card nor verbal or other written instructions describing under what conditions to discontinue the drug.

Unaware of the information contained in the approved drug labeling to discontinue the medication at the onset of symptoms of "anxiety, depression, restlessness, or confusion," he continued to take mefloquine for two additional weeks after the onset of his symptoms, for a total of five doses.

Following his discontinuation of the drug, his psychiatric symptoms gradually improved and he subsequently received a diagnosis of PTSD. Meanwhile, his physical symptoms including photophobia, accommodative dysfunction, vertigo, and disequilibrium became more prominent. On subsequent evaluation, an ear, nose, and throat specialist documented nystagmus, and he was diagnosed with a vestibular injury and "likely [mefloquine] toxicity." Brainstem injury was suspected.

Upon learning that mefloquine could have been the cause of the soldier's behavior, the legal team proposed exposure to the drug as a defense against the charges of cowardice. The soldier's use of mefloquine was initially challenged by the US Army owing to lack of documentation of its prescription (an unfortunately common occurrence). However, the US Army conceded exposure to the drug when the soldier was able to demonstrate possession of his remaining tablets.

On being informed of the diagnosis of vestibular injury, in June 2004 the US Army terminated all legal action against the soldier.

Although causal attribution to mefloquine was never formally acknowledged, in April 2005 the soldier was temporarily medically retired. In August 2006, he was formally medically retired for his vestibular disorder and with a diagnosis of PTSD.

In subsequent years, many of his chronic symptoms of disequilibrium gradually improved following physical and vestibular rehabilitation, but over a decade after onset, he complains of being occasionally short-tempered and irritable and experiencing intermittent vertigo and photophobia.

19.2 Diagnostic Challenges

This case, widely covered in the contemporary media [6–9], vividly illustrates the challenges faced in correctly diagnosing acute mefloquine intoxication, given that its symptoms may readily mimic those of acute stress reaction or other disorders attributable to deployment stressors. To avoid missed diagnosis, mefloquine intoxication or its prodrome must be considered in any psychiatric differential diagnosis where mefloquine exposure is a possibility. As no available biomarkers, imaging, or objective testing modality has sufficient sensitivity to identify mefloquine intoxication in every setting, clinicians must be prepared to rely on details of history, clinical presentation, and the ruling out of other similar disorders for diagnosis.

In particular, in order to avoid a delayed or missed diagnosis and to minimize the risk of continued dosing seen in this case, providers should become familiar with the full range of symptoms associated with acute intoxication and its prodrome, and if these are observed, be prepared to immediately discontinue the medication and consider additional steps in management to mitigate the risk of lasting sequelae.

In retrospective cases, diagnosis may be aided through additional testing and specialist referrals as necessary, which may reveal objective and convergent evidence of chronic sequelae. Certain of these tests may be difficult to obtain except at specialized clinics, therefore frequently necessitating tertiary referral. While the chronic sequelae of mefloquine intoxication may potentially confound diagnosis of PTSD and other chronic neuropsychiatric disorders, particularly with the benefit of specialized testing certain presentations may provide sufficient specificity so as to confidently permit assigning the diagnosis even in the presence of these and other comorbidities, as described below.

19.2.1 Symptomatology

Accumulated experience suggests that where the presentation of mefloquine intoxication is not fulminant as in this case, intoxication may begin with a subtle prodrome that may present with a sense of unease [10] or impending doom and restlessness [11, 12], personality change [10], agoraphobia [13], or other phobias [14]. Prodromal symptoms of intoxication may also include vivid dreams [15], nightmares [15], or sleep disturbances [16], including hypersomnia and often-severe insomnia [17]. Such symptoms may not be easily recognized, or may be misattributed to other causes including common stressors [18].

Over time these prodromal symptoms may progress to a more acute intoxication. Commonly reported symptoms of acute mefloquine intoxication include anxiety [19], paranoia [19] and persecutory mania [20–24], panic attacks [25–27], emotional lability [12], and aggression [28]. Patients may also experience symptoms of psychosis [29] including magical thinking [30] and grandiose [31], persecutory [32] or religious [17, 33] thoughts and delusions, and auditory [10, 20, 33, 34], visual [15, 19, 34–36], and olfactory [37] hallucinations, although as with the case, not infrequently with some degree of preserved insight.

Where insight is preserved, certain patients, particularly within military or other occupational settings, may initially fail to report even very severe symptoms of psychosis, out of concern for stigma, loss of fellow unit members' confidence, or as demonstrated in this case, concern for legal or administrative repercussions, such as potential loss of security clearance.

Acute intoxication may also manifest as depression [15, 19, 25, 38, 39], with sadness [32], tearfulness [32], fatigue [17], malaise and lethargy [40], confusion [15, 19. 34, 41], and a sense of helplessness, hopelessness, or pessimism [32]. In certain cases, those suffering intoxication may also experience dissociative symptoms[13, 42] including derealization [10, 37, 43] and depersonalization [36, 43, 44].

Acute mefloquine intoxication may also manifest with temporospatial disorientation [10, 15, 36, 45–47], and explicit memory impairment, including retrograde and anterograde amnesia [48], and particularly with impairment of short-term, working, and verbal memory [19, 42], with corresponding disturbances in attention or concentration.

With implicit memory typically preserved [48], those affected by explicit memory impairment from mefloquine intoxication may nonetheless be able to continue to participate in complex learned actions [49]. In certain cases, patients may even demonstrate improved performance during certain rote tasks [50], but may later experience profound amnesia to their actions or to events occurring during their period of intoxication [48]. Symptoms of memory impairment may also limit the reliability and completeness of reporting of prodromal symptoms preceding acute intoxication, or limit the reliability of history on initial examination [36].

In certain patients, symptoms of intoxication may quickly progress to a profound delirium [51], which may result in the patient requiring intensive medical care. Intoxication may also present in a fulminant manner as seizures [52]. Each presentation may potentially mask other psychiatric symptoms of intoxication [53].

This accumulated experience with its symptomology further suggests that on initial presentation, those suffering from mefloquine intoxication may often appear to be suffering from a potentially bewildering range of plausible disorders spanning the psychiatric nosology, including acute anxiety, dissociative, depressive, manic, bipolar, psychotic, personality, conversion, and factitious disorders [1, 10, 54].

Rather than reflecting a purely psychiatric disorder triggered or unmasked by the drug, these symptoms of mefloquine intoxication and its prodrome should be considered as organic manifestations of an underlying progressive toxic encephalopathy affecting particularly the limbic system and brainstem [10]. While potentially acutely reversible, this encephalopathy may be associated with a risk of chronic psychiatric effects [30, 55] as well as additional neurological effects likely due to central nervous system (CNS) injury [4].

These neurological effects most typically include dizziness, vertigo, and nystagmus, but not uncommonly also include sleep disorders, photophobia, accommodative disorders, dysesthesias, paresthesias, and occasionally myoclonus or dyskinesias, dysarthrias, dysautonomias, central apnea, and esophageal and gastrointestinal dysmotility, many of which have been observed from brainstem toxicity in closely related quinoline-based drugs [4].

Recognition of these chronic sequelae, through the use of appropriate specialist referrals where necessary, may aid the psychiatrist in disentangling symptoms due to mefloquine from those due to common confounding and comorbid psychiatric disorders that may be prevalent in military and veteran populations.

19.2.2 Biomarkers

Notwithstanding previous creative theories to the contrary [56, 57], neither abnormal liver enzymes, thryoid hormone levels, nor levels of certain common metabolites reliably correlate with risk of intoxication.

Although dose-dependent mefloquine CNS toxicity may be predicted on theoretical grounds based on an abundance of in vivo and in vitro data [58, 59–63], no studies have directly correlated CNS effects with concentrations in brain, nor have threshold toxic CNS concentrations been clinically identified, although physiologically relevant effects may be expected even at the low CNS concentrations that may result from administration of as little as a single tablet.

Additionally, as would be expected of a drug with highly variable neuropharmacokinetics [64], both blood [65, 66] and cerebrospinal fluid [67] (CSF) levels of the drug correlate poorly with those in CNS, and blood levels of mefloquine are not strongly correlated with risk of intoxication [45, 68–70].

For these reasons, quantitative determination of mefloquine concentrations in body fluids, including blood and CSF, should be considered useful only in ruling in exposure [54]. Owing to the extreme lipophilicity of the drug [71, 72], the relative quantitative insensitivity of many assays, and the drug's tendency to pool in organ tissue including brain [62, 73, 74] relative to body fluids, a negative mefloquine serum level may not rule out current or recent intoxicating concentrations in CNS.

Conversely, measurement of mefloquine metabolite levels in blood is not directly relevant clinically, as systemic metabolism may not directly predict CNS concentrations of the drug [74, 75]. Similarly, although genotyping, particularly of drug metabolic and transport enzyme genes [76], may be clinically useful to guide pharmacotherapy in the management of mefloquine intoxication, the genetic epidemiology of intoxication remains uncertain [54], and no gene, genotype or haplotype has yet been linked in confirmatory analysis to a risk of intoxication, despite promising early studies [77] and anecdotal clinical observations [78] implicating possible involvement of the *MDR1 (ABCB1)* gene in predicting susceptibility.

19.2.3 Imaging

No imaging modality has yet been identified that can reliably diagnose mefloquine intoxication [54]. Conventional neuroimaging such as computed tomography (CT) and magnetic resonance imaging (MRI) will typically be normal during acute intoxication [10, 54], although there is insufficient published evidence with functional MRI (fMRI) to rule out this modality being of utility [79]. Limited published evidence also suggests advanced imaging techniques such as single-photon emission tomography (SPET) or positron emission tomography (PET) may reveal evidence of abnormal brain functioning during acute intoxication [30, 80].

In retrospective diagnoses, particularly in cases with neurological sequelae where brain or brainstem injury may be suspected, structural imaging including higher-resolution MRI may eventually hold promise, although neurohistopathological evidence from animal models [63] and from earlier experience with related quinoline drugs [81] suggests neurotoxic injury from mefloquine, when it occurs, is likely to be microscopic and may affect only scattered regions of the CNS, possibly in a cell-type specific manner [4]. Normal results on routine brain imaging should therefore not be considered as ruling out prior intoxication or its chronic sequelae.

19.2.4 Neuropsychological Testing

Although clearly difficult to administer during acute intoxication, detailed neuropsychological testing may be useful in the differential diagnosis of prodromal symptoms of intoxication, and in retrospective diagnoses where chronic psychiatric neurocognitive sequelae may be predominant. Absent baseline testing prior to exposure, the interpretation of single test results either during the prodrome, acute intoxication, or most commonly in retrospective diagnosis, may prove challenging. Serial testing, particularly during the subacute period, may demonstrate mild improvements, although with potentially lasting deficits in tests of attention and concentration, auditory and visual memory, information processing speed, coordination, construction, verbal learning, and productivity [10, 15, 19].

19.2.5 Neurological, Neuro-Otologic, and Neuro-Optometric Testing

Although similarly difficult to administer during acute intoxication, when symptoms dictate, careful evaluation by specialists either during the prodromal period or more commonly during retrospective diagnosis may reveal objective evidence consistent with focal CNS toxic injury. Although gross neurologic motor and sensory evaluation by neurologists in most cases of intoxication is typically normal, evaluation by neuro-otologists, neuro-optometrists, neuro-ophthalmologists, or otorhinolaryngologists may reveal objective evidence consistent with central vestibular or oculogyric dysfunction [10].

Similarly, while surface electroencephalography (EEG) is typically normal after administration of mefloquine [82] and may even be normal in acute intoxication [36], there may be evidence of deep epileptiform or other abnormal activity [46, 83–85]. Similarly, advances in quantitative EEG and deep brain or limbic EEG modalities may hold promise in identifying changes in electrical activity during the prodrome, or associated with possible seizure foci related to neurotoxic injury to the brainstem and subcortical regions in retrospective diagnosis [86].

19.2.6 Additional Testing

When indicated, particularly during retrospective diagnosis, sleep studies may reveal evidence of central apnea or parasomnias [15]. Similarly, in patients with altered speech [15] or esophageal dysmotility, evaluation by speech language pathologists may be appropriate. Insufficient evidence exists to recommend routine neuroendocrine screening, although the drug's accumulation [74] and physiological activity on the hypothalamus [87] provides a plausible mechanism for certain chronic endocrine disorders that may develop after mefloquine exposure.

19.2.7 Coding and Documentation

Acute mefloquine intoxication does not yet have a unique diagnostic code, either in the International Classification of Diseases (ICD) version 9 Clinical Modification (ICD-9-CM) or version 10 Clinical Modification (ICD-10-CM), creating challenges both for the proper coding and documentation of the disorder, and in its surveillance using administrative data systems, such as those commonly used in the military [88].

In the ICD-10 coding system, the series of codes T37.2X5 ("Adverse effect of antimalarials and drugs acting on other blood protozoa"), including T37.2X5S ("sequela"), are technically accurate as primary diagnoses both for acute and subacute intoxication and its chronic effects, but each code may fail to adequately communicate the clinical nature of the intoxication. This lack of specificity may require additional coding to specify the effects of mefloquine acting as a psychoactive substance. Owing to the complexity of the ICD-10 coding system, particularly for drug adverse event reporting [89], further discussion of or recommendations for such coding is deferred.

In contrast, in legacy coding systems, any of the small range of ICD-9-CM codes specified under ICD-9-CM series 292 ("Drug-induced mental disorders") may be appropriate for use as a primary diagnosis, depending on the nature of observed symptoms. For example, ICD-9-CM 292.84 ("Drug-induced mood disorder") or ICD-9-CM 292.11 ("Drug-induced psychotic disorder with delusions") may each be appropriate for diagnosis, depending on the presentation of the acute intoxication. Similarly, subacute or chronic effects may be specified through the use of ICD-9-CM 909.5 ("Late effect of adverse effect of drug, medicinal or biological substance").

However, as these codes are not specific to antimalarials or to mefloquine, in order to aid in surveillance, and to acknowledge the imperfectly specified nature of existing diagnoses assigned to the condition, the ICD-9-CM E-code E931.4 ("Antimalarials and drugs acting on other blood protozoa causing adverse effects in therapeutic use") should also be considered for patients in whom intoxication is suspected.

Although many of the symptoms of mefloquine intoxication may mimic a range of psychiatric disorders, regardless of the coding system used, care should be taken in documentation to not to assign a secondary psychiatric diagnosis where this is excluded by current criteria. For example, a significant change to the diagnostic criteria for PTSD in DSM-5 now excludes the diagnosis if it may be "attributable to the physiological effects of a substance (e.g., medication, alcohol) or another medical condition" [90]. As many of the acute and chronic effects of mefloquine intoxication may mimic almost perfectly this condition [1], the psychiatrist should only consider documenting the diagnosis of PTSD if there is clear evidence of an adequate external traumatic etiology separate from the frequently traumatic effects of mefloquine intoxication.

Similarly, while other formal psychiatric diagnoses without such clear exclusion criteria may appear appropriate, assigning certain of these diagnoses risks confusion in communicating etiology, which may result in inappropriate or ineffective attempts at treatment. Until consensus is achieved in defining formal diagnostic criteria for the intoxication syndrome, the psychiatrist evaluating a patient with mefloquine intoxication or its chronic sequelae should select only those additional psychiatric diagnoses (frequently, those "not otherwise specified") that adequately describe the observed phenomenology while emphasizing its organic etiology.

19.3 Prevention

Presumably in recognition of the lasting risks associated with acute intoxication, ever since the drug's initial licensing in 1989, the US mefloquine product insert has included language warning that "if signs of unexplained anxiety, depression, restlessness, or confusion are noticed, these may be considered prodromal to a more serious event," and has cautioned that should these prodromal symptoms occur, "[i]n these cases, the drug must be discontinued" [54].

Certain users of mefloquine will discontinue use of the drug at the onset of the unsettling prodromal symptoms of intoxication, thus minimizing the number of cases of acute intoxication experienced during prophylactic use. However, as documented rates of discontinuation in military cohorts are significantly lower than the proportion reporting prodromal symptoms [91], military cohorts may be at particular risk of acute intoxication and its chronic sequelae.

For example, among those with a history of certain preexisting neuropsychiatric disorders [92], these symptoms may be erroneously attributed to such disorders or be obscured or confounded by psychotropic drug use [15]. Since 2002, mefloquine has therefore been absolutely contraindicated among those with a current or recent history of psychiatric illness [93], as these users may be at greater risk of failing to discontinue mefloquine as the product insert directs. The manufacturer has similarly cautioned that mefloquine "should not be prescribed for prophylaxis in patients with active depression, a recent history of depression, generalized anxiety disorder, psychosis, or schizophrenia or other major psychiatric disorders" [94]. However, in a recent military cohort, the prevalence of these and other neuropsychiatric contraindications to mefloquine use was approximately one in ten [92], and among these, approximately one in seven may have nonetheless been prescribed the drug [95].

Even among those without contraindications, patients must be clearly informed that neuropsychiatric symptoms that develop during mefloquine use could be evidence of a progressive intoxication that requires the immediate discontinuation of the drug. Prior to the black box warning, such neuropsychiatric symptoms were commonly attributed by influential authorities to other causes and not always appreciated as evidence of toxicity [18, 96–99]. However, even often subtle or overlooked symptoms such as nightmares or vivid dreams [100, 101], and sleep disturbance or insomnia [102] have been listed on various mefloquine product inserts or prescribing guidance as requiring the immediate discontinuation of the medication. Current US guidance makes it clear that "if psychiatric or neurologic symptoms occur, the drug should be discontinued" [103].

According to recent guidance provided by the manufacturer [104], symptoms of abnormal dreaming or disturbed sleep may occur in greater than 10% of the users, and symptoms of depression or anxiety may occur in 1–10% of the users. In randomized controlled trials, neuropsychiatric symptoms that were consistent with prodromal symptoms of intoxication occurred in 29% of the users [105]. In contrast, military guidance as recently as 2009 erroneously stated, the risk of "psychiatric symptoms" with mefloquine use was only "1 per 2000–13,000 persons" [106], or over 1000 times lower than the true value, further complicating compliance with product insert guidance in military settings.

As symptoms of mefloquine intoxication or its prodrome may progress to include anxiety and paranoia [10], in settings such as the military where drug adherence has traditionally been emphasized, such symptoms of anxiety and paranoia may heighten fear of malaria or of judicial and nonjudicial penalties for nonadherence. As a result, even patients who have received adequate education who experience intoxication may fail to comply with product insert guidance to discontinue the medication, and may continue taking the drug despite the awareness of toxicity.

Similarly, as symptoms of confusion may make remembering and complying with mefloquine product insert guidance challenging [48], in military settings, the prescribing clinician should complement patient counseling by ensuring that the patient's military chain of command, particularly those individuals in the deployed environment, is trained in the recognition of the signs and symptoms of mefloquine intoxication, which in prior military settings, as illustrated in the case, have been incorrectly attributed to cowardice or to potentially stigmatizing conditions.

As some prodromal intoxication may be identified during early use of the drug [107], the prescribing clinician should strongly consider a "test prescription" of mefloquine by limiting initial prescription of the drug to a small number of tablets. During this period, prior to prescribing the remaining tablets for deployment [108], the patient should be evaluated regularly and carefully for the development of prodromal symptoms. Where deployment dates are known in advance, and as mefloquine can take 7–10 weekly doses to build protective and steady-state serum concentrations [109], such a period of pre-deployment dosing with careful observation should be considered both to minimize the risk that intoxication may occur and be unrecognized during remote deployments, as well as to improve the effectiveness of the drug.

Even with such precautions, both the clinician and the chain of command must be aware of the possibility that the service member may need to immediately discontinue the medication while remotely deployed. Under the current US military policy that restricts the use of mefloquine to a "drug of last resort" [110, 111], typically no other prophylactic medications would be available to switch to in the event where prodromal symptoms develop. In areas that are highly endemic for malaria, this may require the patient's evacuation to minimize risks when mefloquine is discontinued. Although in remote malaria-endemic areas, it may seem appealing for the chain of command or the clinician to recommend continuing the use of mefloquine even in the presence of prodromal symptoms, the risks articulated in the US product insert of serious and long-lasting psychiatric symptoms and permanent neurological effects with continued dosing make such a recommendation distinctly unwise [103].

Although appropriate recognition and management of prodromal symptoms is a critical component in the prevention of acute intoxication, symptoms consistent with acute intoxication, its prodrome, and its chronic sequelae have been reported after only a single 250-mg tablet [10, 112]. Therefore, even such careful steps will merely minimize, but will not eliminate, the risk of adverse effects from the drug, and clinicians choosing to administer mefloquine must be prepared to recognize and appropriately treat and manage acute cases of intoxication when they occur.

19.4 Management

The management of acute mefloquine intoxication relies on proper diagnosis and should primarily be conservative in nature. The goals of such management should be to encourage the elimination of the drug while minimizing the risk of further acute harm that may occur through psychopolypharmacy or through inattention to appropriate care precautions. Similarly, in subacute to chronic cases, management should also be conservative, with goals focused on rehabilitation and management of disability and avoidance of inappropriate, ineffective, or potentially harmful treatments that may arise through missed diagnosis.

19.4.1 Pharmacotherapy of Acute Intoxication

There are no clinical trials reported in the medical literature investigating management of acute intoxication, although typical case reports describe attempts at treatment primarily with antipsychotic drugs [34, 37, 42, 49]. Psychotic symptoms may be the most striking observed during acute intoxication and may appear to indicate treatment with antipsychotics. However, as the most severe psychotic symptoms associated with cases of acute intoxication appear to be mostly self-limiting even without medication [28, 29, 37, 113], and as psychopolypharmacy may carry a risk of further harm, conservative management may be a more appropriate management strategy.

Specifically, the indiscriminate use of antipsychotic drugs may be problematic owing to the potential for drug–drug interactions. As growing evidence implicates abnormal mefloquine neuropharmacokinetics in the etiology of intoxication [64], drugs that may affect metabolism of mefloquine, or that may risk slowing or delaying its efflux from brain [65], may plausibly increase the risk of chronic sequelae.

For these reasons, as with intoxication with related quinoline antimalarials [114], avoidance of antipsychotics which are substrates of common CNS drug transport and metabolism enzymes appears warranted except in cases where their likely benefits clearly exceed these plausible risks.

Point-of-care pharmacogenetic testing [76], which may identify abnormal drug metabolism and transport phenotypes [115, 116], may provide clinicians information to guide the safer use of such drugs. However, as the pathophysiology of mefloquine intoxication is likely multifactorial rather than strictly limited to isolated dopaminergic dysfunction, the desire for rational drug therapy and the avoidance of psychopolypharmacy may make other treatments more desirable.

For example, as mefloquine and its metabolite are primarily excreted in bile and feces, with very little excreted in urine [71–73, 117], a very rational management strategy for mefloquine intoxication is the promotion of rapid bile excretion to produce a consequent reduction in body stores of the drug. Bile acid sequesterants such as cholestyramine and colesevalem, which would be expected to significantly reduce the enterohepatic recirculation of mefloquine and promote its fecal excretion, should be considered early in therapy to reduce total body drug burden.

Similarly, the use of rifampin to promote the drug's metabolism and transport from brain may be argued both on empirical and theoretical grounds. Rifampin significantly reduces concentrations of mefloquine in blood [118], suggesting efficacy in speeding overall metabolism or excretion. Rifampin is also a known inducer of permeability glycoprotein (P-gp), a major mefloquine drug transporter [65, 119] at locations including within the blood–brain barrier [120]. Rifampin is also an inducer of various cytochrome P450 (CYP) enzymes including CYP3A4 involved in the drug's metabolism [118]. Induction of these pathways through the use of rifampin may therefore act to speed the overall elimination of mefloquine from CNS.

Any therapy aimed at encouraging the drug's excretion, transport, and metabolism in this manner should be accompanied as much as is practicable by avoidance of other P-gp and CYP substrates that may compete for transport of the drug across the blood–brain barrier or compete for its metabolism, as well by avoidance of inhibitors which might antagonize induction and action of P-gp [65, 121]. Although many psychotropic drugs fall into this category [122, 123], other nonpsychiatric drugs, in particular loperamide and other opioids [124], certain other anti-infectives [125, 126], and most other quinoline-derivative antimalarials [127, 128] should be avoided as much as is practical for the duration of acute intoxication.

Where psychopharmacotherapy is deemed necessary for management of behavior or symptoms, among the most interesting potential targets for therapy may be the central cholinergic system. Mefloquine inhibits cholinesterases [129], and a limited number of case reports describe the successful and very rapid reversal of symptoms of acute mefloquine intoxication and intoxication with related quinoline drugs with physostigmine [51, 130]. Similarly, although typically used only in response to mefloquine seizures, valproic acid may be more broadly considered for use in management for its demonstrated efficacy in managing agitation and psychotic symptoms associated with acute confusional states [131, 132], and for its potential neuroprotective properties [133, 134].

19.4.2 Care Precautions During Acute Intoxication

Acute mefloquine intoxication is associated with a morbid curiosity towards violence and death [135]. Together with symptoms of mania, dissociation, and psychosis, these effects may explain the strong association of acute mefloquine intoxication with reported acts of violence [136, 137], compulsive suicidal ideation [25], and impulsive [138] and particularly grizzly acts of suicide [139]. Acute intoxication must therefore be considered a potentially life-threatening condition [140]. Particularly during acute intoxication where symptoms of psychosis, dissociation, confusion, and impaired memory may be present, patients should be closely supervised in an inpatient setting with appropriate care precautions until these symptoms have been deemed to be fully resolved on careful serial evaluation.

19.4.3 Subacute Intoxication and Chronic Sequelae

Insights from regulatory post-marketing surveillance [108, 141], as well as case reports [10, 30, 112, 142] and published cohort studies [55] clearly establish the presence of a period of subacute intoxication and a risk of chronic sequelae that outlast the drug's likely continued presence in the body. Although certain subacute symptoms may be due to the drug's prolonged retention in CNS, chronic psychiatric symptoms, particularly lasting cognitive impairment [55], almost certainly share a mechanism in common with those of other neurotoxicants in reflecting changes in CNS structure and function [4], rather than a persistent directly intoxicating effect of the drug.

Results of studies of related quinoline drugs suggest the possibility of injury to the hippocampus [143, 144], development of temporal lobe epilepsy [145], and injury to regions of the brainstem including the vestibular nuclei [81, 146–148], all of which may plausibly contribute to psychiatric symptoms. The pathophysiology of certain other chronic symptoms, such as dissociation [44], nightmares [55], and changes in personality [10], is less clear but likely also shares a common etiology. Knowledge of the common presentation of subacute and chronic symptoms may aid the clinician in disentangling those due to other potentially confounding neuropsychiatric disorders including PTSD from those due to mefloquine intoxication, and may assist the clinician in ensuring their more appropriate management.

In particular, the chronic central vestibular dysfunction not uncommonly caused by mefloquine can be both diagnostic, and particularly disabling, and thus should be considered early in the evaluation and management of patients [10]. Even when obvious vestibular symptoms are not acutely present, subtle vestibular dysfunction may result in cognitive deficits [149] and anxiety [150], and may result in agoraphobic avoidance of certain environments that may trigger vestibular symptoms and subsequent panic [151, 152].

Common triggers may include flashing or fluorescent lights, rapid vertical or horizontal visual motion which may occur with certain head movements or in busy crowds, and during certain forms of travel such as overbridges or in airplanes, where visual flickering or loss of a visual horizon may be acutely destabilizing. Common comorbid visual disorders including accommodative dysfunction and photophobia may also contribute to this morbidity, as may chronic sensory abnormalities including paresthesias and dysesthesias. For these reasons, definitive diagnosis of any central disorders and subsequent consultation with an experienced vestibular rehabilitative specialist with experience with acquired injury may assist the patient in learning to recognize such triggers, and in developing strategies to mitigate their effects. In certain cases, relatively simple interventions, such as wearing sunglasses, or walking with a cane, may significantly decrease anxiety and irritability associated with this dysfunction.

Where chronic psychopharmacotherapy is considered necessary to complement these more conservative management strategies, the clinician should bear in mind that although the symptoms of chronic sequelae may be similar to those of certain psychiatric disorders, their underlying pathophysiology may be quite distinct from that of the disorder for which a particular drug is indicated to treat. The clinician should also recognize the possible contribution of the patient's genotype, particularly of drug metabolic and transport enzyme genes [77], in contributing to the etiology of the original intoxication, and the possible impact of polymorphisms in these genes also affecting treatment response and tolerability.

19.5 Conclusions

This chapter has demonstrated that mefloquine intoxication may mimic a number of neuropsychiatric disorders common among recent veterans, including PTSD. While exposure to traumatic events that may induce these disorders can seem ubiquitous in combat settings, in many deployed environments, the prevalence of such exposures may be less than the prevalence of exposure to mefloquine, significantly affecting diagnostic considerations.

Specifically, in settings where mefloquine exposure cannot be ruled out, any appropriate psychiatric or neurological symptoms that develop approximately coincident with mefloquine use, or that evolve in the months following exposure, should be considered possible evidence of prior intoxication, even if prodromal symptoms are not documented or remembered by the patient. Conversely, in cases where exposure to traumatic events has been ruled out, but where certain chronic symptoms appear to mimic those of PTSD, the clinician must avoid hastily assigning a diagnosis of malingering, or conversion or factitious disorder, which may have been considered to explain previously unexplained symptoms.

The known deleterious population effects of other neurotoxicants raise questions as to whether even subclinical intoxication with mefloquine, or seemingly inconsequential symptoms of prodromal intoxication, such as vivid dreaming, may also be associated with a risk of chronic sequelae independent of the development of more serious prodromal or acute effects. Although published reports describing lasting symptoms from mefloquine typically only report prior symptoms consistent with acute intoxication, this association may merely reflect the effects of ascertainment bias. Mefloquine has been a common exposure among deployed military personnel since the drug's widespread use beginning in the early 1990s, but the potential effects of exposure and subclinical intoxication on patterns of outpatient care or on measures of psychological health have not previously been evaluated in population-based studies.

Mefloquine intoxication stands to emerge as a significant potential confounder in understanding the health effects of recent wars, and should be considered alongside PTSD as an additional signature disorder of this era. In light of the recent boxed warning, clinicians and researchers in the field must ensure that a thorough mefloquine exposure assessment is conducted during encounters with veterans from this period, and that the acute, subacute, and chronic effects of the drug are properly and fully explained to the veteran, and considered both during clinical evaluation and care, and in research studies of chronic neuropsychiatric health problems affecting this population.

References

1. Nevin RL. Mefloquine and posttraumatic stress disorder. In: Ritchie EC, ed. Textbook of military medicine. Forensic and ethical issues in military behavioral health. Washington, DC: Borden Institute; 2015:277–96.
2. Magill A, Cersovsky S, DeFraites R. Special considerations for US military deployments. CDC Yellow Book—Travelers' Health Chapter 8. http://wwwnc.cdc.gov/travel/yellowbook/2014/chapter-8-advising-travelers-with-specific-needs/special-considerations-for-us-military-deployments (2014). Accessed 8 May 2015.
3. Walter Reed Army Institute of Research. Neurotoxicity associated with mefloquine, an anti-malarial drug: small business technology transfer (STTR) solicitation topic number A06-T034 (Army). http://www.dodsbir.net/sitis/archives_display_topic.asp?Bookmark=28959. (2006). Accessed 8 May 2015.
4. Nevin RL. Idiosyncratic quinoline central nervous system toxicity: historical insights into the chronic neurological sequelae of mefloquine. Int J Parasitol Drugs Drug Resist. 2014;4(2):118–25.
5. U.S. Food and Drug Administration. Release P03–52. FDA creates medication guide for Lariam. 2003.
6. Laskas JM. The coward. Gentlem Q. 2004;74:106–112, 159–161.
7. Fleet M. Case dropped against U.S. soldier initially accused of cowardice. CNN.com. http://edition.cnn.com/2004/US/07/15/army.dropped.charges/. (2004). Accessed 8 May 2015.
8. Brant M. War stories: drugging the troops. Newsweek. 2004 Jan 9. Accessed 8 May 2015.
9. Associated Press. Hallucinations linked to drug given to troops. MSNBC.com. February 14. http://www.nbcnews.com/id/6947472/ns/health-mental_health/t/hallucinations-linked-drug-given-troops/. (2005). Accessed 8 May 2015.
10. Nevin RL. Limbic encephalopathy and central vestibulopathy caused by mefloquine: a case report. Travel Med Infect Dis. 2012;10(3):144–51.
11. Clattenburg RN, Donnelly CL. Case study: neuropsychiatric symptoms associated with the antimalarial agent mefloquine. J Am Acad Child Adolesc Psychiatry. 1997;36(11):1606–08. Accessed 8 May 2015.
12. Kukoyi O, Carney CP. Curses, madness, and mefloquine. Psychosomatics. 2003;44(4):339–41.
13. Barrett PJ, Emmins PD, Clarke PD, Bradley DJ. Comparison of adverse events associated with use of mefloquine and combination of chloroquine and proguanil as antimalarial prophylaxis: postal and telephone survey of travellers. BMJ 1996;313(7056):525–8.
14. Colebunders R. Cured of fear of flying. Travel Med infect Dis. 2011;9(2):82.
15. Peterson AL, Seegmiller RA, Schindler LS. Severe neuropsychiatric reaction in a deployed military member after prophylactic mefloquine. Case Rep Psychiatry. 2011;2011:350417.
16. Van Riemsdijk MM, van der Klauw MM, van Heest JA, et al. Neuro-psychiatric effects of antimalarials. Eur J Clin Pharmacol. 1997;52(1):1–6.
17. Tran TM, Browning J, Dell ML. Psychosis with paranoid delusions after a therapeutic dose of mefloquine: a case report. Malar J. 2006;5:74.
18. Schlagenhauf P, Steffen R. Neuropsychiatric events and travel: do antimalarials play a role? J Travel Med. 2000;7(5):225–6.
19. Javorsky DJ, Tremont G, Keitner GI, Parmentier AH. Cognitive and neuropsychiatric side effects of mefloquine. J Neuropsychiatry Clin Neurosci. 2001;13(2):302.
20. Gascón J, Almeda J, Corominas N, Corachán M. Severe neuropsychiatric reaction following mefloquine use. Med Clin. 1993;101(13):515–6.
21. Tor PC, Lee HY, Tan CH. Mefloquine-induced mania in a 22-year-old Chinese man. Singap Med J. 2006;47(6):549–50.
22. Piening RB, Young SA. Mefloquine-induced psychosis. Ann Emerg Med. 1996;27(6):792–3.
23. Eaton L. Adverse reactions. Nurs Times 1996;92(24):16–7.
24. Thapa R, Biswas B. Childhood mefloquine-induced mania and psychosis: a case report. J Child Neurol. 2009;24(8):1008–9.

25. Caillon E, Schmitt L, Moron P. Acute depressive symptoms after mefloquine treatment. Am J Psychiatry. 1992;149(5):712.
26. De Gennes C, Colas C, Nollet D, et al. Panic attack after therapeutic administration of mefloquine. Ann Med Interne. 1991;142(8):631.
27. Borruat FX, Nater B, Robyn L, Genton B. Prolonged visual illusions induced by mefloquine (Lariam): a case report. J Travel Med. 2001;8(3):148–9.
28. Amraoui A, Burgos V, Alexandre JY. Acute psychosis following mefloquine therapy: a case report. Med Mal Infect. 1998;28:678–9.
29. Sowunmi A, Adio RA, Oduola AM, Ogundahunsi OA, Salako LA. Acute psychosis after mefloquine. Report of six cases. Trop Geogr Med. 1995;47(4):179–80.
30. Meszaros K, Kasper S. Psychopathological phenomena in long-term follow-up of acute psychosis after preventive mefloquinine (Lariam) administration. Nervenarzt. 1996;67(5):404–6.
31. Brumbaugh M, Price P, Fagan N, Hsieh H. Psychotic mania associated with mefloquine in a bipolar patient. South Med J. 2008;101(5):550–1.
32. Lebain P, Juliard C, Davy JP, Dollfus S. Neuropsychiatric symptoms in preventive antimalarial treatment with mefloquine: apropos of 2 cases. Encephale. 2000;26(4):67–70.
33. Croft AM, World MJ. Neuropsychiatric reactions with mefloquine chemoprophylaxis. Lancet. 1996;347(8997):326.
34. Folkerts H, Kuhs H. Psychotic episode caused by prevention of malaria with mefloquine. A case report. Nervenarzt. 1992;63(5):300–2.
35. Stuiver PC, Ligthelm RJ, Goud TJ. Acute psychosis after mefloquine. Lancet. 1989;2(8657):282.
36. Recasens C, Zittoun C, Féline A. A psychotic episode in a patient coming home from Africa: the possible role of mefloquine. Ann Psychiatry. 1993;8(2):100–3.
37. Hollweg M, Soyka M, Greil W. Mefloquine-induced psychoses—problems in etiologic classification based on 2 case reports. Psychiatr Prax. 1995;22(1):33–6.
38. Even C, Friedman S, Lanouar K. Bipolar disorder after mefloquine treatment. J Psychiatry Neurosci. 2001;26(3):252–3.
39. Oueriagli Nabih F, Touhami M, Laffinti A, Abilkacem L. Mood disorder after malaria prophylaxis with mefloquine (two case reports). Encephale. 2011;37(5):393–6.
40. Perry IC. Malaria prophylaxis. BMJ. 1995;310(6995):1673.
41. Minei-Rachmilewitz T. Neuropsychiatric side effects of malarial prophylaxis with mefloquine (Lariam). Harefuah. 1999;137(1–2):25–7, 87.
42. Krüger E, Grube M, Hartwich P. Acute paranoid hallucinatory psychosis following mefloquine prophylaxis (Lariam). Psychiatr Prax. 1999;26(5):252–4.
43. McEvoy K, Anton B, Chisolm MS. Depersonalization/derealization disorder after exposure to mefloquine. Psychosomatics. 2014;56(1):98–102.
44. Nevin R. Organic depersonalization as a chronic sequela of mefloquine intoxication. Psychosomatics. 2015;56(1):103–5.
45. Hennequin C, Bourée P, Bazin N, Bisaro F, Feline A. Severe psychiatric side effects observed during prophylaxis and treatment with mefloquine. Arch Intern Med. 1994;154(20):2360–2.
46. Marsepoil T, Petithory J, Faucher JM, Ho P, Viriot E, Benaiche F. Encephalopathy and memory disorders during treatments with mefloquine. Rev Med Interne. 1993;14(8):788–91.
47. Carme B, Nevez G, Peguet C, Bories C, Andrejak M. Neuropsychiatric intolerance during mefloquine prophylaxis. 5 case reports. Med Mal Infect. 1996;26:728–9.
48. Nevin RL. A Memoir of Mefloquine Amnesia: a review of the answer to the riddle is me by David Stuart MacLean. AJOB Neurosci. 2014;5(4):88–91.
49. Fuller SJ, Naraqi S, Gilessi G. Paranoid psychosis related to mefloquine antimalarial prophylaxis. P N G Med J. 2002;45(3–4):219–21.
50. Vuurman EF, Muntjewerff ND, Uiterwijk MM, et al. Effects of mefloquine alone and with alcohol on psychomotor and driving performance. Eur J Clin Pharmacol. 1996;50(6):475–82.
51. Speich R, Haller A. Central anticholinergic syndrome with the antimalarial drug mefloquine. New Engl J Med. 1994;331(1):57–8.
52. Gobbi F, Rossanese A, Buonfrate D, Angheben A, Postiglione C, Bisoffi Z. Epilepsy triggered by mefloquine in an adult traveler to Uganda. World J Clin Cases. 2014;2(1):12–5.

53. World Health Organization. Central nervous system reactions related to the antimalarial drug, mefloquine. WHO/MAL/89/1054; 1989:1–20.
54. Ritchie EC, Block J, Nevin RL. Psychiatric side effects of mefloquine: applications to forensic psychiatry. J Am Acad Psychiatry Law. 2013;41:224–35.
55. Ringqvist A, Bech P, Glenthøj B, Petersen E. Acute and long-term psychiatric side effects of mefloquine: a follow-up on Danish adverse event reports. Travel Med Infect Dis. 2015;13(1):80–8.
56. Mawson A. Mefloquine use, psychosis, and violence: a retinoid toxicity hypothesis. Med Sci Monit. 2013;19:579–83.
57. Croft AM, Herxheimer A. Adverse effects of the antimalaria drug, mefloquine: due to primary liver damage with secondary thyroid involvement? BMC Public Health. 2002;2:6.
58. Nevin RL. Mefloquine neurotoxicity and gap junction blockade: critical insights in drug repositioning. Neurotoxicology. 2011;32(6):986–7.
59. Hood JE, Jenkins JW, Milatovic D, Rongzhu L, Aschner M. Mefloquine induces oxidative stress and neurodegeneration in primary rat cortical neurons. Neurotoxicology. 2010;31(5):518–23.
60. Dow GS, Hudson TH, Vahey M, Koenig ML. The acute neurotoxicity of mefloquine may be mediated through a disruption of calcium homeostasis and ER function in vitro. Malar J. 2003;2:14.
61. Milatovic D, Jenkins JW, Hood JE, Yu Y, Rongzhu L, Aschner M. Mefloquine neurotoxicity is mediated by non-receptor tyrosine kinase. Neurotoxicology. 2011;32(5):578–85.
62. Dow GS, Milner E, Bathurst I, et al. Central nervous system exposure of next generation quinoline methanols is reduced relative to mefloquine after intravenous dosing in mice. Malar J. 2011;10:150.
63. Dow G, Bauman R, Caridha D, et al. Mefloquine induces dose-related neurological effects in a rat model. Antimicrob Agents Chemother. 2006;50(3):1045–53.
64. Nevin RL. Neuropharmacokinetic heterogeneity of mefloquine in the treatment of progressive multifocal leukoencephalopathy. Intern Med. 2012;51(16):2257–7.
65. Barraud de Lagerie S, Comets E, Gautrand C, et al. Cerebral uptake of mefloquine enantiomers with and without the P-gp inhibitor elacridar (GF1210918) in mice. Br J Pharmacol. 2004;141(7):1214–22.
66. Jones R, Kunsman G, Levine B, Smith M, Stahl C. Mefloquine distribution in postmortem cases. Forensic Sci Int. 1994;68(1):29–32.
67. Pham YT, Nosten F, Farinotti R, White NJ, Gimenez F. Cerebral uptake of mefloquine enantiomers in fatal cerebral malaria. Int J Clin Pharmacol Ther. 1999;37(1):58–61.
68. Hessén-Söderman A, Bergenius J, Palme I, Bergqvist Y, Hellgren U. Mefloquine prophylaxis and hearing, postural control, and vestibular functions. J Travel Med. 1995;2(2):66–9.
69. Jaspers CA, Hopperus Buma AP, van Thiel PP, van Hulst RA, Kager PA. Tolerance of mefloquine chemoprophylaxis in Dutch military personnel. Am J Trop Med Hyg. 1996;55(2):230–4.
70. Schwartz E, Potasman I, Rotenberg M, Almog S, Sadetzki S. Serious adverse events of mefloquine in relation to blood level and gender. Am J Trop Med Hyg. 2001;65(3):189–92.
71. Rozman RS, Molek NA, Koby R. The absorption, distribution, and excretion in mice of the antimalarial mefloquine, erythro-2,8-bis(trifluoromethyl)-alpha-(2-piperidyl)-4-quinolinemethanol hydrochloride. Drug Metab Dispos. 1978;6(6):654–8.
72. Mu JY, Israili ZH, Dayton PG. Studies of the disposition and metabolism of mefloquine HCl (WR 142,490), a quinolinemethanol antimalarial, in the rat. Limited studies with an analog, WR 30,090. Drug Metab Dispos. 1975;3(3):198–210.
73. Chung H, Jimmerson VR, Rozman RS, Sanders JE. Disposition of the diastereoisomer of mefloquine in mice. Pharmacology. 1982;24(5):267–74.
74. Baudry S, Pham YT, Baune B, et al. Stereoselective passage of mefloquine through the blood-brain barrier in the rat. J Pharm Pharmacol. 1997;49(11):1086–90.
75. Schwartz DE, Weber W, Richard-Lenoble D, Gentilini M. Kinetic studies of mefloquine and of one of its metabolites, Ro 21–5104, in the dog and in man. Acta Trop. 1980;37(3):238–42.

76. Burmester JK, Sedova M, Shapero MH, Mansfield E. DMET microarray technology for pharmacogenomics-based personalized medicine. Method Mol Biol. 2010;632(1):99–124.
77. Aarnoudse ALHJ, van Schaik RHN, Dieleman J, et al. MDR1 gene polymorphisms are associated with neuropsychiatric adverse effects of mefloquine. Clin Pharmacol Ther. 2006;80(4):367–74.
78. Zaigraykina N, Potasman I. Polymorphism at the MDR1 locus as a cause of mefloquine-induced psychosis. Harefuah. 2010;149(9):583–4, 620, 619.
79. Van Essen TA, van der Giessen RS, Koekkoek SKE, et al. Anti-malaria drug mefloquine induces motor learning deficits in humans. Front Neurosci. 2010;4:191.
80. Ries S. Cerebral spasm during malaria prophylaxis with mefloquine. Dtsch Med Wochenschr. 1993;118(51–52):1911–2.
81. Loken AC, Haymaker W. Pamaquine poisoning in man, with a clinicopathologic study of one case. Am J Trop Med Hyg. 1949;29(3):341–52.
82. Potasman I, Juven Y, Weller B, Schwartz E. Does mefloquine prophylaxis affect electroencephalographic patterns? Am J Med 2002;112(2):147–9.
83. Bernard J, Le Camus J, Sarrouy J, et al. Toxic encephalopathy caused by mefloquine? Presse Med. 1987;16(33):1654–5.
84. Rønn AM, Bygbjerg IC. Acute brain syndrome after mefloquine treatment. Ugeskr Laeger. 1994;156(41):6044–5.
85. Lapras J, Vighetto A, Trillet M, Garin JP. Transient disorders of memory after a malaria attack. Caused by mefloquine? Presse Med. 1989;18(15):776.
86. World Health Organization. Neurotoxicity risk assessment for human health: principles and approaches. Environmental health criteria series, No. 223. World Health Organization. 2001.
87. Ohbuchi T, Yokoyama T, Saito T, et al. Possible contribution of pannexin channel to ATP-induced currents in vitro in vasopressin neurons isolated from the rat supraoptic nucleus. Brain Res. 2011;1394:71–8.
88. Rubertone MV, Brundage JF. The Defense Medical Surveillance System and the Department of Defense Serum Repository: glimpses of the future of public health surveillance. Am J Pub Health. 2002;92(12):1900–4.
89. Hohl CM, Karpov A, Reddekopp L, Stausberg J. ICD-10 codes used to identify adverse drug events in administrative data: a systematic review. J Am Med Inform Assoc. 2014;21:547–57.
90. American Psychiatric Association. Trauma- and stressor-related disorders. Diagnostic and statistical manual of mental disorders. 5th edn. Washington, DC: American Psychiatric Association; 2013.
91. Boudreau E, Schuster B, Sanchez J, et al. Tolerability of prophylactic Lariam regimens. Trop Med Parasitol. 1993;44(3):257–65.
92. Nevin RL, Pietrusiak PP, Caci JB. Prevalence of contraindications to mefloquine use among USA military personnel deployed to Afghanistan. Malar J. 2008;7:30.
93. Wooltorton E. Mefloquine: contraindicated in patients with mood, psychotic or seizure disorders. CMAJ. 2002;167(10):1147.
94. Hoffman-La Roche F. Dear Pharmacist Letter. September. http://www.fda.gov/downloads/Safety/MedWatch/SafetyInformation/SafetyAlertsforHumanMedicalProducts/UCM170905.pdf. (2002). Accessed 8 May 2015.
95. Nevin RL. Mefloquine prescriptions in the presence of contraindications: prevalence among US military personnel deployed to Afghanistan, 2007. Pharmacoepidemiol Drug Saf. 2010;19(2):206–10.
96. Lobel HO. Adverse health events and malaria prophylaxis. Healthwise (A newsletter for peace corps medical officers worldwide). 1996;5(2):1, 3–4.
97. Schlagenhauf P, Lobel H, Steffen R, et al. Tolerance of mefloquine by SwissAir trainee pilots. Am J Trop Med Hyg. 1997;56(2):235–40.
98. Schlagenhauf P. Mefloquine for malaria chemoprophylaxis 1992–1998: a review. J Travel Med. 1999;6(2):122–33.
99. Schlagenhauf P. Mefloquine, methodologies, and the media. J Travel Med. 1996;3(4):197–9.

100. Hoffman-La Roche F. Lariam patient monitoring card. France. August 7, 2013.
101. Hoffman-La Roche F. Lariam Guide to Healthcare Professionals. Ireland. July, 2013.
102. Hoffman-La Roche F. Lariam Dear Doctor Letter. Ireland. July, 2013.
103. U.S. Food and Drug Administration. FDA Drug Safety Communication: FDA approves label changes for antimalarial drug mefloquine hydrochloride due to risk of serious psychiatric and nerve side effects. July 29. http://www.fda.gov/Drugs/DrugSafety/ucm362227.htm. (2013). Accessed 8 May 2015.
104. Hoffman-La Roche F. Lariam Product Insert. Ireland, July 2013.
105. Overbosch D, Schilthuis H, Bienzle U, et al. Atovaquone-proguanil versus mefloquine for malaria prophylaxis in nonimmune travelers: results from a randomized, double-blind study. Clin Infect Dis. 2001;33(7):1015–21.
106. U.S. Army Office of the Surgeon General. Memorandum. Subject: Updated Guidance on the Use of Mefloquine for Malaria Prophylaxis. February 2. http://www.pdhealth.mil/downloads/DASG_Memorandum.pdf. (2009).
107. Stürchler D, Handschin J, Kaiser D, et al. Neuropsychiatric side effects of mefloquine. New Engl J Med. 1990;322(24):1752–3.
108. Levin A. FDA warning highlights mefloquine's mental health risks. Psychiatr News. 2013;48(18):1.
109. Whitman TJ, Coyne PE, Magill AJ, et al. An outbreak of *Plasmodium falciparum* malaria in U.S. Marines deployed to Liberia. Am J Trop Med Hyg. 2010;83(2):258–65.
110. Woodson J. Memorandum. Subject: Notification for Healthcare Providers of Mefloquine Box Warning. August 12, 2013.
111. Woodson J. HA Policy Memorandum 13–02: Guidance on Medications for Prophylaxis of Malaria. April 15. http://health.mil/libraries/HA_Policies_and_Guidelines/13-002.pdf. (2013). Accessed 8 May 2015.
112. Grupp D, Rauber A, Fröscher W. Neuropsychiatric disturbances after malaria prophylaxis with mefloquine. Aktuelle Neurol. 1994;21:134–6.
113. Sowunmi A. Acute psychosis after mefloquine: a case report. East Afr Med J. 1994;71(12):818–9.
114. Maxwell NM, Nevin RL, Stahl S, et al. Prolonged neuropsychiatric effects following management of chloroquine intoxication with psychotropic polypharmacy. Clin Case Rep. 2015;3(6):379–387.
115. De Leon J, Susce MT, Pan R-M, Fairchild M, Koch WH, Wedlund PJ. The CYP2D6 poor metabolizer phenotype may be associated with risperidone adverse drug reactions and discontinuation. J Clin Psychiatry. 2005;66(1):15–27.
116. Yoo H-D, Lee S-N, Kang H-A, Cho H-Y, Lee I-K, Lee Y-B. Influence of ABCB1 genetic polymorphisms on the pharmacokinetics of risperidone in healthy subjects with CYP2D6*10/*10. Br J Pharmacol. 2011;164(2b):433–43.
117. Jauch R, Griesser E, Oesterhelt G. Metabolism of Ro 21-5998 (mefloquine) in the rat. Arzneimittelforschung. 1980;30(1):60–7.
118. Ridtitid W, Wongnawa M, Mahatthanatrakul W, Chaipol P, Sunbhanich M. Effect of rifampin on plasma concentrations of mefloquine in healthy volunteers. J Pharm Pharmacol. 2000;52(10):1265–9.
119. De Lagerie SB, Fernandez C, German-Fattal M, Gantier J-C, Gimenez F, Farinotti R. Impact of cerebral malaria on brain distribution of mefloquine. Drug Metab Lett. 2009;3(1):15–7.
120. Bauer B, Yang X, Hartz AMS, et al. In vivo activation of human pregnane X receptor tightens the blood-brain barrier to methadone through P-glycoprotein up-regulation. Mol Pharmacol. 2006;70(4):1212–9.
121. Henry M, Alibert S, Rogier C, Barbe J, Pradines B. Inhibition of efflux of quinolines as new therapeutic strategy in malaria. Curr Top Med Chem. 2008;8(7):563–78.
122. Linnet K, Ejsing TB. A review on the impact of P-glycoprotein on the penetration of drugs into the brain. Focus on psychotropic drugs. Eur Neuropsychopharmacol. 2008;18(3):157–69.

123. O'Brien FE, Dinan TG, Griffin BT, Cryan JF. Interactions between antidepressants and P-glycoprotein at the blood-brain barrier: clinical significance of in vitro and in vivo findings. Br J Pharmacol. 2012;165(2):289–312.
124. Skarke C, Jarrar M, Schmidt H, et al. Effects of ABCB1 (multidrug resistance transporter) gene mutations on disposition and central nervous effects of loperamide in healthy volunteers. Pharmacogenetics. 2003;13(11):651–60.
125. Khaliq Y, Gallicano K, Tisdale C, Carignan G, Cooper C, McCarthy A. Pharmacokinetic interaction between mefloquine and ritonavir in healthy volunteers. Br J Clin Pharmacol. 2001;51(6):591–600.
126. Ridtitid W, Wongnawa M, Mahatthanatrakul W, Raungsri N, Sunbhanich M. Ketoconazole increases plasma concentrations of antimalarial mefloquine in healthy human volunteers. J Clin Pharm Ther. 2005;30(3):285–90.
127. Rijpma SR, van den Heuvel JJ, van der Velden M, Sauerwein RW, Russel FG, Koenderink JB. Atovaquone and quinine anti-malarials inhibit ATP binding cassette transporter activity. Malar J. 2014;13(1):359.
128. Kerb R, Fux R, Mörike K, et al. Pharmacogenetics of antimalarial drugs: effect on metabolism and transport. Lancet Infect Dis. 2009;9(12):760–74.
129. McArdle JJ, Sellin LC, Coakley KM, et al. Mefloquine inhibits cholinesterases at the mouse neuromuscular junction. Neuropharmacology. 2005;49(8):1132–9.
130. Summers WK, Allen RE, Pitts FN. Does physostigmine reverse quinidine delirium? West J Med. 1981;135(5):411–41.
131. Alam A, Puri NV. Inefficacy of antipsychotics in treatment of delirium and agitation in two cases of Bickerstaff brainstem encephalitis. J Neuropsychiatry Clin Neurosci. 2014;26(2):176–8.
132. Bourgeois JA, Koike AK, Simmons JE, Telles S, Eggleston C. Adjunctive valproic acid for delirium and/or agitation on a consultation-liaison service: a report of six cases. J Neuropsychiatry Clin Neurosci. 2005;17(2):232–8.
133. Lai JS, Zhao C, Warsh JJ, Li PP. Cytoprotection by lithium and valproate varies between cell types and cellular stresses. Eur J Pharmacol. 2006;539(1–2):18–26.
134. Monti B, Gatta V, Piretti F, Raffaelli SS, Virgili M, Contestabile A. Valproic acid is neuroprotective in the rotenone rat model of Parkinson's disease: involvement of alpha-synuclein. Neurotox Res. 2010;17(2):130–41.
135. Burke BM. Mefloquine. Lancet. 1993;341(8860):1605–6.
136. Prescrire International. Medication-induced violence towards others. Prescrire Int. 2014;23(150):153–5.
137. Moore TJ, Glenmullen J, Furberg CD. Prescription drugs associated with reports of violence towards others. PLoS ONE. 2010;5(12):e15337.
138. Scrip. Roche's Lariam linked to a suicide in UK. Scrip 1998;(2331):23.
139. Jousset N, Rougé-Maillart C, Turcant A, Guilleux M, Le Bouil A, Tracqui A. Suicide by skull stab wounds: a case of drug-induced psychosis. Am J Forensic Med Pathol. 2010;31(4):378–81.
140. Pharmaceutical Journal. BNF updates "suicide" warnings for mefloquine. Pharm J. 2013;291:620.
141. Prescrire International. Mefloquine: persistent vestibular disorders. Prescrire Int. 2014;23(150):157.
142. Lobel HO, Coyne PE, Rosenthal PJ. Drug overdoses with antimalarial agents: prescribing and dispensing errors. JAMA. 1998;280(17):1483.
143. Ismail T, Mauerhofer E, Slomianka L. The hippocampal region of rats and mice after a single i.p. dose of clioquinol: loss of synaptic zinc, cell death and c-Fos induction. Neuroscience. 2008;157(3):697–707.
144. Takeda a, Takada S, Ando M, et al. Impairment of recognition memory and hippocampal long-term potentiation after acute exposure to clioquinol. Neuroscience. 2010;171(2):443–50.

145. Ferrier TM, Schwieger AC, Eadie MJ. Delayed onset of partial epilepsy of temporal lobe origin following acute clioquinol encephalopathy. J Neurol Neurosurg Psychiatry. 1987;50(1):93–5.
146. Schmidt IG, Schmidt LH. Neurotoxicity of the 8-aminoquinolines; lesions in the central nervous system of the rhesus monkey induced by administration of plasmocid. J Neuropathol Exp Neurol. 1948;7(4):368–98.
147. Schmidt IG, Schmidt LH. Neurotoxicity of the 8-aminoquinolines; reactions of various experimental animals to plasmocid. J Comp Neurol. 1949;91(3):337–67.
148. Schmidt IG, Schmidt LH. Neurotoxicity of the 8-aminoquinolines. III. The effects of pentaquine, isopentaquine, primaquine, and pamaquine on the central nervous system of the rhesus monkey. J Neuropathol Exp Neurol. 1951;10(3):231–56.
149. Hanes DA, McCollum G. Cognitive-vestibular interactions: a review of patient difficulties and possible mechanisms. J Vestib Res. 2006;16(3):75–91.
150. Redfern MS, Furman JM, Jacob RG. Visually induced postural sway in anxiety disorders. J Anxiety Disord. 2007;21(5):704–16.
151. Jacob RG, Furman JM, Durrant JD, Turner SM. Panic, agoraphobia, and vestibular dysfunction. Am J Psychiatry. 1996;153(4):503–12.
152. Yardley L, Britton J, Lear S, Bird J, Luxon LM. Relationship between balance system function and agoraphobic avoidance. Behav Res Ther. 1995;33(4):435–9.

Polytrauma with Sexual Dysfunction in a Female Soldier Following IED Blast Exposure

20

Jonathan R. Dettmer, Shannon C. Ford and Kyle J. Gray

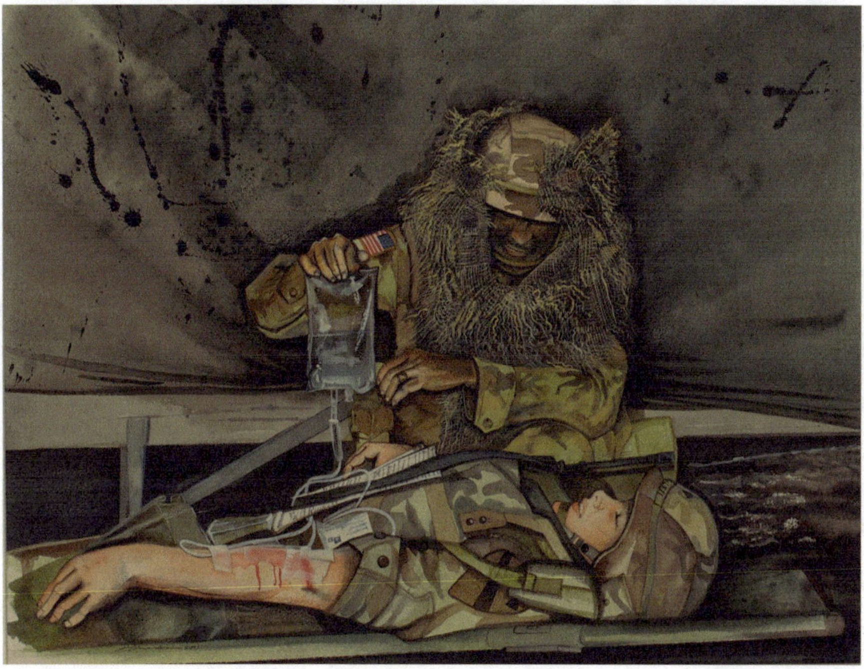

Combat Medic, by Msg. Henrietta Snowden, courtesy of the Army Art Collection, US Army Center of Military History.

J. R. Dettmer (✉)
2d Marine Regiment Psychiatrist, Camp Lejeune, Jacksonville, NC, USA
e-mail: dr.jdettmer@gmail.com

S. C. Ford · K. J. Gray
Department of Psychiatry, Walter Reed National Military Medical Center, Bethesda, MD, USA

E. C. Ritchie (ed.), *Posttraumatic Stress Disorder and Related Diseases in Combat Veterans,* DOI 10.1007/978-3-319-22985-0_20

Historically men comprised an overwhelming majority of military forces. As recently as the Vietnam conflict, only 2% of active duty forces were female [1]. In 2010 that figure had risen to approximately 15% [1, 2]. The 1994 Department of Defense Direct Ground Combat Definition and Assignment Rule (DGCDAR) prohibited women from serving in infantry or special operations units until recently [2]. So, despite the marked increase in female service members, women's specific exclusion from serving in units whose primary mission included combat jobs would lead one to expect the morbidity and mortality rates for women to remain very low. However, the amorphous battle space and guerilla techniques used during the Operation Iraqi Freedom and Operation Enduring Freedom (OIF/OEF) conflicts exposed personnel in supporting roles to more combat [1, 3]. In fact, over 160 casualties and 1000 wounded service members from the OIF/OEF conflicts have been women as a result of these shifts in service demography and fighting tactics [4].

Perineal injury and lower limb amputation have been described as the "signature injury" of veterans of the conflict in Afghanistan [5]. The injury pattern has replaced the more historic genitourinary injury of renal trauma in part due to the successful introduction of torso personal protective equipment and the coincident rise in improvised explosive device (IED) utilization by enemy forces [6]. While these injuries have been investigated in male soldiers to some degree, it has yet to be well examined in females. In this chapter, we use a case to discuss how amputation, perineal trauma, and genital injury may affect female veterans. Additionally, we explore the existence and characterization of gender differences in psychological symptoms secondary to combat experiences.

20.1 Case Presentation/History

A 22-year-old single female Army soldier with no prior psychiatric history presented with posttraumatic stress and depressive symptoms in the context of severe physical injuries. Private First Class (PFC) Anderson, a pseudonym, was in her usual state of good psychological health until riding in a convoy that was struck by an IED. She sustained immediate traumatic amputation of her distal lower extremities and injuries to her perineum. She reported a clear recollection of the events. Documentation after the blast indicates that she did not lose consciousness or show signs of altered mental status, until chemically sedated in the field prior to transport. Management of her wounds during progression of the medical evacuation system resulted in bilateral above the knee amputations and pelvic injuries. She had genital scarring but her urinary tract was repaired with only mild residual pelvic floor instability.

Surgical management and stints in the intensive care unit characterized the first two months after injury. During lucid periods she was stolid though adequately participative in care. However, at a major medical center 3 months post-injury, the surgical team managing her care noted low mood, poor participation in physical therapy, crying episodes, variable appetite, irritability, hopelessness, nightmares, irregular sleep cycles, intrusive recollections of the IED blast, and avoidance of reminders associated with the day of injury. She frequently asked her parents to leave her room and angrily refused their help with transfers and other activities despite continued limitations imposed by her injuries.

At the time of consultation she was taking calcium, vitamin D, pregabalin, acetaminophen, and oxycodone as needed for pain, which she described as well managed. Prosthetics had not yet been fitted due to continued wound healing. She later resumed menstrual cycles, although it was unclear if she retained reproductive capacity. The psychiatric consultation team was asked to evaluate PFC Anderson and specifically tasked with managing the psychological symptoms interfering with optimal participation in rehabilitative services.

PFC Anderson had previously been without other medical conditions. She denied a family history of psychiatric disorders. She grew up as the fourth of seven children to an intact family in the Western USA. She denied a history of physical, sexual, or emotional abuse. Among her hobbies, she had enjoyed staying active by jogging and participating in yoga. She completed high school on time with excellent grades. Immediately after graduating she enrolled in community college and worked as a yoga instructor. Her aspirations included becoming an athletic trainer, but first she wanted to attend university to receive her degree in a related field.

Due to the cost of college and her extended family's history of military service, she enlisted in the Army two years after high school to save money and gain access to education benefits. She intended to complete her initial four-year obligation and then get out of the service in order to raise a family.

This was her first deployment and she had no problems in her unit. She had two previous sexual partners in the context of committed relationships but was not dating at the time of her injury.

Mental status exam revealed a supine female with appropriate hygiene dressed in hospital attire. There were no alterations in her sensorium or abnormal behaviors. She displayed a dysthymic and restricted affect and minimal eye contact. She denied suicidal or homicidal ideations. Labs were normal, including hemoglobin, estrogen, cortisol, and thyroid stimulating hormone (TSH) levels.

20.1.1 Clinical Pearls

1. Establishing rapport is paramount in a consultative role. When a patient has been decimated by injuries, it would seem natural and appropriate to immediately focus on these. Rather, first inquire into and acknowledge their military service as a way of gaining rapport, especially if the mental health provider does not have a military background [7]. Chossing initial topics such as the service member's branch of service, military occupational specialty, and previous duty stations can facilitate history gathering.
2. A comprehensive assessment of mental health issues in women post-deployment should include asking about physical injuries as well as explicit evaluation for thoughts about suicide, depression, anxiety, PTSD, alcohol use, sleep disturbances, and military sexual trauma (MST) [2]. As with men, women might not volunteer information unless specifically asked.

20.1.2 Potential Pitfalls

1. Avoiding sensitive topics out of discomfort or fear of causing increased psychological injury. It is important to evaluate the whole person, including a discussion about sexual activity. Although not extensively studied in veteran populations with genital injury, women with injuries impacting sexual functioning generally expect sex education during rehabilitation [8].
2. Assuming that because the patient is female she has not been exposed to combat or gone through a life-changing experience. Deployment, separation from family, combat exposure, and a heightened concern of MST are all issues that commonly affect female veterans [2].

20.2 Assessment/Diagnosis

20.2.1 Somatic Polytrauma and the Respective Psychological Implications

Though the full extent of PFC Anderson's somatic injuries and their sequelae were uncertain, her case represented an increasingly common injury pattern.

20.2.1.1 Perineal injury

In American forces perineal injury from IED blast exposure has yet to be well studied. Prevalence data for this specific injury in the US military population is not readily available. An epidemiological study of musculoskeletal combat wounds from conflicts in Iraq and Afghanistan between 2005 and 2009 does not specifically quantify genital or perineal trauma, but found that soft tissue injuries to nearby regions of the thigh/hip and buttock accounted for 8.6 and 1.3 % of total musculoskeletal combat injuries, respectively [9]. Furthermore, this study found that pelvic fractures, which are often associated with perineal injury, combined with spinal fractures comprised 16.8 % of the total fractures sustained during combat.

One of the many obstacles PFC Anderson faced has been researched in civilians. Perineal injury can result in pelvic floor disorders that seem to have a dynamic relationship with depression and anxiety. For instance, in patients with pelvic organ prolapse, prevalence of depressive symptoms are reportedly high, while body image and multiple measures of quality of life have been found to be low [10–12]. These mental health implications also appear to adversely affect treatment outcomes. A study of 108 women in the UK observed that patients who benefitted most from the intervention of pelvic floor muscle training displayed absent or minimal anxiety or depression using subjective and objective measures of psychological health [13].

20.2.1.2 Sexual/Reproductive Functioning

The psychological impact of genital injuries has also yet to be adequately addressed in the literature. The few articles that address the mental health consequences of genital or perineal injuries exclusively examined men. For example, Lucas and colleagues interviewed thirteen male patients who suffered some degree of genital trauma while serving the British Army in Afghanistan between 2009 and 2011 (eleven with bilateral or triple amputations). Eight of the thirteen described their genital injury as more important than losing their legs. The authors explained this finding by noting that those eight patients felt a loss of gender identity associated with the loss of their testicles [14]. Additionally, the patients' ability to cope with these injuries depended on whether or not their fertility was preserved, either through sexual intercourse or artificial methods. Also highlighted were the expectations patients had to discuss their genital injuries with health-care professionals, despite the sensitivity of the topic [14].

While the literature on traumatic genital injury in women is lacking, research has shown that patients with spinal cord injury (SCI) face multiple barriers to sexual activity. In their study on Malaysian women with SCI, Julia and Othman noted that psychological factors such as perceived unattractiveness, lack of self-confidence, feelings of dependence, and concerns over satisfying their partners have been found to limit sexual activity more than physical impairments [8].

That study and the Lucas publication on male genital trauma both indicate that patients desired more information on sexually related matters such as fertility. In addition to recommending increased sexual counseling by health-care professionals, Julia and Othman described peer support groups as a "necessary" coping strategy due to the role models for recovery and decreased embarrassment while sharing intimate subjects with women managing the same problems [8].

20.2.1.3 Traumatic Amputation

As of 2014 more than 1500 US military personnel lost limbs in Iraq and Afghanistan [15]. The vast majority of amputees have been men, but dozens of women have also suffered from these injuries [7]. A qualitative study conducted by Cater has begun to shed some light on how women may cope with being affected by traumatic amputation. In her interviews with six soldiers who lost one or more limbs, four psychosocial adjustment variables were identified as important: grieving, body image, personal safety factors, and coping with the attitudes of others. These themes should be explored in patients like PFC Anderson. Factors that appear to aid in recovery included positive attitude, social support, personal courage, resiliency, military training, humor, and finding meaning in her limb loss [7].

While global quality-of-life measures are on average lower in the amputee community, the Cater study also touched upon the idea that traumatic limb loss is not necessarily a net negative experience for patients [7]. Several women reported that surviving the loss of a limb gave them new courage and made them stronger. Similarly, Benetato explored posttraumatic growth (PTG)—a positive psychological change experienced as a result of a struggle with a difficult life challenge—among OIF/OEF veterans who suffered combat-related amputation. She found a small but statistically significant correlation with higher levels of social support and a moderate-sized correlation between PTG and "rumination," defined as the "process of re-examining the beliefs that characterize one's assumptive world in light of an unexpected trauma [16]." Thus, fostering a supportive environment, in which the patient is encouraged to cognitively process the traumatic event and the resulting injury, is considered an important element of recovery and growth. As will be discussed in the treatment course, the consulting team's formulation of this patient directly informed the role of facilitated rumination for PFC Anderson.

Mental health professionals working with amputees should also be familiar with the process of emotional adaptation to limb loss. As noted by Belon and Vigoda in their review on this topic, grief is a natural and normal emotional response experienced by all amputees [17]. As such, grief resolution is a primary area of focus in treatment. They endorse the following coping strategies: relaxation training, proper diet and exercise, having an adequate support network, developing awareness of and addressing negative self-talk, and pacing physical recovery.

It is noteworthy that the authors proposed eye movement desensitization and reprocessing (EMDR)—an APA-endorsed treatment strategy for patients with PTSD—as a self-talk technique for reducing the power of emotionally charged memories [18]. Two small, uncontrolled studies have also demonstrated promising effects for using EMDR in the treatment of phantom limb pain [19, 20]. In patients with comorbid PTSD, traumatic amputation and phantom limb pain, EMDR is a reasonable treatment choice.

20.2.2 Gender Differences with PTSD

As previously noted the OIF/OEF conflicts represent the first time that military men's and women's occupations have overlapped to such an extent that their post-traumatic stress characteristics could be effectively compared. Overall, the limited number of available studies in veterans or active duty personnel have shown few consistent conclusions about gender differences in the development and manifestations of PTSD. The studies tend to be hampered by limitations, including using self-report data collection and cross-sectional design. Furthermore, while statistically significant differences have been noted, the clinical relevance of the variations is debatable. Table 20.1 summarizes recent findings comparing the etiology, rate of development, and presentation of PTSD symptoms for military personnel.

In the current military population, women are more likely than men to develop PTSD as a result of sexual assault, while men are comparatively more likely to have combat exposure as their index trauma [21, 22]. MST can be defined as "sexual harassment and sexual assault that occurs in the military environment," and meets the "A" criterion for PTSD when accompanied by violence or a threat of violence. A threat of violence may be more common in MST because military personnel often have combat training and access to firearms.

After leaving the service, 22 % of women noted being victimized from MST versus approximately 1 % for males [21]. Women that screen positive are five to nine times more likely to meet criteria for PTSD than those without MST [21, 22]. While the prevalence of MST among women appears to be increased compared to men, unexplored findings indicate that exposure to MST causes a comparatively higher rate of PTSD development in men versus women in the active duty population, but not the veteran population [21, 23].

Table 20.1 Suggested but inconclusive gender differences in PTSD trauma, susceptibility, and manifestations for veterans and military service members

	Women	Men
Primary trauma(s)	Sexual trauma, including MST [2, 21, 22]	Combat exposure/violence [22]
	Combat exposure [2]	
Rate of PTSD development	Equal for those with similar levels of overall combat exposure or recent deployment [3, 23, 24]	Active duty has a higher rate for those exposed to military sexual trauma [23]. This has not been the case in veteran populations [21]
	Higher than overall active duty personnel [23]	
Individual PTSD criteria and symptoms of other disorders	Symptoms including concentration problems and reminder distress may be more common [24]	Symptoms including nightmares, emotional numbing, and hypervigilance may be more common [23, 24]
	Higher levels of all factors for those exposed to the most violent aspects of wartime stressors, especially injury [22, 23]	Externalizing behaviors including alcohol abuse is more common [22]

One epidemiologic survey using the civilian PTSD checklist (PCL) included almost 25,000 active duty respondents. The study was conducted by Hourani and colleagues and found that women more frequently met criteria for PTSD and indicated higher distress on all four of the core factors of the disorder: reexperience, avoidance, emotional numbing, and hyperarousal [23]. However, in a *Journal of Abnormal Psychology* article, Vogt et al. identified no significant gender difference in the rate of PTSD development or symptom severity in those within 1 year of returning from an OIF/OEF deployment [3].

Furthermore, multiple studies have shown that when controlling for levels of combat exposure or recent deployment, male and female OIF/OEF veterans reported similar levels of symptoms [23, 24]. In the Hourani study combat exposure was defined as combat patrols, receiving incoming fire, encountering IEDs or mines, personally firing weapons at enemies, witnessing unit members being wounded or killed, suffering casualties within the unit, or knowing someone that was killed [23]. Women still reported significantly higher levels of self-reported symptoms in all four PTSD factors when there was exposure to "violence," which included participating in hand-to-hand fighting, being injured in combat, questioning detainees, or witnessing/engaging in acts of cruelty [23].

Studies have also compared men and women with respect to comorbid mental health disorders and individual symptoms of PTSD in military personnel. These studies have slight variations in the study population and instruments used for measuring severity levels, which might contribute to the differences in the results. Using military-PCL responses controlled for PTSD severity, King and colleagues found that post-deployment OIF/OEF male veterans more frequently suffered nightmares, emotional numbing, and hypervigilance while females had greater reminder distress and concentration problems [24]. Maguen, Luxton, Skopp, and Madden found no gender difference in PTSD symptoms in previously deployed service members, but women manifested higher depressive symptoms while men were found to have more substance abuse [22]. In the previously mentioned Hourani et al. study, men described higher alcohol use while women reported higher distress on 15 of 17 individual PTSD symptoms when exposed to the most violent aspects of war [23].

Even if meaningful gender differences in PTSD vulnerability or symptom manifestation exist, the reasons are not clear. The findings in a study by Nillni et al. imply that menstrual cycles may play a role [25]. Similar correlations between PTSD development and neurohormones released in response to stress show promise and studies are ongoing to investigate these potential relationships [26]. Ultimately, at this time no clear biological or psychological factor has been elucidated that satisfactorily explains these relationships between PTSD symptoms and gender [23]. Final conclusions may be difficult to construct but one hypothesis asserts that women may be more likely to meet DSM criteria because they are more likely to exhibit internalizing symptoms, whereas men more commonly manifest PTSD with externalizing behaviors [22, 23].

Applying these study results to PFC Anderson, they suggest that because of her gender she has a greater degree of suffering than a male would be expected to have in the same situation. This increased distress is not attributable to a difference in her vulnerability or reaction to combat exposure, which would be expected to result in similarly reported distress levels in males. Rather, the fact that she has been injured in a combat situation resulted in increased reported severity versus an equivalently injured male counterpart.

This interpretation is explicitly supported by findings in a 2012 Maguen et al. publication [22]. Additionally, PFC Anderson's depressive symptoms, including appetite disturbances and tearfulness, may be more likely in post-deployment women [2, 22, 26]. This may be partially explained by the hypothesized increase in internalizing tendencies that was previously mentioned.

20.2.3 Case Formulation

No theoretical system holds a monopoly on formulating patient cases. The authors chose to utilize the Biocognitive Model to understand PFC Anderson's psychological functioning. Dr. McLaren's model is elucidated elsewhere [27], but a brief conceptual summary here suggests the reasons for its utility in this case. First, the model proposes that in the absence of structural or physiological disruptions, psychological symptoms must be assumed to be strictly mental. This does not mean that there is no disorder or physiologic changes, but that without a comprehensible or actionable deficit, the etiology and treatment are mental events and not biochemical or anatomical modifications. Second, anxiety and grief can be thought of as normal, evolutionarily adaptive responses to environmental factors. Lastly, humans have a, perhaps, unique ability to have meaningful life events trigger these typically adaptive anxious or depressive symptoms. Whereas primates may have fear responses to visible or audible threats, people have the capacity to perceive danger entirely mentally.

For instance, a weather forecast calling for a flood or hurricane will likely induce an anxious response. In this example a simple piece of information that an imminent but otherwise unperceivable event poses a threat suffices to induce a fear response. Dr. McLaren posits that psychological disorders then can be the result of inappropriate or excessive activation of fear or grief responses based on pieces of information that people believe, either implicitly or explicitly.

The appeal of the Biocognitive Model for PFC Anderson's case then becomes clear. Her premorbid psychological functioning was excellent. She suffered no overt head injuries and did not meet criteria for a traumatic brain injury. Her serum values of TSH, cortisol, hemoglobin, and estrogen were in the normal range. Although the DSM-5 criteria for major depressive disorder and PTSD were met and diagnosed, these offered little in the way of explaining her presentation or guiding the treatment.

Instead, her challenged identity of being a runner, newfound dependence, concerns over her body image, and doubt about her ability to attract a mate resulted in activation of the depressive signs that triggered consultation. She was literally grieving for her losses. The things she both implicitly and explicitly believed about herself were challenged by new internal and external exigencies. Similarly, the hyperarousal, nightmares, and irritability that she displayed resulted from the activation of threat perception. With this broad outline, the treatment team began to elucidate all of the "beliefs" or "rules" that resulted in symptom formation.

20.2.4 Clinical Pearls

1. Gathering symptomatology or having the patient complete a PCL is insufficient for understanding these complex patients. Becoming familiar with a method of formulating patients with PTSD will allow for a thorough assessment. With empathic understanding of patient suffering, as well as an appreciation for the meaning ascribed to their suffering, treatment planning becomes easier.
2. Be sensitive to the potential differences between genders with respect to PTSD presentation. Women may internalize symptoms which align with DSM criteria and may explain why current PTSD criteria are more frequently met by population samples of active duty service members [23]. In contrast, men manifest externalizing behaviors, such as alcohol misuse and hypervigilance [22, 23].

20.2.5 Potential Pitfall

1. Focusing strictly on the patient's completion of specific tasks may lead to misdiagnosis as each gender presents distress differently. Additionally, this can lead to loss of rapport, negative countertransference, and increased resistance by the patient to participate in therapy.

20.3 Treatment/Management

20.3.1 Psychopharmacologic Management

As formulated, the role of psychotropic medications in PFC Anderson's treatment was minimal. The Biocognitive Model does not typically indicate large roles for antidepressants or anxiolytics. However, if initial psychological interventions did not result in a meaningful increase in her rehabilitation participation due to persistent depressive symptoms, a serotonin reuptake inhibitor may have been a reasonable next step based on the practice guideline for treating PTSD [18].

The tremulousness, sweating, and increased heart rate she noted during periods of irritability may have benefitted from an adrenergic agent like a beta-blocker. However, with the potential for further surgical revision and ongoing physiologic adjustment to a lower circulating blood volume, these medications were deferred. Pregabalin, which is used off-label for generalized anxious states, may have provided some anxiolytic benefit but was not temporally related with any significant improvement based on the patient's report [28].

20.3.2 Psychotherapeutic Management

The mental health consult liaison team met 2 or 3 times per week with PFC Anderson for 8 consecutive weeks. Encounter length varied from 15 to 60 min, based mostly on patient availability. The first few sessions were devoted to rapport building and articulating both the conscious and unconscious "rules" that PFC Anderson organized her life with. Despite some uniqueness in formulation secondary to the Biocognitive Model, the treatments informed by our formulation resemble cognitive behavioral therapy interventions of cognitive restructuring and schema therapy [29, 30]. Table 20.2 specifies the beliefs and rules that PFC Anderson held that were suspected sources of conflict for her in her post-injury state.

After developing a preliminary treatment plan, the initial targets of intervention were restoring a sense of safety and self-efficacy. Her bed was moved so that she could easily see all people entering or occupying her room. She was encouraged to discuss the various triggers for increased activation in her room, including unannounced room entry and having people in the room when she woke up.

The consult team facilitated a discussion between the ward staff and her parents to identify specific tasks that PFC Anderson wanted help with, and which she did not. For instance, she wanted to be solely responsible for all of her hygiene, dressing, wheelchair transfers, and propulsion of her wheelchair. After she felt she had regained control and could set limits effectively, it was acceptable to move towards working through the trauma, and the events on the day of injury could be discussed in detail.

The differences between her current hospital environment and the threats she faced in the theater of operations were highlighted. These initial interventions reduced irritability with staff and family, and either time or the guided discussion through her index trauma resulted in a decrease in nightmare frequency.

Table 20.2 Identified conflicts and intervention strategies

Premorbid self-concept	Current belief	Attempted Intervention
"I am a strong, independent person"	"I need my parents and caretakers for everything"	Discuss boundaries, reestablish self-efficacy
"I am safe, and my training will keep me from harm"	"My training couldn't protect me" and "my safety continues to be threatened"	Reassure safety, accurately appraise current threats, emphasize that previous training continues to have a role through recovery
"I am well liked and physically attractive"	"No one will be attracted to me without my legs"	Visits from other amputees and her family, focusing on her attractive attributes that are nonphysical
"My recreational and occupational activities depend on my physical fitness/performance"	"I cannot run and will not enjoy many activities. My desired career is in jeopardy"	Emphasize what she can do and provide examples through other amputees, while defining her "new normal"
"I want to be a wife and a mother"	"I do not know if sex will be pleasurable or if I will be able to have children"	Facilitating her concerns and encouraging open discussion with primary providers

The first column describes the "rules" by which PFC Anderson structured her understanding of herself and the environment she inhabited. The second column shows how these tenets have been challenged by her post-injured world. The last column describes how the treatment team attempted to reduce the conflict created by the discrepant statements

Despite the improvements in irritability and hyperarousal, she continued to resist full participation in physical therapy. She identified several activities, such as trail hiking, that were questionably viable for her to continue to perform, which led to a sense of futility for the patient. At these times, she was encouraged to grieve that potential loss, and there was continued development of her sense of a "new normal" through facilitated rumination.

The treatment team then attempted to aid her exploration of additional fields of interest that may have provided recreational outlets, but little progress was made after multiple sessions. She still reported concern over how she was going to be treated by others and about her ability to participate in physically exerting activities. At that time, other wounded warriors who were further along in recovery were invited to meet with her and discuss her expectations for recovery.

Then, PFC Anderson met two amputees who had married a significant other subsequent to their injuries. Additionally, several of her siblings were finally able to visit, and she relayed that seeing them and having them interact with her like she remembered eased her concerns about feeling accepted. She identified these interactions as restoring hope for her interpersonal and recreational functioning.

Approximately one month prior to the end of her stay in the medical center, she was fitted for prosthetics and her participation in therapy increased substantially. Ultimately, PFC Anderson expressed the desire to serve as an example to others of how one can overcome the physical limitations imposed by such severe orthopedic injuries.

Progress in the final focus of intervention proved elusive in the time available for consultant care, as often happens. Little was known about her reproductive capacity and her concerns regarding sexual functioning which could not be fully addressed in the hospital setting. The treatment team did discuss her hopes for a large family, as well as how safe, loved, and cared for she herself felt growing up in a family of nine.

Discussed with her were alternate methods of reproduction including surrogacy, gestational carriers, and in vitro/intrauterine fertilization [31]. Sexual counseling was recommended as her recovery continued. The primary surgical team and gynecology services were encouraged to frequently invite questions regarding management of menstrual cycles, genital sensitivity, and vaginal lubrication.

20.3.3 Clinical Pearl

1. Establishing a safe environment is necessary before trauma psychotherapy can be conducted. The loss of control needs to be addressed and communication opened so that the patient can discuss underlying issues.
2. Psychological symptoms may result from incomplete care of somatic injuries. Veterans in transition from military care to Veterans Affairs or network care may be establishing new providers. In the case discussed here, sexual counseling will need to occur. It is important that each provider inquires about this and does not assume that it is not a problem or that it has been handled by another provider.
3. By bringing this issue up to the patient first, it mitigates a potentially awkward or uncomfortable topic and normalizes underlying fears. It contributes to a sense of "whole self" by bringing relationships, including the sexual component, to the forefront.

20.3.4 Potential Pitfall

1. Focusing on what the patient does or does not do (in the case of PFC Anderson, it was physical therapy) can create hostility between the consulting mental health provider, the primary team, and the patient. Understanding underlying fears and the patient's experience can lead to a shared picture and goal development. Holding multidisciplinary meetings with the patient and family present (if appropriate) ensures everyone has the same vision for treatment ends.

20.4 Outcomes/Case Resolution

The primary purpose of consultation, which focused on increasing participation in physical therapy, improved alongside the above psychological interventions. Unfortunately, the final outcome information in this case was not available due to transfer from the inpatient ward to a rehabilitation facility, as often happens.

Based on current published studies, there is reason for optimism with respect to her prognosis. Her social support, level of education, continued involvement in military culture, amenability to changes in self-concept, and progress towards carving out meaning for herself post-injury suggest a more favorable outcome [7, 17]. Going forward, the level of recovery from her somatic injuries, as previously discussed, will correlate with her overall mental health. Additionally, community integration to improve connectedness, occupational rehabilitation to avoid unemployment, and aggressive treatment of any residual anxious or depressive symptoms remain priorities to maximize her psychological functioning [17].

20.5 Conclusion

- Those working with veterans are increasingly likely to interact with women who have experienced combat exposure [26]. In 2012 the DGCDAR was amended, partly due to acknowledgement that combat exclusion restrictions did not prevent female service members from combat exposure. This opened thousands of Army jobs in combat-related occupational specialties to women [2, 23]. Furthermore, women may eventually be allowed to serve in the infantry. Designed to operate for 10 months beginning in October 2014, the Ground Combat Element of the Integrated Task Force was created to "inform the decision-making process on opening ground combat units" to female Marines [32].
- Over 3.5 million living female veterans are expected to be enrolled in VA healthcare by 2016, approximately double the number from 2011 [26]. Therefore, community care accessed by those who share similarities with PFC Anderson is more likely to occur going forward. As discussed, providers should take care to appropriately establish rapport and subsequently address the variety of psychological and physical sequelae of combat-related trauma unique to women.

References

1. Sternke LM. Measurement of military combat exposure among women: analysis and implications. Women's Health Issues. 2011;21(4 Suppl):S160–8.
2. Boyd MA, Bradshaw W, Robinson M. Mental health issues of women deployed to Iraq and Afghanistan. Arch Psychiatr Nurs. 2013;27(1):10–22.
3. Vogt D, Vaughn R, Glickman ME, Shultz M, Drainoni M, Elwy R, Eisen S. Gender differences in combat-related stressors and their association with postdeployment mental health in a nationally representative sample of U.S. OEF/OIF Veterans. J Abnorm Psychol. 2011;120(4):797–806.
4. U.S. military casualty conflicts reports: Defense Casualty Analysis System Web site. https://www.dmdc.osd.mil/dcas/pages/main.xhtml Accessed: 19 Feb 2015.
5. Mossadegh S, Tai N, Midwinter M, Parker P. Improvised explosive device related pelvi-perineal trauma: anatomic injuries and surgical management. J Trauma Acute Care Surg. 2012;73(2 Suppl 1):S24–S31.
6. Sharma DM, Webster CE, Kirman-Brown J, Mossadegh S, Whitbread T. Blast injury to the perineum. J Royal Army Med Corps. 2013;159(Issue Suppl 1):i1–3.

7. Cater JK. Traumatic amputation: psychosocial adjustment of six Army women to loss of one or more limbs. J Rehabil Res Dev. 2012;49(10):1443–56.
8. Julia PE, Othman AS. Barriers to sexual activity: counselling spinal cord injured women in Malaysia. Spinal Cord. 2011;49:791–4.
9. Belmont PJ Jr, McCriskin BJ, Hsiao MS, Burks R, Nelson KJ, Schoenfeld AJ. The nature and incidence of musculoskeletal combat wounds in Iraq and Afghanistan (2005–2009). J Orthop Trauma. 2013;27(5):e107–13. doi:10.1097?BOT.0b013e3182703188.
10. Ghetti C, Lowder JL, Ellison R, Krohn MA, Moalli P. Depressive symptoms in women seeking surgery for pelvic organ prolapse. Int Urogynecol J. 2010;21(7):855–60.
11. Jelovsek JE, Barber MD. Women seeking treatment for advanced pelvic organ prolapse have decreased body image and quality of life. Am J Obstet Gynecol. 2006;194(5):1455–61.
12. Zeleke BN, Ayele TA, Woldetsadik MA, Bisetegn TA, Adane AA. Depression among women with obstetric fistula, and pelvic organ prolapse in northwest Ethiopia. BMC Psychiatry. 2013;13:236.
13. Khan ZA, Whittal C, Mansol S, Osborne LA, Reed P, Emery S. Effect of depression and anxiety on the success of pelvic floor muscle training for pelvic floor dysfunction. J Obstet Gynaecol. 2013;33(7):710–4.
14. Lucas PA, Page PRJ, Phillip RD, Bennett AN. The impact of genital trauma on wounded servicemen: qualitative study. Injury (Int J Care Injured). 2014;45(5):825–9.
15. Fisher H. A guide to U.S. military casualty statistics: Operation Inherent Resolve, Operation New Dawn, Operation Iraqi Freedom, and Operation Enduring Freedom. Congressional Research Service. https://www.fas.org/sgp/crs/natsec/RS22452.pdf Published November 20, 2014. Accessed: 16 Feb 2014.
16. Benetato BB. Posttraumatic growth among operation enduring freedom and operation Iraqi freedom amputees. J Nurs Scholarsh. 2011;43(3):412–20.
17. Belon HP, Vigoda DF. Emotional adaptation to limb loss. Phys Med Rehabil Clin N Am. 2014;25:53–74.
18. Practice Guideline for the Treatment of Patients with Acute Stress Disorder and Posttraumatic Stress Disorder. Arlington, VA: American Psychiatric Association Practice Guidelines; 2004.
19. de Roos C, Veenstra AC, de Jongh A, den Hollander-Gijsman ME, van der Wee NJA, Zitman FG, van Rood YR. Treatment of chronic phantom limb pain using a trauma-focused psychological approach. Pain Res Manag. 2010;15(2):65–71.
20. Schneider J, Hofmann A, Rost C, Shapiro F. EMDR in the treatment of chronic phantom limb pain. Pain Med. 2008;9(1):76–82.
21. Kimerling R, Gima K, Smith MW, Street A, Frayne S. The Veterans Health Administration and military sexual trauma. Am J Public Health. 2007;97:2160–6.
22. Maguen S, Luxton DD, Skopp NA, Madden E. Gender differences in traumatic experiences and mental health in active duty soldiers redeployed from Iraq and Afghanistan. J Psychiatr Res. 2012;46:311–6.
23. Hourani L, Williams J, Brav R, Kandel D. Gender differences in the expression of PTSD symptoms among active duty military personnel. J Anxiety Disord. 2015;29:101–8.
24. King MW, Street AE, Gradus JL, Vogt DS, Resick PA. Gender differences in posttraumatic stress symptoms among OEF/OIF Veterans: an item response theory analysis. J Trauma Stress. 2013;26:175–83.
25. Nillni YI, Pineles SL, Patton SC, Rouse MH, Sawyer AT, Rasmusson AM. Menstrual cycle effects on psychological symptoms in women with PTSD. J Trauma Stress. 2015; epub ahead of print, published online January 22, 2015. doi:10.1002/jts.21984.
26. Resnick EM, Mallampalli M, Carter CL. Current challenges in female veteran's health. J Women's Health. 2012;21(9):895–900.
27. McLaren N. The mind-body problem explained: the biocognitive model for psychiatry. Ann Arbor: Future Psychiatry Press; 2012.

28. Stahl SM. Stahl's essential psychopharmacology: the prescriber's guide. 3rd ed. New York: Cambridge University Press; 2009.
29. Ehlers A, Clark DM. A cognitive model of posttraumatic stress disorder. Behav Res Ther. 2000;38:319–45.
30. Westbrook D, Kennerley H, Kirk J. An introduction to cognitive behavioral therapy: skills and applications. 2nd ed. London: Sage; 2011.
31. Burns LH. Psychiatric aspects of infertility and infertility treatments. Psychiatr Clin North Am. 2007;30:689–716.
32. About Ground Combat Element Integrated Task Force. Marines.mil Web site. http://www.gceitf.marines.mil/About.aspx. Accessed: 16 Feb 2015.

A Community Building Approach to PTSD Using the Arts in a Military Hospital Setting

21

Seema Reza, Kerrie Earley and Matthew St Laurent

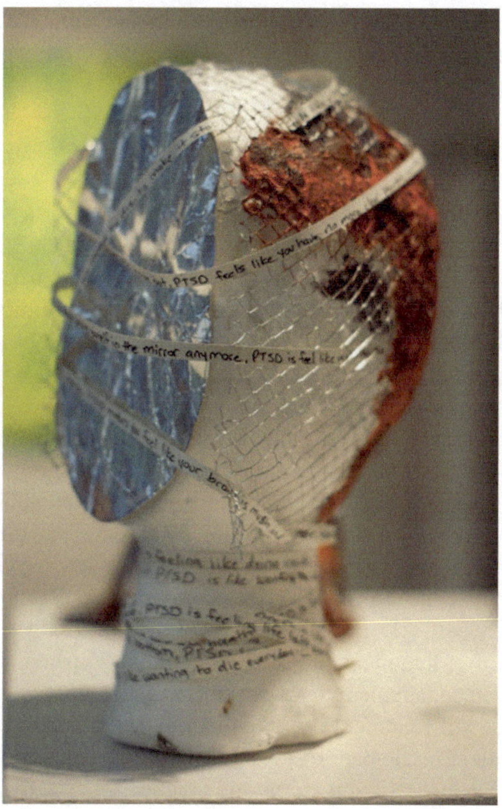

PTSD Feels Like, Mixed Media Sculpture by Cpt Rina Shah (USA, ret) exhibited at Lorton Workhouse Arts Center in Lorton, Virginia, 2011.

S. Reza (✉) · M. St Laurent
Department of Rehabilitation, Walter Reed National Military Medical Center, 8901 Wisconsin Avenue, Bethesda, MD 20889, USA
e-mail: seema.b.reza.ctr@mail.mil

E. C. Ritchie (ed.), *Posttraumatic Stress Disorder and Related Diseases in Combat Veterans,* DOI 10.1007/978-3-319-22985-0_21

Social support plays an integral role in the management of the negative impact of stress upon health and recovery from trauma [1]. Sufferers of combat-induced posttraumatic stress disorder (PTSD) frequently complain of feelings of isolation, loss of identity, and a decreased ability to connect with and empathize with others, including loved ones. The stigma of mental illness, internal and external pressure to uphold the dominant narrative of the invulnerable hero, and the complexity of emotions toward the combat experience are among the barriers to honest communication and reintegration into civilian society [2]. But trauma and the resultant fragmentation of memory provides an opportunity for patients to rebuild identity and meaning through the regular construction of narratives—not once, but on a regular basis, as circumstances evolve [3]. Encouraging individuals to independently and interdependently engage in the arts as an occupation [4, 5] through which to actively reevaluate relationships with themselves, their memories, and their loved ones empowers them to become active participants in their treatment, and can improve outcomes across the continuum of care.

21.1 History and Overview

In 2011, during Base Realignment and Closure (BRAC) the arts program operating out of the Morale, Welfare, and Recreation (MWR) Arts and Crafts Center at Forest Glen, a satellite facility of Walter Reed Army Medical Center, became a program of the Department of Rehabilitation at Walter Reed National Military Medical Center (WRNMMC) in Bethesda, Maryland. Since then, the program has expanded, offering 17 weekly recurring programs for patients and families (not including bedside visits and one-on-one co-treatment sessions) at both WRNMMC and Fort Belvoir Community Hospital (FBCH) in Virginia. More than 600 patients and family members participate in recreational arts activities through the program each month.

The WRNMMC Department of Rehabilitation's Occupational Therapy Service provides recreational arts activities, facilitated by artists, through multiple departments, including psychiatric partial hospitalization, inpatient psychiatry, pediatrics, oncology, and others. These programs are offered as: (1) treatment directed sessions, (2) voluntary/self-selecting sessions, and (3) weeklong workshops, which include a mixture of in-treatment and self-selecting participants. In all of these sessions, the focus is on engagement in art-making as an occupation which aids transitions through phases of treatment (i.e. inpatient to outpatient, active duty to civilian), increasing patient/participant responsibility for care, creating opportunities for healthy socialization, and providing tools and practice for effective communication. Participants are introduced to a wide range of art forms including writing, visual arts, music, and performing arts.

Further explanation of the primary components of the arts activities is given below:

K. Earley
Psychiatry Continuity Service, Walter Reed National Military Medical Center, 8901 Wisconsin Avenue, Bethesda, MD 20889, USA

1. *In-treatment sessions* are held in collaboration with partial-hospitalization/intensive outpatient programs, as well as some inpatient programs primarily in group settings. In addition to physical injuries, these individuals may be in treatment for mental illness, trauma-related stress, substance dependency, or a combination. Attendance in recreational arts activities is mandatory, often in spite of initial trepidation, and participation is documented by or under the supervision of a licensed clinician.
2. *Open sessions*, held on the hospital campus, are by and large, not treatment-directed, though many participants were initially referred or made aware of the sessions from occupational therapists and behavioral health providers. Participants choose to attend and work on projects of their choice. At one table, people explore self-portraits, soapstone carving, knitting, painting, and more. The atmosphere is social conversation, laughter, coffee drinking, coming and going. A flattened hierarchy is maintained in these groups—all first names, regardless of rank. The sessions take place at set times and locations, and last for 2 h or more. Participants are not required to arrive on time or stay for the entire session. This accommodates busy schedules and makes it easy for individuals to remember and return to the sessions after an absence. These sessions include patients from all over the hospital, inpatients, and family members.
3. *Weeklong workshops* are art, writing, film, music, or combination workshops culminating in a performance that is open to the public. The daily sessions are held at the USO Warrior and Family Centers at Bethesda and Ft Belvoir, and are facilitated in collaboration with contemporary, professional civilian, and veteran artists. As a group, participants work through the week to plan and complete their portion of an exhibit or performance. Each individual is completing a personal work of art, but is simultaneously working as an interdependent group, supporting and propelling one another forward. Participants leave with a completed "product"—a piece of writing, a short film, a piece of artwork, or a recorded track of music and the culminating performance. This product represents successful participation and an opportunity to step out and claim their narratives.

It is important to note that these arts activities are presented as an occupational therapy modality rather than art therapy—meaning that *occupation* in these activities is considered both process and product [4]. Through the process of creating art within the group context, participants both directly and indirectly address the issues of isolation, stigma, and loss of identity as they connect with people with shared experiences rather than in individual doctor's offices or isolated behind closed doors at home. Participants learn to make sense of their emotions, history, experiences, and stories, understand and empathize with those around them, and consider ways of connecting with civilians, family members, and fellow service members. Many of these participants have experienced a significant life changing event due to service-related injuries and, as a result, often an unplanned and challenging transition from military to civilian life. They must manage these obstacles in addition to coping with the avoidance, re-experiencing, alterations to mood and thoughts, heightened arousal and reactivity, and often co-occurring family and social discord that come with PTSD. By engaging in the creation of art, which provides in the most basic sense a chance to use coping skills and practice effective communication, participants are also empowered to build new skills and identities during their treatment and recovery.

There is much overlap in the benefits and approach of these activities with more traditional therapies; however, these sessions differ from traditional clinical arts therapy or psychotherapy support groups in these key ways:

- Inclusivity: Mixed groups of participants may include combat- or noncombat-deployed service members, veterans from various eras, physically or mentally ill patients, traditional military dependents and nonmedical attendees.
- Participant led: While project ideas or writing prompts are available, participants are not required to respond to a specific topic or directive, but instead are encouraged to direct themselves based on individual interests.
- Emphasis on independence/community reintegration: Participants begin tasks that are unlikely to be completed in the course of one session and are encouraged and enabled (through availability of materials and access to community resources) to continue to pursue these interests outside of sessions, on their own or with peers.
- Nondiagnostic: The artwork produced is not assigned meaning by a therapist; instead the process is used by the participant to construct his or her own subjective meaning, and given the opportunity to explain that meaning in a social setting.
- Active facilitator engagement: Participants and facilitators are engaging in the art-making process simultaneously in an environment of flattened hierarchy.
- Duration and frequency of participation are not pre-determined, but have organic ebb and flow dictated by individual needs—participants may suffer setbacks such as re-hospitalization or difficulties within personal relationships and find a need to attend more frequently or conversely, may gain employment or leave the military health system, but may choose to attend public events and openings. This is key, as participants need continued support as they move through the system and reintegrate back into their chosen communities.
- Continuity of facilitators—participants are able to build and maintain rapport with facilitators as they move through phases of treatment, creating a relational bridge that helps individuals who struggle with change and mistrust to push themselves creatively while feeling a sense of social support.

The cases presented below are composite case histories based on the hundreds of participants in the arts programs. Care has been taken to protect the identities of participants while demonstrating realistic treatment courses based on common symptom profiles and outcomes.

21.2 Case 1

21.2.1 History/Presentation

Susan is a 28-year-old African–American female army combat medic, married with children, with two combat deployments. Susan endured childhood trauma, including abandonment, sexual trauma, the loss of a sibling, and a suicide attempt. Susan first sought treatment in March 2012 after being assigned to work at WRNMMC and noticing difficulty functioning in her personal and professional lives. Susan began with weekly therapy appointments in the outpatient behavioral health clinic, and was prescribed medication for anxiety, depression, and panic. After 2 months, Susan received a referral to the Psychiatry Continuity Service (PCS), an intensive outpatient psychiatric program.

Initially referred for her childhood experiences, it was soon determined that due to significant combat trauma during her first 15 month deployment (including responding to mass casualties, treating gunshot wounds on Iraqi children, and recovering severed body parts), Susan would benefit from taking part in the trauma recovery program, the track for individuals suffering from combat related PTSD. She described "panic attacks," feeling as though she could not breathe, crying, and an overwhelming need to leave the situation triggered by crowded spaces and loud noises. Each attack was followed by a sense of shame and fear that she would never recover or be able to function as she did before her deployments, leading to further isolation and decreased interest in activities she had previously enjoyed.

21.2.2 Intervention

21.2.2.1 May 2012

Susan attended weekly writing groups with the recreational arts program during her stay in the partial hospitalization program. Susan was quiet at first, very obviously skeptical of the process, but during her third session, she shared a piece of writing that was honest and clear, acknowledging struggling with feelings of inadequacy as a mother. She wove together multiple narratives—the neglected child, the witness to the horrors of war, the parent who missed so many of her children's birthdays. Sharing it was obviously difficult, and Susan had to pause multiple times during the reading to collect herself, but she completed reading and began to share her writing regularly thereafter.

Afterward, Susan indicated that she had never written or enjoyed reading poetry (unless it was by Dr Seuss). But the sessions exposed her to a wide range of writing styles and authors and she found a "new way to express myself."

21.2.2.2 June 2012

Susan took part in a weeklong veteran-led workshop in writing and making paper out of military uniforms at Pyramid Atlantic Art Center in Silver Spring, Maryland. The weeklong workshop, led by veteran artists and a facilitator familiar to the participants, guides participants through a technique of making paper out of used military uniforms and then putting art and writing on the paper. Susan made a series of four panels, which facilitators helped her screen print with the names of over 80 fallen comrades. At the culminating exhibit, Susan participated in a performance piece in front of an audience where she cut a fellow soldier out of his uniform to symbolize his retirement from the military, while a third soldier read a poem.

When Susan had first cut into the uniforms to make paper, she said she was reminded of cutting uniforms off of soldiers as a medic. After the performance at the art gallery, Susan indicated that cutting the uniform as an act of "freeing a Soldier from combat, into their own life, in front of an audience put a different spin on that experience."

21.2.2.3 August 2012

Susan attended a therapeutic outing to the American Visionary Art Museum. During this trip she experienced another of her panic attacks while in the crowded gift shop. The old worries that "she may never recover, never return to her old self, never be able to go places with her family" came flooding back. After using coping skills learned through treatment and with support of peers, she was able to regain composure and process the progress made, and the accomplishment of attending the outing and returning to the museum after the panic attack.

21.2.2.4 September 2012

Upon discharge, Susan discovered that she could continue to work on art and writing. She began to attend open art and writing sessions two or three times weekly. The options of recreational/community reintegration activities available to her, as a soldier not assigned to a WTU (Warrior Transition Unit) were limited, so she had concerns about how to productively fill her time.

21.2.2.5 December 2012

Susan took part in another weeklong workshop, the music and words workshop, facilitated by civilian artists. In this workshop, participants work with two contemporary award-winning musicians, an accomplished writer, and a facilitator they are familiar with to write a poem to be made into a song for performance (Fig. 21.1). On day 1 of the workshop, Susan expressed some misgivings about working with "civilians" who would not "get it." By the end of the 4-day workshop, Susan performed two songs she wrote in front of an audience, one an ode to her weapon and the other a poem dedicated to the artists.

21.2.2.6 February 2013

A sculpture of Susan's was included in an exhibition at Lorton Workhouse Arts Center.

21.2.2.7 September 2013

Susan's husband and children moved into their new home while she remained in the Washington, DC area awaiting her medical evaluation board, an assessment of a service member's ability to continue military service, compensation, and treatment after separation. While she was awaiting final separation from the military, Susan stayed with an oncology patient she met at the art table.

Susan spent more than 1 year in the medical board process and found the unpredictability of the process extremely frustrating. The separation from the support of her family was difficult. Susan said, "But you know what? I'm okay, because next Tuesday I have art in the morning and afternoon writing." I have something to look forward to. I may not be healed, and the path ahead is still a long and hard one but at least now I've found a reason to travel it."

21.3 Case 2

21.3.1 History/Presentation

Sara is a 33-year-old divorced Latina senior noncommissioned officer in the Marine Corps with one combat deployment. Sara sought treatment for suicidal ideation linked to recurring flashbacks, intrusive thoughts, and depressed mood upon returning from deployment. While many of her symptoms were linked with her combat experiences, she was significantly troubled by a resurgence of memories from her own childhood abuse triggered by discovering the abuse of her child while she was deployed. She was hospitalized twice before her first enrollment in PCS where she attended the intensive outpatient program for issues related to her diagnosis of PTSD and depression. After PCS, she continued outpatient appointments weekly but was still troubled by chronic suicidal ideation, so was referred for additional

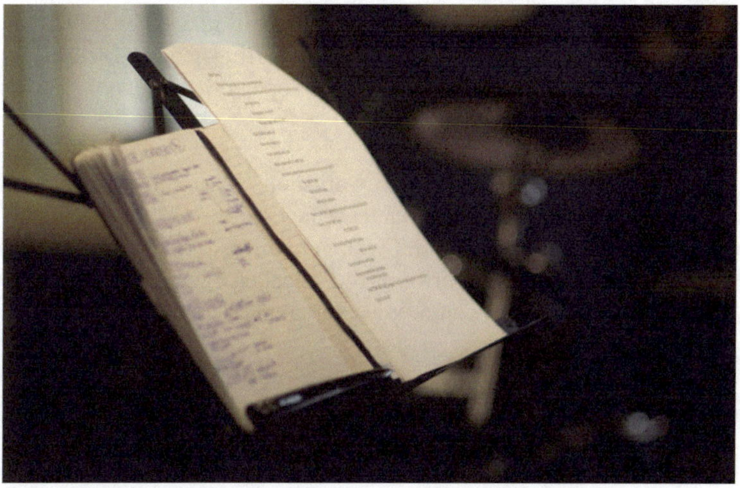

Fig. 21.1 Participant writing alongside musician's notes during music and words workshop. (Courtesy of SGT Timothy Brown, USMC (ret))

PCS treatment a year and a half post injury. She felt that she was no longer able to function at work as a top performer. Her irritability, difficulty concentrating, and high levels of anxiety and depression impaired her to the point of seeking medical assistance. She continued to be troubled by guilt and self-blame. She believed the world was unsafe and felt that she had to control and plan for as many things in her life as possible to protect her and her family. She had established a new relationship with a same sex partner, but was experiencing strain in the relationship due to emotional distance and poor communication.

During her first round of treatment, Sara was quiet and reserved, admitting later that she was still trying too hard to manage her symptoms and her presentation of "having it together." She still wanted to be perceived as a person others could count on, so did not let on how much she was struggling despite having flashbacks and heightened anxiety when driving, hearing children cry and dogs barking, or when her partner touched her. As a result, she was not able to take full advantage of programs offered the first time through treatment. Despite sleep disturbances and pain associated with back, knee, and hip issues, she declined medication out of worries she would not be able to waken or react in the event of an emergency.

21.3.2 Intervention

21.3.2.1 April 2014

During her second round of treatment at PCS, Sara took part in twice weekly writing groups, one 90 min group and another 30 min skill-building. Though unwilling to share her writing, she expressed that the groups were helpful to her and shared her writing with her therapist during individual sessions. After approximately 3 weeks, Sara shared her initial piece of writing with the group.

Afterward, Sara said that in the writing groups she began to allow herself to interpret the prompts/writing offered and write about it in a different way than the others in the group. "Rather than worrying that my writing made no sense, just write it, share it. For me overcoming that fear began to open other doors."

21.3.2.2 May 2014

Sara attended a 4-day music and words workshop with civilian musicians. Sara made a great deal of personal effort to attend the entire workshop, including altering her schedule and bringing her child with her when she had difficulty acquiring childcare. After the culminating performance, attended by approximately 35 members of the military and civilian community, Sara remarked that she "hadn't realized that so many people want to hear our stories."

21.3.2.3 June 2014

After attending the workshop, Sara continued treatment in PCS. She attended a group outing to the Museum of Health and Medicine, and was noticeably more actively engaged in conversations with others. Her contributions in groups increased.

She showed a sense of greater relaxation and began to joke more easily and develop a rapport with participants and facilitators.

As she prepared for discharge from PCS to return to ongoing outpatient therapy, she continued to grapple with whether or not to continue on her planned trajectory to complete her 20 years of service for military retirement, or separate from the military to focus on her family, her recovery, and a career that involved fewer pressures. This was the first time she had considered that her plan and identity did not have to revolve solely around her military service, recognizing that she was only 33 and had many options.

In her last few weeks of PCS treatment before returning to outpatient weekly appointments, she was confronted by a suicide attempt by her parent. While this was extremely difficult for her, she was still able to manage both to provide support and set boundaries with her family. She was able to effectively communicate and seek support from her partner. This helped her remain focused on her own gains in treatment. She used journaling, a skill she learned in the arts program, as a way to cope.

21.4 Case 3

21.4.1 History/Presentation

Sam is a 33-year-old Caucasian male, married, with multiple combat deployments. During his most recent deployment, he suffered a physical injury that required extensive physical therapy. Sam had been attending weekly outpatient treatment without much benefit, and was sent to WRNMMC for intensive PTSD treatment and was awaiting his MEB. Sam lived in barracks/dormitory on base separated from his family and other natural supports while attending full-day treatment. He was experiencing nightmares, irritability, hypervigilance, recurrent flashbacks and intrusive thoughts, and isolation and detachment from others. During group therapy, he sat on the periphery of the group, back against the wall, scanning the room throughout the sessions. He was the last one in and first one out of each group and said nothing, shaking his head when asked a direct question other than his name.

21.4.2 Intervention

21.4.2.1 June 2012

Sam's experience with the arts program began with weekly attendance in the writing groups. The first several weeks, he sat by the door scanning the room as he did in all his therapy groups, headphones in but not on as was usually the case. Facilitators handed him notebooks which sat on his lap unopened for the hour and a half sessions, until one day he picked up the pen and started writing. Within a few short weeks, he was arriving on time, with his own notebook and pen. He started inching toward the table finally leaving his coveted spot by the door for a seat at the table.

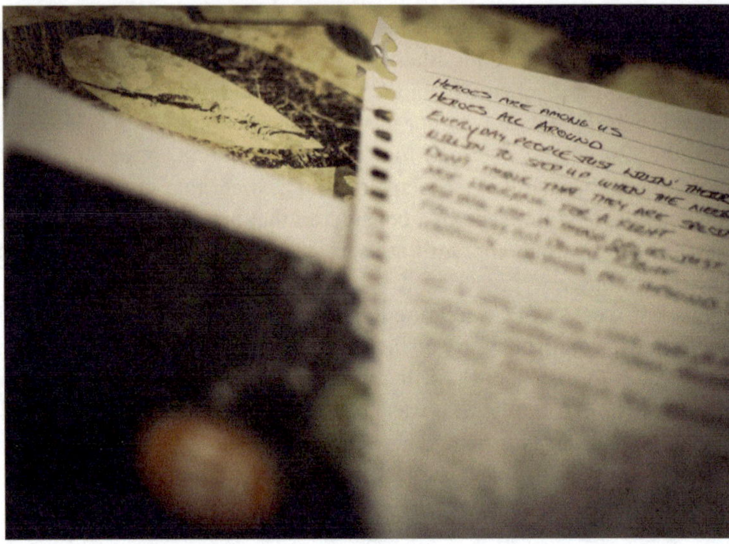
HEROES ARE AMONG US
HEROES ALL AROUND
EVERYDAY PEOPLE JUST

Fig. 21.2 Participant writing during music and words workshop recording session. (Courtesy of SGT Timothy Brown, USMC (ret))

A few weeks into treatment, during writing group, Sam volunteered to read his writing to the group, sharing stories from his family's past and fond memories from his childhood. He smiled as he spoke more than two words for the first time in the group setting. Sam expressed that in writing and art he discovered a way to express himself without having to talk, which was a great relief for him.

21.4.2.2 September 2012

Sam voluntarily participated in a weeklong workshop, making paper from military uniforms. Though his interaction with the facilitators and the group was limited, he contributed a piece of writing and two pieces of artwork to the culminating exhibit. Sam attended the exhibit but declined to read his work aloud or even enter the room in which the exhibit was being held, leaving before the reception was over. Sam's writing did not acknowledge his own complicated feelings about war, but instead he wrote a piece about the "enemy" feeling his "wrath and vengeance."

21.4.2.3 October 2012

Sam was discharged from PCS groups and continued in individual therapy.

21.4.2.4 November 2012

Sam participated in a 4-day music and words workshop (Fig. 21.2). At the close of the first day, the group was given a writing assignment to complete independently. Sam arrived the following morning with a blank notebook. When asked, he reported that he had been writing and then erasing his work, feeling repeatedly that it was not "quite right." Sam spent the first half-hour of that day's workshop in an indi-

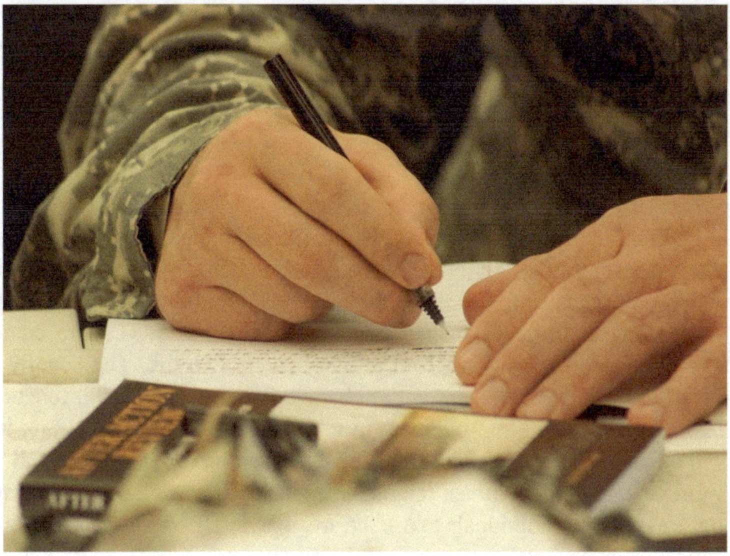

Fig. 21.3 A soldier participates in a writing workshop. (Courtesy of SFC Willie Young, US Army (ret).)

vidual session with the musicians. He emerged ready to write, and sat at the table and filled three pages of his notebook. Though in the beginning Sam contributed to casual conversation only when addressed directly, by day 3 he volunteered a funny observation to one of the facilitators he had grown comfortable with. At the culminating performance, Sam offered, "I don't have much to say, but if I mess up, it's their fault," and pointed behind him at the musicians. In front of an audience at a theater in Arlington, Virginia, Sam sang a piece about "Coming home to a foreign land," in which he expressed his frustration and confusion since returning to the USA after his deployment.

21.4.2.5 December 2012–February 2013

Facilitators arranged for Sam to continue with biweekly sessions with the musicians from the workshop. Sam attended these sessions regularly, and continued to attend writing groups on the unit despite having been discharged.

21.4.2.6 February 2013

Sam attended another paper making workshop (Fig. 21.3), working more independently on artwork and writing and showing an increased interest in craft/editing. Sam's family travelled to the area to attend the culminating performance, which took place in an art gallery in Rockville, Maryland. Sam sang a song a capella in front of an audience of 80 people. The song was about the feelings of grief and loss he experienced when he lost comrades at war. He stayed until the end of the reception, socializing with audience members and others.

21.4.2.7 April 2013

Sam was assigned to a Warrior Transition Brigade closer to his family to finish out his medical retirement process.

21.5 Outcomes

It would be great to report that patients who have participated in the arts program have achieved resolution of all PTSD, depressive, and anxiety symptoms. This unfortunately is not the case for many of the participants of these programs who are likely to face ongoing effects of their exposure to trauma for years to come and often have to adapt to transitions from military to civilian life. The benefits from participation in these programs are better characterized by changes in functioning, reduction in isolation, and improvement in relationships. The arts program invites patients to engage in personally meaningful activities that offer experiential learning to improve social interactions, relationships, and expression of self to improve function. Empowering individuals to use the arts to actively reevaluate relationships with themselves, their memories, and their loved ones provides them with the skills to address the challenges that they will continue to face after the formal treatment groups, the medical boards, the transition from the military, and the ongoing tests of life.

Patients such as Susan tend to see benefit by a reduction of symptoms. While they may continue to experience anxiety and mistrust, the negative impact on day-to-day functioning becomes reduced, allowing increased participation in community activities, engagement with family, and the building of new relationships. Making it through the checkout line at a grocery store instead of leaving a cart in the aisle is a huge functional success. Confidence in making new friends and discovering new skills, counters the negative impact trauma has on individuals attempting to reintegrate and participate in a community, or accomplish personal goals.

Patients such as Sara may continue to have passing thoughts of suicide, but those are more quickly replaced by problem-solving with other options such as validation of emotions or confidence that negative thoughts will pass or can be managed. These patients learn to set boundaries within relationships and consider an identity that includes, but is not exclusively tied to military culture or success. They can leave children with a babysitter while out to dinner and develop relationships as a part of an adult life. Medication becomes an acceptable option to improve sleep. Confidence in skills will help make challenging decisions on how to balance life in the military with her own self-care and the care of her family, or start a new civilian life and go back to school.

Patients such as Sam experience reduction in isolation. While they may continue to enter a room and scan for exits and potential threats, it no longer prevents social engagement, or taking part in activities that interest him. He can communicate and may once again employ humor to connect. Confidence and willingness to express his struggles using the arts first to himself, then to others close to him begin to emerge. Building an identity for himself that includes, but is not limited to, a role in the military becomes acceptable.

21.6 Challenges

Patients and mental health providers alike may have reservations about addressing extensive histories of trauma in unstructured ways that the arts can promote. Fears of opening Pandora's box, inability to contain difficult emotions that are triggered by recounting traumatic events, and uncertainty about how to process the thoughts and beliefs that contribute to ongoing distress without re-traumatizing the individual are but a few of the worries that need to be addressed for a population that often uses avoidance of the thoughts and memories of trauma as means of coping. By beginning to explore the arts for healing within a structured program with the support of mental health providers, participants can explore tools and techniques that are safe for them within the context of community support from peers with shared experiences and with follow up with mental health professionals. As they transition from a structured setting, the connections made with others similar to them, promote positive peer pressure for ongoing self-care, healthy recreation, participation, and medication management, etc.

The above factors, arguably the strength of this approach as an adjunct to traditional therapies are challenging to study scientifically. Further, the frequency of phone calls, social visits, help with childcare and tasks that stem from these activities are difficult to measure. The authors' belief that anecdotal experiences are objective indicators that PTSD patients benefit from the arts interventions and that additional study and exploration in this area could expand the field, attract funding sources, and provide continued opportunities for healing.

References

1. Wilcox S. Social relationships and PTSD symptomatology in combat veterans. Psychol Trauma: Theory Res Pract Policy. 2010;2(3):175–82. doi:10.1037/a0019062.
2. Hoge CW. Once a warrior, always a warrior navigating the transition from combat to home—including combat stress, PTSD, and mTBI. Guilford: GPP Life, 2010.
3. Crossley ML. Narrative psychology, trauma and the study of self/identity. Theory Psychol. 2000;10(4):527–46. doi:10.1177/0959354300104005.
4. Roley SS, DeLany JV, Barrows CJ, Brownrigg S, Honaker D, Sava DI, Talley V, Voelkerding K, Amini DA, Smith E, Toto P, King S, Lieberman D, Baum MC, Cohen ES, Cleveland PA, Youngstrom MJ. Occupational therapy practice framework: domain and process. 2nd Ed. Am J Occup Ther. 2008;62:625–83.
5. Paquin JD, Kivlighan DM, Drogosz LM. If you get better, will I? An actor–partner analysis of the mutual influence of group therapy outcomes. J Couns Psychol. 2013;60(2):171–9. doi:10.1037/a0031904.

Part V
Cultural Competence/Special Populations

Mental Health Care of Special Operations Forces

22

Paul Sargent

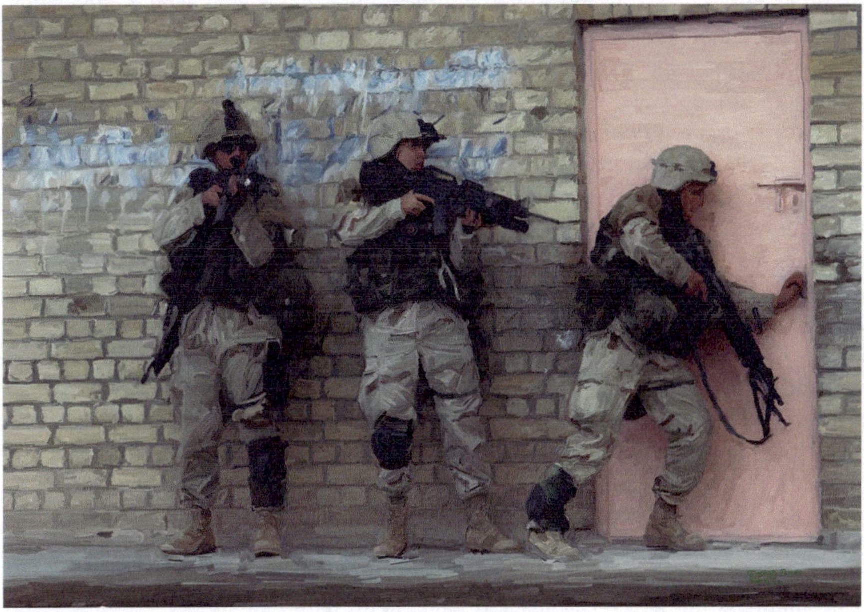

What Is Behind the Pink Door?, Darrold Peters, courtesy of the Army Art Collection, US Army Center of Military History.

"Terrorism and extremism are problems that we will have to deal with for some time to come. We face unprecedented challenges from an increasingly complex operating environment filled with agile, rapidly adapting belligerents—adversaries that we expect to be even more innovative and asymmetric in their approach to conflict in the years ahead."
-Wm McRaven Posture Statement before the 113th Congress, House Armed Services Committee

P. Sargent (✉)
LOGSU Medical Department, Naval Special Warfare Group ONE. 2424 Rendova Road San Diego CA 92155
e-mail: Paul.d.sargent8.mil@mail.mil

E. C. Ritchie (ed.), *Posttraumatic Stress Disorder and Related Diseases in Combat Veterans*, DOI 10.1007/978-3-319-22985-0_22

22.1 The Organizational Context of Special Operators

Providing optimal care for special operations forces (SOF) requires familiarity with the organizational culture and the operational job requirements of this group; yet there is very little written in the psychiatric literature which would prepare a provider for this challenge. The US Special Operations Command (USSOCOM or SOCOM) is the Unified Combatant Command which oversees the various Special Operations Component Commands of the Army, Air Force, Navy, and Marine Corps. Each Component Command of USSOCOM has its distinct cultural mores and areas of expertise, but it can also be said that the Special Operations Commands (SOCOM) are more similar to each other than they are to their conventional counterparts. It may not be possible for a clinician to become culturally adept in the jargon and practices of each service, but there are some tenants which universally apply, which distinguish this group from other military organizations.

These commands hold the following five "Special Operations Forces (SOF) Truths" as core doctrinal of their organizations.

Truth 1: *Humans are more important than hardware*. People—not equipment—make the critical difference.

Truth 2: *Quality is better than quantity*. A small number of people, carefully selected, well trained, and well led, are preferable to larger numbers of troops, some of whom may not be up to the task.

Truth 3: *Special Operations Forces cannot be mass produced*. The personnel who make up SOF units are highly screened and selected for competence. Only a few will make the cut.

Truth 4: *Competent Special Operations Forces cannot be created after emergencies occur***.** Employment of fully capable special operations capability on short notice requires highly trained and constantly available SOF units in peacetime.

Truth 5: *Most special operations require non-SOF assistance*. The operational effectiveness of deployed SOF forces cannot be, and never has been, achieved without being enabled by their joint service partners.

Clearly, the focus of these "truths" is on the primacy of the people and the teams who complete the missions over the technology they employ. SOF training and missions require a high level of physical and psychological resilience that is not consistently found in conventional military members.

In order to select the very best personnel, psychological health is one factor carefully assessed. This process includes initially "screening out" candidates for special operations duty that includes significant character pathology, emotional problems, poor interpersonal skills, low stress tolerance, and limited intelligence.

Despite this, there is no ideal special operations profile. To the contrary, heterogeneity among personnel often leads to creative improvements in how things are done [1]. The process of assessment does not end with the mental health staff, but usually concludes with some type of selection board in which all the available information is reviewed and a final decision is made by an experienced special operations personnel.

Once the assessment and selection is complete, the selected individuals begin the high attrition training process that will allow a very few to become special operators. The early training process for these special operators is arduous and can be dangerous in and of itself. In Navy Basic Underwater Demolition School (BUD/S), the motto is "The only easy day was yesterday."

Despite every effort to conduct safe training, injuries are commonplace in early training and frequently result in an early attrition rate of over 70 %. Those who make it through this selection process must also have high psychological resilience and must be able to experience intense suffering, yet continue to pursue their objective.

The high value placed on persistence and resilience is reflected in the adage that "the more you sweat in training, the less you bleed in combat." In each service branch, the process to achieve the basic qualification as a special operator is over a year. This is, however, just to build the requisite skills to join a team as a "new guy."

During their career, special operators will be deployed for 6 out of every 24 months. Over a full career they may accrue between six and ten deployments on average. This can make history taking a challenge for the provider as there are often multiple exposures to combat, as well as head trauma, which need to be explored.

Special operators (US Navy SEALs, US Army Special Forces, US Air Force Combat Controllers and Pararescuemen, and US Marine "Raiders") highly value independent and "irregular" approaches to problem solving. According to Col David Hackworth, "If you find yourself in a fair fight, you didn't plan your mission properly."

This independence of thought may lead to them being misunderstood by the public, as well as by other members of the military. Calculated risk taking and innovation are highly valued among this group of "unconventional" warriors. Their operations "differ from conventional operations in the degree of physical and political risk, operational techniques, mode of employment, independence from friendly support, and dependence on detailed operational intelligence and indigenous assets" [2].

Special Operations Commands (SOCOM) conducts several types of missions to include counter-terrorism, direct action, special reconnaissance, foreign internal defense, and unconventional warfare. These operations may occur during the times of war or times of peace, and are often done with great secrecy. Special operators take pride in being "quiet professionals." They feel uncomfortable talking about themselves and may minimize the amount of trauma they have endured.

Much of what they do remains classified, and they sign "Non-Disclosure Agreements," which may prevent them from discussing certain details related to their deployment experiences. Nevertheless, over time as trust is established, it may be possible for the provider to understand some general scenarios which have occurred, as long as specific details are not revealed by the operator.

Maintaining apparently intact social and occupational function despite a high symptom burden could be considered a hallmark of this group. This makes diagnosis using traditional criteria from the *Diagnostic and Statistical Manual* challenging. The special operator with more than one deployment has typically spent a great deal of time living and working in a high-threat environment.

Some of their instinctive physical and autonomic responses as well as cognitive patterns have adapted to that high-threat environment. The operator may endorse a belief that they only feel normal when they are deployed, or that they can no longer relate to anyone who is not an operator. The provider should be patient, but also persistent in eliciting information related to psychologically troubling experiences. With time and trust, enough information will be presented to clarify the diagnosis.

A provider working within a Special Operations Commands (SOCOM) should take every opportunity to build relationships within the organization. It will be invaluable to identify loci of authority and influence that may not be perceptible to an outsider. From these sources, the command culture can be ascertained, and more optimal advisement can be given to the client on how to navigate their challenges.

If the provider finds themselves working with a prior special operator in a veteran's administration or civilian clinic, time should be taken to ask about the relationships with other people in the patient's previous chains of command. Knowing the names and dynamics between the patient and their teammates will build rapport and facilitate taking an accurate history.

22.2 Case Study

22.2.1 Initial Patient Encounter

It was nearing 17:00 (5 pm) as Dr. Smith sat at his desk, catching up on his daily notes. He was so focused on his work that he almost did not hear the quiet knock at his door followed by a deep but familiar voice asking, "Hey Doc, you got a second?" He looked up to see Senior Chief Petty Officer Gerald Erickson standing in his doorway.

Dr. Smith had been aware of Jerry for the past year as an irregular presence during staff meetings, in which they both occupied seats in the "back row" of the Commodore's conference room. Until now, Jerry has been polite but reserved, rarely speaking or offering opinions in the meetings, and seeming uncomfortable in the spotlight.

He was not a large man and would not likely attract much notice in public place. On the afternoon he walked in, he was wearing sweaty PT gear as if he just worked out and then, perhaps as an afterthought, decided to stop by for a quick psych consult. He was lean and fit, much more so than might be expected for a 35-year-old man. He awaited the answer to his question with tension in his jaw, and dark circles under his eyes. He clearly had not shaved for a few days, and Dr. Smith guessed he has not slept much either.

"Sure Jerry, come on in," Smith offered. With a look of relief, Jerry came in and slowly lowered himself into the recliner just inside the door. Dr. Smith asked, "Door open or closed?" and Jerry reached out with one hand to nudge the door shut. There was an awkward pause as Jerry stared blankly for a moment not knowing where to start.

Dr. Smith knew this was a common, but uncomfortable, starting place for a SEAL operator. He may be a master of tactics and small unit combat, yet remain uncomfortable and out of his element when seeking help. He knew Jerry felt exposed, or "skylined," in the office. Dr. Smith knew that in order to help him, his first job is to establish rapport, and trust. "It's good to see you, Jerry, how can I help?"

"I'm honestly not sure you can," replied Jerry. "I just don't know where else to turn right now, and the command master chief (CMC) mentioned that you might be helpful. I…I…I guess it's a problem at work mostly. I found out Friday that I am being relieved as Troop SEA (Senior Enlisted Advisor). My guys have lost confidence in me and the Commanding Officer (CO) has decided to let me go."

His eyes were downcast, and he looked ashamed. "It's been getting worse and worse for the past few months as we get through work ups. I don't blame the CO. He and the CMC have talked with me before about problems, and I just can't seem to fix them. Really it's all on me, and I don't know why I just can't get my shit together this time." He leaned forward in his chair, wringing his hands.

Dr. Smith looked at this man, so accustomed to violence, and yet so unnerved by the threat of dishonor, and disappointment. He noticed the tattoos encasing both forearms, starting from the wrists and disappearing up under both T-shirt sleeves. Jerry wore a black metal wrist band on his right wrist, and though he could not make out the words, Dr. Smith knew it was inscribed with the name of a fallen teammate. "That sounds rough, Jerry, what do you think is going on?"

"Well, I think it's really about the guys. When I moved into this job, I was excited to get back to the Team. I thought I was ready, but now I think I bit off more than I can chew. I have been having trouble keeping training events organized and scheduled, maintaining performance standards, and keeping morale up. My troop just completed their Land Warfare block, and nearly failed. If my platoon chiefs hadn't stepped up, it would have been a shit show, and pretty much all my fault. After that, the Officer In Charge (OIC), the mess, and all the guys started to see me as a weak link. I have never failed like this before. I don't want to quit, but I also don't want to put anyone else at risk because I can't get organized. I feel like I'm in some kind of daze."

Dr. Smith noticed the wedding band on Jerry's finger, and commented, "I've got some ideas about things we can check out for you Jerry, but first tell me how things are going at home, any better there?"

"Not really, Doc. I haven't been living with my wife for the past 3 months. She is a good woman, but work has been keeping me so busy, I haven't made the time to be with her or the kids. It's not like I was much fun even when I was around. She said I wasn't reliable, and that I forget everything she tells me, because I just don't care. She says I'm either completely disconnected or totally enraged. Either way, it doesn't help our kids, and I agree. I want to be a good dad, but I think the family does better when I'm not at home."

"They have gotten used to me being gone over the years anyway, so I just grabbed a sleeping bag. I now crash out in the back of my truck when I get done at work. It's not like I was sleeping well at home anyway. Staying in the parking lot overnight isn't such a big deal, and it keeps me off the roads. Sometimes I want to kill people when its gets bad on the roads…."

As he sat with Jerry and thought about his story, Dr. Smith knew that he could help him, but he also knew it is going to take a lot more than one quick visit. Smith was not sure how much interaction this man would tolerate before fading in to the background of the teams again, so he asked Jerry if he was willing to work with him for a few sessions and Jerry agreed. "Anything to get back on track, Doc."

Dr. Smith reviewed the boundaries of informed consent for treatment, and Jerry was hesitant but agreed. Dr. Smith knew now that he had enough trust to begin to take a history. However, he also knew that building trust does not just happen over the first 5 min of the encounter. Rather, trust was built up over months of sitting in that conference room, establishing good relationships in the command, and coming to understand something of the culture in which both the doctor and the SEAL found themselves.

22.2.2 History of Present Illness

Gerald "Jerry" Erickson was a 35-year-old separated Caucasian male Navy E-8 SEAL with 15 years of continuous active duty. He had no prior mental health history and was now presenting for depressed mood, low energy, feelings of irritability, excessive guilt, sadness, insomnia, difficulties with attention, concentration, and short-term memory for the preceding 12 months. He also reported that the symptoms had become much worse in the last 2 weeks in the context of occupational problems.

Nothing he had tried had alleviated his symptoms, and yet he continued to "push through the pain." He kept a regular gym schedule of at least 5–6 days per week and described his workouts as his main outlet for stress. He consistently came to work, but the quality of his work was seen by those around him as poor. He reported that his sleep was often fragmented, and he believed his total sleep time is between 5 and 6 h per night. He did endorse some combat-related nightmares which occurred one night per week on average.

He also reported that he liked to stay busy because when he remained still for too long he found himself thinking of his best friend Steve who was killed by an IED on their last deployment. Jerry had escorted Steve's body back, and felt ashamed when he lost his composure during the memorial service.

While he was able to acknowledge that he typically felt "lousy" after each of his five earlier deployments, Jerry never had the negative emotions persist like they had since his last deployment. He denied any history of manic episodes, psychosis, or chemical dependency, though he had been told by his wife to cut back on his alcohol intake. He had never taken any psychotropic medications, and had never been hospitalized for psychiatric reasons. He adamantly denied suicidal or homicidal ideation. He was highly motivated to return to duty as soon as possible, and did not want to lose his chance to deploy again with "his guys."

22.2.2.1 Family Psychiatric History

The patient had no history of family psychiatric illnesses.

22.2.2.2 Past Medical History

Jerry reported multiple orthopedic problems, most notably shoulder and knee pain. He already had two shoulder surgeries (bilateral superior labral tears) and one knee surgery (anterior cruciate ligament repair) as a result of occupational injuries. When asked about his previous history of concussions, Jerry revealed that he has had multiple head traumas during his life. They are listed in Table 22.1.

Jerry had previously completed neurocognitive baseline testing as part of his routine medical screening. His scores revealed some downward trends that had not previously been identified. Over the past 5 years, his verbal memory has declined from the 66th percentile to the 12th. His visual memory has declined from the 78th percentile to the 14th. His visual motor speed has remained constant around the 50th percentile, and his reaction time has slowed from the 80th percentile to the 35th percentile.

A review of systems revealed daily headaches which were worst in the morning when he woke up, mild hearing loss in his left ear, and occasional dizziness after staring at a computer screen for more than an hour. He also reported some erectile dysfunction for the prior 2 years which was responsive to phosphodiesterase medication.

22.2.2.3 Substance History

From the end of his last deployment, until 6 months prior to the evaluation (about a 1-year period), Jerry reported a history of binge drinking up to 8–10 drinks per night. He endorsed tolerance during that period, but denied withdrawal. His wife has been bothered by his drinking, but he felt that he was consuming about the same amount as his friends and never attempted to cut back until his job performance began to suffer. He currently drinks less than 1 day per week, and then limits himself to two 12 oz beers until his work performance improves. He endorsed using chewing tobacco, consuming about 2 cans per week. He denied any history of illicit drug use.

22.2.2.4 Military History

Jerry enlisted in the Navy at age 19. He completed Basic Underwater Demolition/SEAL (BUD/S) training on his first try, despite sustaining a concussion. His first deployment was in 2003 during the initial invasion of Iraq. He then completed a second deployment to Iraq in 2006, during which he fought in and around the town of Ramadi. He described this as his most combat-intensive deployment, but also the one he felt proud of. He was deployed subsequently three more times to Afghanistan in 2008, 2010, and 2012.

After his last deployment, he was assigned as an instructor at the Training Detachment (TRADET). He negotiated this transfer in order to have time to be with his family, and try to "pull it together" after losing his friend Steve to an IED. He negotiated a transfer from TRADET back to his team in order to prepare for one

Table 22.1 Lifetime history of patient's head injuries

	Age	LOC	AOC	PTA	Focal neuro	Imaging
Motocross racing	16	Approx 1 min	12 h	None	None	Negative CT in the ER
Basic Underwater Demolition/SEAL (BUD/S) boat dropped on his head	20	No	12 h	None	None	None
Lead breacher (2nd deployment) 3–4 concussions	28	No	5–6 h each	48 h	None	None
Parachute hard landing (training prior to 4th deployment)	31	5 min	48 h	48 h	None	Negative CT in ER

more deployment. He has always received favorable evaluations and has consistently been promoted on time. He has multiple individual medals including three Bronze Stars with Valor.

22.2.2.5 Developmental History

Jerry was the second of two children born into an intact union and raised in suburban Seattle, Washington. He was frequently left on-his-own and became very independent as a child. He enjoyed outdoor activities and spent many hours playing in the woods behind his home. He denied any history of physical, emotional, or sexual abuse. In high school, he won the state wrestling championship in his weight class. He reported that discovering "beer and girls" in college led to him failing out after only 1 year. He then decided to join the Navy and become a SEAL because he wanted to maintain a fast-paced lifestyle. He has been married for the past 10 years and has two daughters age 8 and 6. Jerry reported that his wife had grown more frustrated with him over the past 2 years. She is not sure the marriage will survive even if he does get help. Jerry's professional plan was to complete 20 years in the Navy. He reported that he has "no idea" what he will do for a job after leaving the military. With a tense, halfhearted smile, he asked, "Think I'm too old to be a fireman, Doc?"

22.2.2.6 Mental Status Examination

Jerry was a very fit, but mildly disheveled man who appeared about his stated age. He was cooperative with evaluation, and made good eye contact. He had dark circles under his eyes and appeared tired. He was initially tense but his sense of humor was preserved and he made jokes at several points in the evaluation but without lightening his affect. His speech was regular rate and rhythm. His stated mood was "worried" and his affect was tense at first but then became slightly more open, as rapport was established. His thought process was linear, logical, and goal directed, and his thought content revealed no suicidal or homicidal ideation or perseveration. His insight and judgment were good and his impulse control appeared to be intact.

22.2.2.7 Assessment/Diagnosis

Jerry has a history of multiple mild concussions and two moderate concussions. From his initial screening, it is likely that he also has posttraumatic stress disorder (PTSD), but before arriving at a definitive diagnosis, other possibilities will need to be explored within a differential diagnosis. These possibilities include anxiety disorder secondary to a general medical condition (TBI), major depressive disorder, and cognitive disorder due to a general medical condition (TBI, sleep deprivation, or endocrine abnormality). Less likely possibilities include adjustment disorder (he has a history of significant resilience under stress), and alcohol dependence (he certainly meets some of the criteria and may be minimizing his current drinking).

His initial workup revealed normal vital signs, but on neurological exam he had a positive Rhomberg test (a standing test of proprioception which is considered positive if a person cannot maintain their balance with their eyes closed and arms spread). A laboratory evaluation was completed which revealed a normal CBC, chemistry panel, liver function panel, and thyroid function panel. Because of his history of head trauma followed by erectile dysfunction, his pituitary function was assessed with labs for prolactin, follicle stimulating hormone, leutinizing hormone, testosterone, and sex hormone binding globulin. This workup revealed hypogonadism with a total testosterone of 150 ng/dl (Normal range 270–1070 ng/dl). Subsequent brain imaging with an MRI revealed a normal appearing sella (an area of the skull normally containing the pituitary gland which will appear "empty" if the pituitary is damaged), but several small frontal lobe lesions at the gray matter/white matter junction of undetermined significance, but possibly consistent with diffuse axonal injury, related to head trauma.

Jerry was referred for a formal neuropsychological evaluation. His results were considered valid and he demonstrated good effort in test taking. His objective report described moderate difficulty with sustained attention and processing speed. Also delayed recall was mildly below expectations for his age and education level. His language, visuospatial, and motor function were grossly intact. His PHQ-9 score was 10 suggesting moderate depression, and his PCL-M score was 62, consistent with a diagnosis of PTSD. While Jerry's objective neurocognitive scores were somewhat below what would be expected for a man of his age, it is also more difficult to interpret them in the context of a SOF Operator who very likely was above average in all of those categories earlier in his career.

No baseline testing had been completed prior to his enlistment, and therefore a true baseline did not exist for comparison. This is often the case when evaluating SOF operators. When reviewing objective test results in this population it may be appropriate to consider the existence of a "relative deficit," in the context of low-normal scores.

Due to his history of head injury, cognitive problems, disrupted sleep, and early morning headaches, he was referred for a formal sleep evaluation. His polysomnography (PSG) study revealed mild obstructive sleep apnea (OSA) and he was recommended for treatment with CPAP. This device would be difficult for Jerry to use while sleeping in his truck; a plan was made for him to talk with his wife about him coming home while he got his treatment started.

Jerry was reluctant to discuss this issue with her, due to his concern that if he was in the home, they would start arguing again. He agreed to see a couple's counselor, but only on the condition that he gets to see someone who has experience "working with guys like him." He was referred to the Families Overcoming Under Stress (FOCUS) project office which was located close to his base.

This program has been available to teach communication and family resilience skills to service members since 2009, and has become very familiar with treating SOF personnel. Once Jerry agreed to participate in couples counseling, and sleep in the spare bedroom, his wife was amenable to this plan.

22.2.2.8 Treatment/Management

Jerry agreed to a multidisciplinary treatment plan which would include interventions by his psychiatrist, endocrinologist, sleep specialist, and vestibular rehabilitation specialist. From a nonmedical standpoint, he also agreed to consult with his physical trainer about a modified exercise regimen, and a dietitian who could make recommendations on his diet. He was initially concerned that attending all these appointments would be impossible for him while also completing his workup for the next deployment. He agreed to have his psychiatrist discuss his treatment plan with his CO, to see what accommodations could be made.

It was explained to the CO that Jerry's cognitive problems were service connected and probably related to multiple concussions, and possibly sleep problems, or PTSD. The CO was relieved to hear about the progress that had been made in Jerry's assessment, now understanding that this SEAL was not failing at his job due to incompetence or lack of effort, but rather because of a previously undiagnosed medical problem. It was decided that the best way for Jerry to have a successful deployment with the team in the future, was to sit out this deployment and focus on his treatment. This would allow him to be better prepared for the next deployment cycle with either his team or another team.

Jerry was assigned a nurse case manager to help him coordinate a variety of appointments and stay engaged in treatment. However, it is often psychologically difficult for special operations personnel to remain in the "sick role." As individuals, they will habitually direct their energy toward "completing the mission" or improving performance. This means that habits of self-care and allowing for recovery time may be underdeveloped.

They may become frustrated with the "slow and steady" pace offered through many rehabilitation protocols, and then become noncompliant as they attempt to accelerate their recovery on their own terms. Regular interaction with a qualified nurse case manager to set goals, review milestones, and reinforce medical recommendations is highly advisable when caring for patients with multidisciplinary care plans.

For his PTSD and stress management, his psychiatrist recommended that Jerry start with psychotherapy to discuss the loss of his best friend and also target his distorted beliefs related to perfectionism and overly high expectations for himself leading to a chronic sense of disappointment. Jerry and his therapist would also engage in some grief work around the loss of his best friend, Steve, and work to consider how to best honor his memory.

Jerry would also likely benefit from a low-dose selective serotonin reuptake inhibitor (SSRI). It was explained to him that the Navy Bureau of Medicine and Surgery (BUMED) now allowed special operators to have up to 6 months of treatment with an SSRI before requiring a waiver to continue serving in that capacity (Manual of the Medical Department NAVMED P-117. 2012). Nevertheless, Jerry asked that this decision be deferred until after the psychotherapy, CPAP, and testosterone therapy had a chance to work. Finally, a plan was made to observe Jerry for symptom improvement and repeat a PCL-M in 1 month. If his score on the instrument was still above 50 then he would be started on a course of cognitive processing therapy (CPT) (one of the three most extensively researched treatments for PTSD).

After his initial evaluation at the sleep clinic, Jerry had difficulty with compliance with the CPAP device due to noise and discomfort. After some training in relaxation skills, however, his compliance improved and he stopped waking up with headaches. He noticed his energy throughout the day was improving, and he was less irritable in the evenings with his family.

His endocrinologist then started him on 30 mg of testosterone injected intramuscularly weekly. He reported improved energy and a little better strength in the gym, despite cutting back to only 3 workout days per week (his physical trainer had also mentioned to him that like many athletes, he may have been overtraining and should include recovery days into his regular plan). His libido improved, leading to more contention with his wife who was not interested in reciprocating his ardor yet. Jerry attended vestibular rehabilitation once per week, and engaged in exercises at home to help improve his balance, as well as his ability to sit in front of the computer screen without becoming dizzy.

22.2.2.9 Outcome/Resolution

After 1 month of abiding by his treatment plan, Jerry experienced a rapid improvement in mood anxiety, but his concentration problems persisted. Objective neuropsychological reassessment confirmed this finding. His psychiatrist again discussed his results with him and rather than starting on an antidepressant, they discussed the possibility of a low-dose stimulant to target attention problems.

Jerry gave informed consent with the understanding that such medication can sometimes worsen anxiety, and he would need to closely follow up with his psychiatrist for several months. He was started on long-acting methylphenidate, 18 mg daily. This was increased to 36 mg daily, when he reported no subjective benefit after 2 weeks.

Jerry's vital signs remained stable, and on his second follow-up appointment, he reported significant improvement in his ability to follow conversations, and stay focused while reading. He also noticed less fatigue by the end of the day, feeling that he had more energy for his family. He was less irritable at home, and felt those relationships were improving as a result of the medical treatment as well as the couples counseling work.

Jerry was given temporary orders to work as an instructor, while his team was deployed. His new CO was briefed regarding his case and agreed to continue observing his performance in the workplace and to defer any determination whether or not Jerry should return to a deploying unit. Jerry worked well in his new unit and 6 months into treatment was felt by his treatment team as well as his chain of command to be fit for duty.

However, due to his medical conditions and ongoing treatment with stimulant medication, he was considered "not physically qualified" for special operations duty as per US Navy Instructions. As a part of his full return to deployable status, a waiver request would have to be submitted on his behalf to the Bureau of Medicine and Surgery.

22.3 Discussion

22.3.1 Psychological Resilience of Special Operators

Early research on highly resilient individuals focused on personality factors using the five-factor model. One study involving SEALs revealed that they have higher than average extraversion (indicating more social engagement and excitement seeking) and conscientiousness (indicating more organization and persistence) but lower than average agreeableness (indicating more ability to function autonomously). "These characteristics indicate that SEALs are more likely to be forceful, energetic, and to become leaders than men of the general population" [3]. While this profile of an assertive, goal-directed, yet novelty-seeking individual correlated with high psychological resilience, it remained unclear what mediated the relationship.

More recent studies have looked for quantifiable biomarkers of psychological resilience. Several studies have implicated differences in neurotransmitter levels between normal soldiers and SOF assets, most notably high levels of Neuropeptide Y (NPY) being released under stress [4, 5]. This factor also appeared to correlate with good performance under captivity and decreased risk of dissociation [6]. Other biochemical studies on resilience have implicated higher levels of dihydroepianosterone (DHEA), and also homozygosity for the long allele of the serotonin transporter protein (5HTTLPR) may be associated with higher levels of resilience [7].

Neuroimaging has also recently identified differences in brain structure between elite performers (Elite Adventure Racers, Navy SEALs) and normal controls [8, 9]. One consistent finding from these fMRI-based studies has been that the right insular cortex is differentially activated or attenuated based on the stimuli presented. It is therefore hypothesized that interoceptive ability (somatic awareness) is enhanced in elite performers. This "interoceptive tuning" directs mental resources differentially when needed and conserves or attenuates them during exposure to nonthreatening or non-salient stimuli. This tuning leads to more efficient use of mental resources and possibly greater ability to tolerate aversive stimuli.

One question which remains unanswered is how these CNS findings manifest themselves in operational scenarios. Is there a significant difference in the way successful SOF operators balance sympathetic and parasympathetic nervous systems which may not only make them more impervious to stress, but also improve their tactical performance in high threat situations?

22.3.2 Traumatic Brain Injury and Neuroendocrine Dysfunction

Blast exposure is known to be a common cause of traumatic brain injury (TBI) in service members [10]. One important factor to consider is the frequency with which special operators may be exposed to low-level blast in a training environment. Although the intensity of each blast may be relatively low, it is not yet well understood if there is a detrimental effect from exposure to multiple low-level blasts repeatedly in over a short (less than 24 h) period of time. Special operators regularly train with explosives and heavy weapons, and may be exposed to hundreds of these blasts over the course of their careers. Providers who are planning to care for this type of patient should become familiar with neurocognitive assessment and management of TBI.

The sources of TBI include many of the commonly seen incidents such as motor vehicle accidents (MVIs), and improvised explosive devices (IEDs), also planned explosions during training (breaching, heavy weapons use), or rapid acceleration/deceleration scenarios including fast boat maneuvers, hard parachute openings, and even combative (hand to hand) training.

On the battlefield, exposure to a large blast is not uncommon. Patients should be asked about blast exposures, and even if loss of consciousness (LOC) is not endorsed, the patient should be further questioned about whether or not alteration of consciousness (AOC) occurred.

A careful history will reveal that many special operators have experienced several hours of altered consciousness after blast exposure, which should elevate the need for objective assessment in the provider's mind. TBI is notoriously difficult to diagnose in the field and may also be missed during evaluations at higher echelon military medical facilities [11]. TBI may not even be visible on initial neuroimaging. And therefore, a careful history along with neurocognitive testing may be more helpful in detecting cases that have previously not come to attention. Cognitive complaints after repeated blast exposure became so prevalent that in 2009 the US Army Special Operations Command adopted the ImPACT Neurocognitive Assessment to provide baseline measurements of all personnel prior to their deployments [11].

The ImPACT test is well validated in civilian concussion research, and has been useful as a screening tool for mental health providers who are interested in rapidly assessing their patients for cognitive dysfunction. The test takes about 30 min to complete on almost any web-enabled computer. If the test subject has previously completed a baseline exam, the results can be quickly compared to determine if there is a change, but there are also normative values presented along with the subject's scores in the areas of verbal memory, visual memory, visual motor speed, and reaction time.

If there is a significant decline from baseline performance, or if several scores are below one standard deviation from the mean, it may indicate the need for referral for formal neuropsychological testing. Used in this way it enables the clinician to more adeptly screen patients and select those who are more likely to benefit from time consuming and expensive testing resources.

Often TBI is comorbid with PTSD and the symptoms can be difficult to distinguish. Indeed some have suggested that there are overlaps at the level of neuropathology as well, with one recent study showing elevated plasma levels of S100B (a marker of blood brain barrier disruption) having been found in psychologically traumatized children who had not previously experienced head trauma [12]. S100b is a well validated marker of neurotrauma [13], and this finding in both conditions blurs the line between our understanding of psychological and physical brain injury.

Nevertheless, the treatment of TBI can be quite different from that of PTSD, and the patient should be evaluated for both. This starts with a thorough history and neurological exam looking for qualitative findings of vestibular dysfunction, or ocular symptoms. Further, a brief neurocognitive evaluation (RBANS, ImPACT or similar), and laboratory studies to include evaluation of the hypothalamic-pituitary-adrenal axis is useful.

Pituitary dysfunction is prevalent after TBI [14], and most commonly manifests as growth hormone deficiency. In addition to the physical findings of decreased lean body mass, decreased bone density, and fatigue, the psychological manifestations of growth hormone deficiency include poor memory, social withdrawal, and depression. There are a variety of other hormonal abnormalities which may be screened for in patients who fail to recover from TBI at the expected rate, or who manifest chronic symptoms many months after the exposure.

Powner and colleagues report that pituitary dysfunction is often missed as a cause for persisting symptoms after a TBI incident [15]. The general incidence of neuroendocrine abnormalities within the first 90 days after injury has been estimated at 30–50% [15, 16] and may persist for over 1 year. It is prudent for a psychiatrist suspecting an endocrine abnormality to consult with an endocrinologist. If the psychiatrist would like to start the evaluation prior to the referral, then commonly utilized screening labs include a chemistry panel, thyroid function tests, early morning testosterone, follicle stimulating hormone, leutinizing hormone, prolactin, and IGF-1 levels. If an abnormality is found, then a more complete referral can be made, and if none is present, it is unlikely that any referral will need to be made.

Treatment of TBI-related complaints is often symptom focused, and this is not unique to SOF communities. There are two important factors to consider when considering the use of psychotropic medication. The first is that not all medications will allow the operator to be eligible for a waiver to continue in special operations duty. While having a symptomatic TBI condition will be disqualifying in and of itself, it may be difficult to achieve a waiver with certain medications. Often SSRI or SNRI use will be granted a waiver, but more powerful antidepressants might not (Tricyclic antidepressants (TCAs), Mono-Amine Oxidase Inhibitors (MAOIs), or Apripiprazole).

The mental health provider should communicate with the special operator's primary care physician (often embedded in their unit), and consider alternative treatments before prescribing any medication. A second consideration is the possibility of lowering the seizure threshold. Conditions such as TBI may increase a person's risk for seizure and the medications used to treat the TBI may increase the risk as well. Given the extreme and austere environments which a special operator is required to work in, a seizure occurring at a pivotal moment could place the individual, their team, and the entire mission at risk.

In the case presented above, the choice was made to treat the individual with a stimulant medication. There are studies which suggest that sympathomimetic stimulants can increase the risk of seizure, but those studies were primarily completed with amphetamines. There are no conclusive studies which show methylphenidate increases the risk of seizure and to the contrary, there has been one study suggesting that methylphenidate lowers the risk of seizure in some epileptics [17]. Special operators taking stimulant medication for ADHD have been granted waivers in the past. Nevertheless, in the case of TBI, the presentation is so variable,each case will be considered for waiver individually based on its own risk profile.

22.3.3 Sleep Disorders

It has been said, "People sleep peaceably in their beds at night only because rough men stand ready to do violence on their behalf," but what about those rough men? How do they sleep at night? Sleep deprivation is a well-known contributor to problems with cognitive and emotional functioning, metabolic slowing, elevated cortisol levels, decreased testosterone levels, and cardiovascular disease [18–20].

In the special operations community, sleep deprivation is encountered early in the training pipeline and is used as a tool in the selection process. Sleep deprivation in the context may go for several days and is intended to simulate battlefield conditions in which trainees are expected to perform very demanding physical and mental tasks. Instructors then have the opportunity to determine which of these students has the correct mental and physical attributes to succeed in the face of these challenges [21]. However, this early exposure also has an unexpected negative consequence. Some operators come to believe that they can continue to perform without much sleep, and have reported a bias that "sleep is for the weak." Unfortunately, this belief can lead to voluntary sleep restriction and a multitude of adverse health consequences.

The relationship between insomnia and poor health is a complex and nonlinear. For example, insomnia can lead to weight gain, which can in turn contribute to obstructive sleep apnea syndrome. In another example, insomnia can lead to increased anxiety, which can subsequently lead to worse insomnia. Both can be improved with behavioral interventions [22].

There are two underappreciated effects of insomnia which are particularly problematic for the special operator. These problems relate to which phase of the sleep cycle is disrupted. First, it has been demonstrated that the loss of slow-wave sleep early in the sleep cycle is associated with decreased secretion of human growth hormone [23]. It is also well established that wound healing may be slowed in patients with insomnia [24], and growth hormone could play a significant role in that effect. For special operators, wound healing is critical. Allowing insomnia to persist could delay recovery from a variety of injuries and adversely affect military readiness.

The second underreported complication of insomnia is reduction of testosterone for those who are losing REM sleep or loss of sleep late in the sleep cycle [25]. At this time, there have been no published studies demonstrating increased risk for hypogonadism in the special operations community. However, there are studies which demonstrate transient reductions in testosterone from stressful military training [5], and long-term reductions in testosterone after concussions [26].

Special operators should be thought of as athletes, whose sport is war. Like many athletes, they are often looking for a performance edge in their area of expertise. As such they will read and research on their own, and frequently have questions about hormonal effects on performance. It is not uncommon for them to present to their medical department requesting evaluation for hypogonadism in the context of feeling fatigued, losing libido, or losing lean body mass.

There have been many recent advances in the home monitoring of sleep with over the counter smartphone apps, or wearable devices. While these do not currently have the same validity as actigraphy, it is feasible that they could support the evaluation of insomnia with the same level of evidence as a sleep journal [27], and also support greater compliance with treatment recommendations. Data from these devices not only helps to clarify the initial diagnosis of insomnia, but could potentially also provide feedback on the patient's response to an intervention.

The relationship between TBI and insomnia is complex, and the underlying neurological disruptions contributing to insomnia are difficult to evaluate clinically. The provider must start by gathering subjective evidence and then also strongly consider gathering objective evidence from a sleep diary or formal sleep study. Patients with a history of TBI are notoriously poor historians when it comes to their sleep [28], and special operators are no different. It is recommended that the clinician use a sleep diary with patients when evaluating their reports of insomnia [29], but poor patient compliance with such instruments is also well-known [30].

Once the diagnosis is established, the treatment of insomnia in this population is not significantly different than the treatment of insomnia in other populations. The use of non-medication interventions such as sleep hygiene education, or cognitive behavioral therapy for insomnia is preferred. However, if medications are to be used, it is recommended that they be time limited, not habit-forming, or over-sedating. There are many good review articles on pharmacologic approaches to insomnia treatment in people with a history of concussions [31, 32].

It is not clear why concussions and neuroendocrine disorders can initiate or perpetuate sleep disorders. There are many possible etiologies for this association, but the two which have more recently researched include disruptions of hypocretin secretion [33], and reduction in melatonin secretion as a result of damage to the pineal gland [34, 35]. Another theory proposes that TBI disrupts the homeostatic drive for sleep due to changes in mitochondrial function, reduction in ATP metabolism, and therefore, a reduction in adenosine production [36].

22.4 Conclusion

Providing mental health care for SOF operators is a challenging endeavor for any provider who should be so honored as to work among them. One should keep a broad differential diagnosis to include neurological problems, endocrine problems, and sleep disorders which could underlie psychological complaints. Intervening with specificity based on a comprehensive assessment can yield great improvements. In medicine as in combat it can be said, "Delivering modest amounts of fire at the right place and at the right time often determines the outcome of a major engagement" [37]

Treatment planning should emphasize options which are based on solid evidence, and also be flexible to meet with unique occupational demands of the patient. An interdisciplinary approach is usually best. The SOF mental health provider should have advanced knowledge in the areas of sleep disorders, traumatic brain injury, and psychotherapeutic skills, as these patients often are reluctant to take psychotropic medications.

Due to the high degree of autonomy and trust placed in each special operator, it is also very important to engage closely with a patient's chain of command in order to obtain optimal outcomes, and not allow them to be exposed to situations in which they may not be prepared to perform. Creating a good outcome for each individual, multiplies the effectiveness of that team by allowing them to retain their most experienced warriors. Given the nature of our current prolonged asymmetric conflicts, the effectiveness of our special operations teams are vital in supporting our national interests.

References

1. Prusaczyk WK, Goldberg GM. Organizational, psychological, and training aspects of Special Operations Forces. In: Lounsbury DE, editor. Medical aspects of harsh environments. Washington, DC: Department of the Army, Office of The Surgeon General; 2002. pp.1166–93.
2. Joint Chiefs of Staff Publication on Special Operations. Washington DC: Department of Defense; 17 Apr 1998: Chap I: 2–4. Joint Publication 3–05. www.dtic.mil/doctine. Accessed 20 April 2015.
3. Braun DE, Prusaczyk WK, Pratt NC. Personality Profiles of US Navy Sea-Air-Land (SEAL) Personnel. No. NHRC-94-8. NAVAL HEALTH RESEARCH CENTER SAN DIEGO CA, 1994. http://www.dtic.mil/dtic/tr/fulltext/u2/a281692.pdf. Accessed 20 April 2015.
4. Morgan CA, Wang S, Southwick SM, et al. Plasma neuropeptide-Y concentrations in humans exposed to military survival training. Biol Psychiatry. 2000;47(10):902–9.
5. Morgan CA, Wang S, Mason J, et al. Hormone profiles in humans experiencing military survival training. Biol Psychiatry. 2000;47(10):891–901.
6. Morgan CA, Rasmusson AM, Wang S, Hoyt G, Hauger RL, Hazlett G. Neuropeptide-Y, cortisol, and subjective distress in humans exposed to acute stress: replication and extension of previous report. Biol Psychiatry. 2002;52(2):136–42.
7. Southwick SM, Vythilingam M, Charney DS. The psychobiology of depression and resilience to stress: implications for prevention and treatment. Annu Rev Clin Psychol. 2005;1:255–91.

8. Paulus MP, Flagan T, Simmons AN, et al. Subjecting elite athletes to inspiratory breathing load reveals behavioral and neural signatures of optimal performers in extreme environments. PLoS ONE. 2012;7(1):e29394.
9. Simmons AN, Fitzpatrick S, Strigo IA, et al. Altered insula activation in anticipation of changing emotional states: neural mechanisms underlying cognitive flexibility in Special Operations Forces personnel. Neuroreport. 2012;23(4):234–9.
10. Magnuson J, Leonessa F, Ling GS. Neuropathology of explosive blast traumatic brain injury. Curr Neurol Neurosci Rep. 2012;12(5):570–9.
11. Hettich T, Whitfield E, Kratz K, Frament C. Case report: use of the immediate post concussion assessment and cognitive testing (ImPACT) to assist with return to duty determination of special operations soldiers who sustained mild traumatic brain injury. JSOM. 2010;10(4):48–55. https://www.yumpu.com/en/document/view/8175054/fall-united-states-special-operations-command/3.
12. Falcone T, Janigro D, Lovell R, et al. S100B blood levels and childhood trauma in adolescent inpatients. J Psychiatr Res. 2015;62:14–22.
13. Shahim P, Tegner Y, Wilson DH, et al. Blood biomarkers for brain injury in concussed professional ice hockey players. JAMA Neurol. 2014;71(6):684–92.
14. Munoz A, Urban R. Neuroendocrine consequences of traumatic brain injury. Curr Opin Endocrinol Diabetes Obes. 2013;20(4):354–8.
15. Powner DJ, Boccalandro C, Alp MS, Vollmer DG. Endocrine failure after traumatic brain injury in adults. Neurocrit Care. 2006;5(1):61–70.
16. Tanriverdi F, Senyurek H, Unluhizarci K, Selcuklu A, Casanueva FF, Kelestimur F. High risk of hypopituitarism after traumatic brain injury: a prospective investigation of anterior pituitary function in the acute phase and 12 months after trauma. J Clin Endocrinol Metab. 2006;91(6):2105–11.
17. Wroblewski BA, Leary JM, Phelan AM, Whyte J, Manning K. Methylphenidate and seizure frequency in brain injured patients with seizure disorders. J Clin Psychiatry. 1992;53(3):86–9.
18. Hanlon EC, Knutson KL. Sleep deprivation and metabolism. In: Bianchi MT, editor. Sleep deprivation and disease. New York: Springer 2014. pp. 111–29.
19. Short MA, Banks S. The functional impact of sleep deprivation, sleep restriction, and sleep fragmentation. In: Bianchi MT editor. Sleep deprivation and disease. New York: Springer; 2014. pp. 13–26.
20. Wittert G. The relationship between sleep disorders and testosterone in men. Asian J Androl. 2014;16(2):262–5.
21. Lieberman HR, Tharion WJ, Shukitt-hale B, Speckman KL, Tulley R. Effects of caffeine, sleep loss, and stress on cognitive performance and mood during U.S. Navy SEAL training. Sea-Air-Land. Psychopharmacology (Berl). 2002;164(3):250–61.
22. Bowden A, Lorenc A, Robinson N. Autogenic training as a behavioural approach to insomnia: a prospective cohort study. Prim Health Care Res Dev. 2012;13(2):175–85.
23. Sassin JF, Parker DC, Johnson LC, Rossman LG, Mace JW, Gotlin RW. Effects of slow wave sleep deprivation on human growth hormone release in sleep: preliminary study. Life Sci. 1969;8(23):1299–307.
24. Bahammam A. Sleep in acute care units. Sleep and Breathing. 2006;10(1):6–15.
25. Schmid SM, Hallschmid M, Jauch-Chara K, Lehnert H, Schultes B. Sleep timing may modulate the effect of sleep loss on testosterone. ClinEndocrinol (Oxf). 2012;77(5):749–54.
26. Wilkinson CW, Pagulayan KF, Petrie EC, et al. High prevalence of chronic pituitary and target-organ hormone abnormalities after blast-related mild traumatic brain injury. Front Neurol. 2012;3:11.
27. Min YH, Lee JW, Shin YW, et al. Daily collection of self-reporting sleep disturbance data via a smartphone app in breast cancer patients receiving chemotherapy: a feasibility study. J Med Internet Res. 2014;16(5):e135.
28. Ouellet MC, Morin CM. Subjective and objective measures of insomnia in the context of traumatic brain injury: a preliminary study. Sleep Med. 2006;7(6):486–97.

29. Carney CE, Buysse DJ, Ancoli-israel S, et al. The consensus sleep diary: standardizing prospective sleep self-monitoring. Sleep. 2012;35(2):287–302.
30. Broderick JE, Schwartz JE, Shiffman S, Hufford MR, Stone AA. Signaling does not adequately improve diary compliance. Ann Behav Med. 2003;26(2):139–48.
31. Weber M, Webb CA, Killgore WD. A brief and selective review of treatment approaches for sleep disturbance following traumatic brain injury. J Sleep Disorders Ther. 2013;2(110). doi:10.4172/2167-0277.1000110.
32. Chen AJ, Loya F. Mild-moderate TBI: clinical recommendations to optimize neurobehavioral functioning, learning, and adaptation. Semin Neurol. 2014;34(5):557–71.
33. Baumann CR, Werth E, Stocker R, Ludwig S, Bassetti CL. Sleep-wake disturbances 6 months after traumatic brain injury: a prospective study. Brain. 2007;130(7):1873–83.
34. Yaeger K, Alhilali L, Fakhran S. Evaluation of tentorial length and angle in sleep-wake disturbances after mild traumatic brain injury. AJR Am J Roentgenol. 2014;202(3):614–8.
35. Frieboes RM, Müller U, Murck H, Von cramon DY, Holsboer F, Steiger A. Nocturnal hormone secretion and the sleep EEG in patients several months after traumatic brain injury. J Neuropsychiatry Clin Neurosci. 1999;11(3):354–60.
36. Verweij BH, Muizelaar JP, Vinas FC, Peterson PL, Xiong Y, Lee CP. Impaired cerebral mitochondrial function after traumatic brain injury in humans. J Neurosurg. 2000;93(5):815–20.
37. Marshall SLA. Men against fire. Gloucester: Peter Smith. McNally; 1978. pp. 138–156.

Treating War-Related Moral Injury and Loss with *Adaptive Disclosure*: A Case Study

23

Alexandra L. Laifer, Amy D. Amidon, Ariel J. Lang and Brett T. Litz

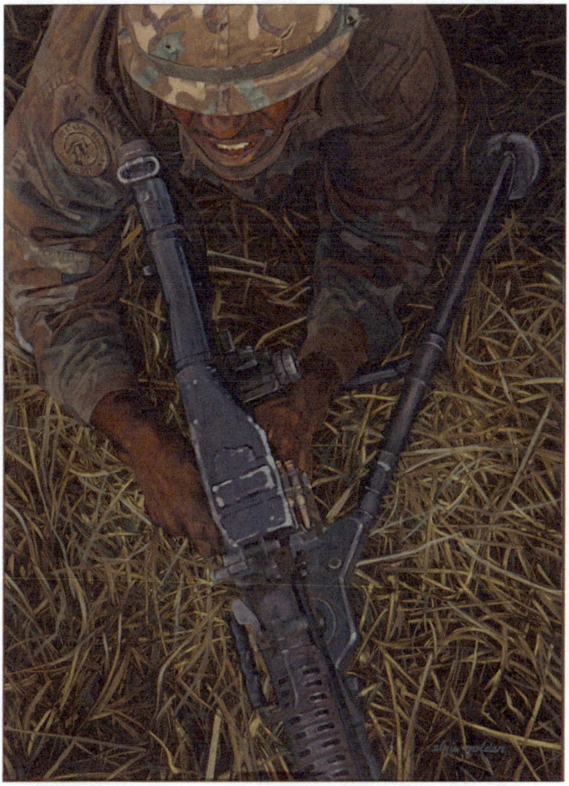

M60 Gunner, by SFC Elzie Golden, courtesy of the Army Art Collection, US Army Center of Military History.

A. L. Laifer (✉)
Veterans Medical Research Foundation,
VA San Diego Healthcare System, San Diego, CA, USA
e-mail: alexandra.laifer@gmail.com

E. C. Ritchie (ed.), *Posttraumatic Stress Disorder and Related Diseases in Combat Veterans*, DOI 10.1007/978-3-319-22985-0_23

Relative to most civilian traumas, war zone exposure has been associated with considerably more enduring psychiatric, social, spiritual, and behavioral problems, as well as with poorer responses to treatment [1–7]. In order to improve the health and welfare of deployed service members and war veterans, it is critical to investigate why this is the case [8]. In doing so, there has been a focus on disaggregating war zone harms and their consequences into what appear to be three broad yet distinct principal types: life-threat (danger), traumatic loss, and moral injury [9].

Existing evidence-based treatments for posttraumatic stress disorder (PTSD) have overemphasized danger-based war zone harms; however, unlike civilian traumatic event contexts, there is good reason to assume that many fear- or danger-based stress reactions are mitigated by military preselection, training in resilience and recovery, and aspects of military culture, such as, leadership, cohesive units, rituals, which can serve as protective factors. By contrast, there are far fewer resources to alleviate and heal the lasting impact of traumatic loss and moral injury, a syndrome of self-handicapping and demoralization that occurs following a perpetration, failure to prevent, or bearing witness to war zone acts that violate deeply held beliefs and expectations about moral and ethical conduct; the crux of moral injury is significant guilt and shame in response to acts of commission or omission that entail culpability from the service member's point of view [9]. It has been argued that because loss and moral injury are inherently *not* fear-based, they each require different ecologically sensitive and valid treatment strategies that are not part of existing treatments for PTSD [9].

Prolonged exposure (PE) [10] and cognitive processing therapy (CPT)[11], generally considered front-line treatments for PTSD, have started to include some content about ways in which guilt from loss and perpetration should be "contextualized" or "processed," but there are no explicit exercises or developed dialogues to illustrate how that might be done. Without the latter, it is unlikely that therapists will know consistently and with confidence what to do when confronted with traumatic loss or moral injury, or whether their approach is replicable based on an operationalized standard. Indeed, these existing treatments for PTSD are well suited to help service members who are haunted by "should haves" (hindsight bias) and who shoulder an excessive amount of perceived responsibility due to a known, unequivocal, noncontingent outcome. However, it is unclear how these therapies specifically address the core elements of loss and moral injury among service members, as outlined above.

In many ways, these existing therapies for PTSD do not sufficiently consider the distinct cultural elements of military trauma or the phenomenology of exposure to

A. D. Amidon
Department of Psychology, Naval Medical Center San Diego, San Diego, CA, USA

A. J. Lang
VA San Diego Healthcare System, University of California, San Diego, San Diego, CA, USA

B. T. Litz
Department of Psychiatry, VA Boston Healthcare System, Boston University, Boston, MA, USA

combat and operational stressors, that is, loss and moral injury. In order to begin to address the gap in the treatment of service members and veterans, a new psychotherapy for PTSD has been developed that is specifically and strategically informed by an understanding of the unique phenomenology of service members' experience, the warrior culture and ethos, and the diverse stressors and conflicts that arise in battle, especially in the context of guerilla wars of insurgency such as those in Iraq and Afghanistan. This therapy is called *adaptive disclosure* [12].

Adaptive disclosure is a relatively brief individual therapy that occurs over eight 90-min weekly sessions and employs different strategies to specifically target the unique phenomenology of danger-, loss-, and moral injury-based principal war zone harms [13, 14]. It is designed to help service members and veterans with PTSD experientially and emotionally process these divergent types of war zone harms, allowing them to gain exposure to corrective and more productive ways of construing the implications of their combat experiences, particularly in terms of their military identity, how they feel about themselves, how they relate to other people, and how they construct a narrative about their future.

Adaptive disclosure was predicated on a number of core assumptions and preconditions. First, adaptive disclosure is specifically designed to train providers in understanding, honoring, and accommodating military culture as well as the unique phenomenology of war trauma. This is particularly relevant when delivered within the context of active-duty military life where service members may be struggling with symptoms yet having to prepare for their next deployment or other military roles. Experienced providers in the military and Veterans Affairs (VA) clinics should be well versed in these matters; however, this may not be the case with trainees or civilian providers outside these contexts.

The assumption is that if all clinicians possess adequate knowledge about military culture, and are prepared to hear about every dimension of war experience without judgment, then service members would be more willing to build trust and have confidence that the intensely emotional and evocative engagement that is required when going through adaptive disclosure would be worthwhile. It is also important to bring military roles and expectations into the therapy room and for clinicians to understand the nature of a service member's job, the degree of leadership responsibility inherent in that role, as well as how all of this may align with their former and current goals and aspirations. This knowledge provides context for clinicians to understand why the service member may be interpreting the events in a particular way as well as allow the clinician to help service members better conceptualize the implications of construing traumatic events with so much condemnation and self-destruction; it may also help inform a more realistic perception of expectations of behavior and responsibility so that service members may reconcile within themselves and move forward in their lives.

Second, the approach is based on the premise that the goal of the therapy should be to create a foundation for healing, repair, and recovery; in other words, treatment serves as an *introduction* to a different way of dealing with the psychological, behavioral, and spiritual legacy of combat and operational events, rather than an end point. Although it is possible for meaningful change to occur over the course of treatment, the brevity of adaptive disclosure and the chronicity of complex PTSD secondary to combat trauma make it unrealistic to assume that all symptoms will be eradicated and maladaptive cognitions and schemas supplanted with more realistic ones upon completion of the therapy. For many service members and veterans, a complete and total cure may not be possible and they should prepare themselves for life-long challenges. Instead, the idea behind adaptive disclosure is to "plant seeds" of healing through a deeper understanding of the context of events, moving toward acceptance of imperfections within oneself and others.

The third assumption is that active-duty service members and veterans who are treatment naïve may not be well versed in sharing and disclosing their experiences. As such, their narratives of shame- or guilt-based experiences may initially be somewhat disorganized and unduly limited; it typically requires time, along with the development of a trusting therapeutic relationship, for narratives to be properly revealed and processed. However, the reality of life for an active-duty service member is such that there is not a lot of time to do preparatory relationship and trust building. Therefore, by honoring and understanding the military ethos, utilizing a "no-nonsense, let's get right to it" experiential approach, and targeting issues that resonate deeply with deployed service members, clinicians can create a trust that would otherwise take much longer to cultivate.

Fourth, given that meaning-making is an essential change agent in all forms of psychotherapy, the developers of adaptive disclosure were especially keen to employ strategies to help service members uncover and clarify the meaning they ascribe to the experiences that haunt them, particularly in terms of their identity and behavior as service members and future veterans, as well as in various interpersonal roles they hold in their lives. Perhaps due to the characteristic stoicism reinforced by military identity and training, many service members and veterans have not sufficiently reflected on the meaning and implications of war zone harms, let alone articulated and shared these ideas prior to treatment. Consequently, it is important that service members engage in evocative experiential strategies to unearth constructions of the meaning and implications of war zone harms.

Finally, as a point of departure from conventional CBT approaches, adaptive disclosure does not assume that anguish, shame, and distress are inevitably caused by distorted thinking. In many instances, self-blame or blame of others is not entirely inaccurate, given the values embedded within military culture and particularly in the context of the codependencies of units in battle. Clinicians need to be aware that military training and culture teach service members that their most treasured moral construct—honor—is earned through actions that are identified as just, moral, and ethical, as well as through noble sacrifices. Consequently, perceived transgression is particularly anguishing and disruptive for a service member; it undermines their moral identity by damaging their ability to trust their sustaining moral values and guiding ideals, or to even abide by them. Therefore, in adaptive disclosure, the goal is not necessarily to have the patient challenge the veracity of these conclusions, but rather to respect and honor the foundation from which they come while promoting more adaptive and sensible future possibilities.

At its core, adaptive disclosure entails exposure-based, experiential, and emotion-focused processing of the principal combat or operational experience and a real-time rendering of constructions about the implications of the event in terms of self-view, professional role, expectations about others, and the future. For all trauma types, similar to other CBT-based approaches, adaptive disclosure provides an opportunity for service members and veterans to realize how they have changed as a result of combat and operational experiences, to reflect upon who they want to be, and to create a path of how to get there. Unlike other therapies for PTSD, adaptive disclosure employs strategies that are specific to each type of principal harm. If the service member endorses life-threat as his or her most currently distressing and haunting war zone experience, then the therapy is similar to PE, given that conceptually and empirically PE has been demonstrated to be the treatment of choice for conditioned fear-based PTSD [15]. If the principal event is related to loss or moral injury, separate break-out strategies are used to foster exposure to corrective experience and new learning specific to these dynamics.

The therapy follows a set structure. Each session includes an intense narrative of the traumatic event followed by raw emotional processing of the meaning and implication of the event and an experiential exercise related to the principal identified harm. The narrative is exposure-based in that it requires the patient to recount the event in real time with eyes closed and in great detail. Unlike traditional exposure therapy for life-threat/danger-based PTSD, where the goal is to extinguish conditioned fear and to modify fear-beliefs, adaptive disclosure uses exposure to bring about emotional activation or a "hot-cognitive" state of mind, in order to facilitate deeper meaning-making processing around loss or moral injury. As such, the trauma is told via exposure only once each session, followed by the other treatment elements. Many times the intensity of these experiences elicits a high level of distress and arousal that requires the inclusion of grounding exercises at the end of the session in order for the patient to be returned to a functional state. Each session also includes a written homework assignment that is either related to the content of the current session or preparation for the following session. Some assignments also include behavioral tasks as well.

In cases where loss is most prominent, the emotions and thoughts that are elicited following the trauma narrative usually involve self-blame and guilt. In order to further process these emotions and thoughts, the accompanying experiential exercise entails an imaginal dialogue with the person who was lost. The idea is for the patient to acknowledge, in real time, how the loss has impacted him, what it might mean to the person who was lost, and then for the patient to voice how that person might respond to the patient's self-destructive ways. The goal is to promote an emotionally charged accommodation of a corrective "message" voiced by the deceased, who would likely only want the patient to live well. In addition to the dialogues in session, the patient is also encouraged to think about and engage in behavioral tasks outside the therapy room that may memorialize the person. This may include going to a specific place that held meaning to the person, visiting a cemetery, reaching out to family members and others who served alongside the person, volunteering for a related cause, or doing an activity that elicits positive associations with that person.

In cases where moral injury is the principal harm, the experiential exercise involves an imaginal "confession" and dialogue with a compassionate, forgiving moral authority or other salient figures (e.g., a subordinate service member or veteran, a "future self," the harmed victim, etc.) in order to begin to challenge and address the shame and self-defeat that accompany such experiences. There are also homework assignments that include behavioral tasks to initiate the process of moral repair, such as giving back to the community or other ways to engage their innate goodness in a way that might be meaningful to them.

The assumption of adaptive disclosure is that the treatment can start, but cannot finish, the moral repair process. It is believed that self-forgiveness and the possibility of living a moral and virtuous life will ultimately require significant life-course changes for most veterans of war. Moreover, the goal is not to attempt to eradicate or fully replace the service member's self-constructions of moral compromise, as this is unlikely to occur within the context of such a short intervention, but rather to foster a more balanced perspective of the event, a deeper understanding of the context of the injury, and forward movement. Adaptive disclosure aims to help the patient accept the part of him or herself that engaged in or was subjected to morally transgressive acts without overly attempting to modify constructions about culpability or the moral implications of the event(s). At the same time, the therapy is designed to help the patient reclaim goodness and humanity and to manifest those parts in his life as prominently as possible.

Here, a case study will be reported in which adaptive disclosure was used to target moral injury in a recently discharged Marine who suffered from combat-related PTSD. This case was treated in a VA outpatient specialty care context.

23.1 Case Study

23.1.1 Case History

"Stew" was a 27 year old, divorced, Native American Veteran who served in the Marine Corps infantry for 8 years. He had two combat deployments to Afghanistan and had been diagnosed with PTSD a few months prior to completing his second enlistment. Stew reported that he joined the military because he had always thought it was "badass" and he wanted more opportunities for himself. He had grown up on a reservation in South Dakota amid a lot of interpersonal chaos; his parents divorced when he was 5 years old and his father was an alcoholic who was physically abusive. Moreover, he experienced a number of significant losses over the course of his life including the suicide of an uncle when he was a teenager as well as the murder of his cousin during the treatment. As such, Stew would often say that he was used to "getting bad news all of the time" and was fearful of looking forward to things because he assumed that anything positive would never come to fruition. His marriage had been unsuccessful as well, ending after he discovered his wife had cheated on him while he was on deployment. Once he left the Marine Corps, he decided to stay in California and at the time of treatment, he was attending a local college.

Stew reported passive-dependent behaviors in terms of the management of his own mental health. Although he had been taking medication for PTSD and depression while on active duty, he had not followed-up with doctors to continue his medication upon discharge because he reportedly "kept waiting for them to contact [him]." Nevertheless, he eventually took it upon himself to come to the VA Mental Health Clinic because he had experienced an increase in symptoms, and it had become difficult for him to complete his schoolwork.

23.1.2 Assessment and Treatment

At the time of his intake, Stew reported significant isolation, numbness, and constant worry. He said that he would "freak out" often and perspire excessively which led him to avoid going places unless it was absolutely necessary; he was particularly avoidant of crowds and had become increasingly hypervigilant. Moreover, he had trouble falling asleep and experienced regular nightmares related to his combat experience. He also reported significant anger, though no physical aggression, and stated that he hated Middle Eastern people.

Stew had been exposed to a number of blasts during his deployments that led to chronic pain as well as some difficulty with short-term memory. Although he had been receiving cognitive rehabilitation services that he reported were helpful, he continued to experience a good deal of anhedonia, lethargy, and general sadness related to his personal actions in combat as well as the loss of fellow Marines who were killed in various combat incidents. He had engaged in daily alcohol use for 5 years while on active duty and had also been arrested for driving under the influence on base during that time. He reported that although he stopped drinking liquor a few months prior to beginning treatment, he would still drink beer occasionally. Moreover, he would use marijuana three or four times per week to control his chronic pain.

The initial session of adaptive disclosure involves a general assessment of current functioning, a discussion comparing and contrasting what the individual was like pre- and post-trauma, and identifying what the person hopes to gain from treatment. It also includes information about the various components of the treatment process, including the trauma narrative and experiential exercises, as well as psychoeducation about the nature of trauma and combat stress. The main goals of adaptive disclosure are presented as follows: learn to talk about what happened in a useful way in order to better understand what is bothering you as well as come to terms with the meaning and implications of the trauma; chip away at rigid interpretations and consider alternative explanations for events; and reclaim good parts of yourself rather than be defined by negative aspects of combat experiences. The final part of the session involves identifying the trauma that will be the focus of treatment.

At the end of the first session, the therapist discusses the role of homework and assigns a *Meaning and Implication of Key Events* form. This form is very similar to the *Impact Statement* used in CPT [11] and is common to many trauma- or adversity-focused therapeutic approaches [16]. In adaptive disclosure, the goal is to establish a baseline of constructions and meanings that the patient can use as a basis of comparison at the end of the therapy. The assignment is designed to have the patient reflect on what he or she believes may have "caused" the trauma (e.g., something he did wrong, something someone else did wrong, something that went wrong, the nature of war itself, etc). It also asks the patient to consider subsequent changes in beliefs about himself, others, and the world that have occurred in response to the trauma. The purpose is to take an inventory of change and to reveal some of the cognitive rigidity that may have developed around the event.

Given the short duration of adaptive disclosure, along with the intensive focus on the trauma, it is always important to set expectations about the process and to communicate that treatment is incremental and healing from trauma takes time along with commitment. Moreover, as the individual begins going deeper into the trauma memory, it is possible the patient will experience more pain and distress before ultimately feeling better. Patients are strongly encouraged to attend sessions regularly and to do their best to override the inevitable urges to avoid the emotional engagement that treatment entails.

Stew presented to his first session in a very anxious state. His hands were shaking, he was looking around the room, and it was difficult for him to maintain eye contact. Despite his anxiety, Stew was able to articulate that he had been depressed with little motivation. He stated that he used to enjoy going out and being sociable but recently, he had been isolating himself from others, including his girlfriend. In addition, his lack of motivation was making it difficult to go to class, and he was having trouble deciding the direction of his studies. As such, he was hoping to break out of the isolation and to regain some clarity about what he wanted in his life.

Although Stew had a number of significant traumas during his two combat deployments, when asked to identify an index trauma, he knew right away what it would be: On his second deployment, he had been called upon by his corpsman and his captain to help an older, wounded Iraqi man but he refused to do so. He said he could not stop thinking about the event and what a terrible person he was because of it. This was a prototypic moral injury. He agreed to complete the written assignment and bring it to the next session.

Session 2 of adaptive disclosure involves an oral reading of the written statement and discussion of the themes. This is followed by the first trauma narrative with subsequent processing of the meaning and implications of it. Stew's written statement included strong themes of failure and a sense that he deserved some recrimination, but he also revealed some ambivalence. He wrote that "karma" was the cause of the event but he also justified what he had done by saying that he could not be sure in that moment that the man had not been the enemy "laying down improvised explosive devices (IEDs) and killing Marines," and that this uncertainty may have motivated his inaction. Still, he felt he was to blame for the "poor choice," that is, allowing a potentially innocent man to suffer and die, and now he was "carrying guilt constantly to make up for it." He stated, "God saw me and felt me refuse to help. People think I'm a hero but I'm not."

Stew was haunted by his apparent failure to act, which violated his values as well as his sense of honor and duty. Those who struggle with moral injury tend to internalize extremely negative ways of thinking in order to cope with the dissonance that is created by their perceived transgression. This may include self-protective denial and numbing or excessive assimilation of the significance of the event into preexisting self-schema, that is, "the Marine Corps is just and good, I am just and good, so what I did must be just and good," leading to negation of wrongdoing and a potentially slippery slope of additional immoral behavior. Alternatively, maladaptive coping may involve over-accommodation of the significance of the incident such that the person allows it to redefine himself as a bad person who deserves to be punished, with no appreciation of anything good he may have done in the past. This is typically accompanied by excessive feelings of shame, guilt, disgust, and self-hatred. Stew clearly fell into this last category and given that he had never had the opportunity to fully process the emotional impact of the event, including the ambivalence he felt about it, he was slowly inhibiting his life in response to the anxiety, distress, and deep pain it was causing.

Following this discussion, Stew moved into the first trauma narrative. He was presented with the rationale for exposure and then instructed to close his eyes and retell the story slowly, with as much detail as possible, in the present tense as if it were happening again while he was imagining it. Stew was very nervous about telling the story, reporting a distress level of 50 (out of 100) before beginning. His narrative included very little detail but recounted how he had been on a mission without sleep for 35 h. He described being "tired, pissed off, and on edge" and having to respond to a call to pick up someone who had been injured. They arrived to the specified location and Stew had to ride with the man back to the base. Although the corpsman was yelling that Stew needed to help tend to the man's wounds, he "didn't want to listen to him." Once on base, people were staring and seemed to think he was a "badass" but the reality was that, "I am not a hero." At the end of the narrative, Stew reported that his distress was up to 85.

Stew was clearly emotionally activated and the therapist moved into further processing the experience. He indicated that the retelling was indeed as difficult as he had anticipated; he was feeling nauseous and sweaty and his head was throbbing, similar to how he had felt at the time of the event. He reiterated how this event had made him hate "Muslim-looking" people and that he avoids being near them. Moreover, he explained that because of the event, he had become uncomfortable whenever he would visit his family for fear that they would think he is a hero. He had never shared the story before and themes of failure and moral injury were abundant. When asked which part of the memory was the most difficult to recount, he stated that riding alongside the man and seeing what was happening to him was the worst part (and indeed that part had been fairly glossed-over in the retelling). At the end of the session, after going through a grounding exercise to help decrease his agitation, he was assigned for homework to reflect upon and identify someone in his life with whom he might feel comfortable sharing the story and to write about how he would share it.

Sessions 3–7 involve a review of homework, engagement in the trauma narrative with subsequent emotional processing of the meaning and implication of it, an experiential exercise targeting the principal harm, and assignment of new homework.

Stew returned for Session 3 the following week and reported that the previous session had been very hard, leading him to continue to think deeply about the event during the subsequent days. He had completed the written homework and read it aloud, indicating he would probably share the story with his girlfriend and his brother but he might not tell them all of the details because he was ashamed. His experience was validated; he was reminded that this was a relatively common response and very understandable given the circumstance, and a discussion ensued about how much he would benefit from working through the shame he was experiencing. The trauma narrative was then revisited. This time, he was instructed to slow down the retelling and go into more detail about riding alongside the man. He reported his distress at 85 (on the PTSD scale) and began to tell the story.

During the exposure, Stew revisited the scene of being notified that he had to pick up someone and further described being on edge due to concerns that there would be an IED during the drive as well as the fact that the casualty was unknown. They arrived in a ditch and discovered that the person who was wounded was an older, heavyset Iraqi man wearing a white robe. The man had been shot in the neck and face and no one wanted to carry him so he was "hot-potatoed," that is, passed around from person to person, until he was finally placed in the truck. During the course of events, Stew's position was shifted so that he ended up having to sit in the back of the truck with the man and the unit corpsman. He narrated:

> My heart is beating really fast, trying to stare out at the surrounding area but also focusing on the guy. There is snot, blood, and vomit coming out of his mouth. The doc is yelling at me and I am yelling back that I don't want to touch him. I feel real gross. Part of me wants to help but I also don't want to. His feet are dirty; his hands are rough and remind me of my dad. I am not thinking about the fact that he might die, just thinking how gross the situation is. We get back to base and I walk away, go to the chow hall. I'm dirty and people are asking me if I helped so I bullshit them and say, Yeah, I helped. Then I start to feel gross. Everything [the man] was going through is still on me, the blood is on my gear, the stain of murder.

Following the narrative, Stew reported his distress at 95 (on the PTSD scale). He discussed how the corpsman had informed him later that day that the man had died. He further described that what he had done was "unforgivable," that he "didn't do anything and should have done more." Most profoundly, he said, "I feel like I lost a piece of myself that day." It was pointed out that the context of the event—the brutality of war, the extreme fatigue—may have impacted his behavior. He remained unconvinced.

After the processing, Stew was moved into the next component of treatment, the breakout experiential exercise. As mentioned earlier, in addition to processing the trauma narrative in depth and providing cognitive restructuring where appropriate, adaptive disclosure addresses moral injury via break-out experiential exercises in which the patient has hypothetical real-time conversations with people who can offer an alternative, compassionate perspective, and/or encourage new ways of thinking. The initial conversation is typically held with a person identified by the patient as someone who serves as a compassionate figure in his life and cares about him deeply. Depending upon the event, subsequent conversations may be held with other relevant figures, including the person who the patient feels he has harmed or others who were present at the event, as a means of determining ways to make amends or, in cases where the patient may be assigning himself a disproportionate amount of blame for what occurred, lessen the burden of responsibility which he may be carrying. Given that adaptive disclosure focuses on the patient moving forward in his life, the conversation could also involve a hypothetical figure who might exist in an imagined future life, that is, a child or a significant other.

These exercises are designed to allow the patient to express his perceived transgression in an authentic, visceral way, akin to a confession, while receiving feedback that can challenge the extreme, rigid ways of thinking about it. The idea is not necessarily to minimize the act but rather to bring awareness to the totality of his experience and incorporate a new, more nuanced way of thinking about the event within the context of his life. Although these exercises are considered to be "conversations" in the sense that the patient shares his thoughts aloud, and provides the feedback he would imagine coming from the other person, it is important to distinguish this experience from an actual conversation that would happen outside the therapy room and to establish for the patient that the purpose is to shift into something "out of the ordinary" in order to gain a different perspective on the trauma. Most importantly, through these hypothetical conversations, the patient is meant to experience a sense that despite his deep feelings of guilt, shame, and failure, he deserves compassion and permission to forgive himself, move forward, and create a life of value and meaning.

This process was described to Stew and he was asked whom he might want to include in the exercise. Based on his homework, the therapist expected him to choose his brother or his girlfriend but instead he immediately identified his grandmother who had been instrumental in raising him and whom he felt he had disappointed the most. It seemed like a good choice so he was asked to close his eyes and tell the therapist about her. He described her as an older, Sioux woman who was very religious and always spoke about God and the Great Spirit. He said that she was "small but powerful" and despite that fact that Stew was quite a bit taller than she, he often found himself intimidated by her even though he also described her as being very warm. He added that she did not speak English, and he did not speak their native language very well, but somehow they managed to communicate.

The therapist told him to imagine she was in the room, sitting in the chair next to him. Once he had conjured that mental image, he was instructed to tell her what had happened in Iraq. He paused for a moment with his hands shaking, mouth clenched, and moisture in his eyes, as he welled up in pain. He suddenly opened his eyes and said he could not do it; he could not tell her what he had done.

The struggle to engage in this exercise is not unusual as it requires a level of vulnerability that is often intolerable to the patient. When this occurs, the therapist will typically normalize the experience, explain once again how it can be helpful to gain a different perspective, and strongly encourage the patient to continue, cheerleading his efforts while pushing him along. This was done to some extent with Stew but it was clear he was paralyzed and unable to get the words out. As such, the exercise was modified a bit and he was simply asked what Grandma would say to him about forgiving himself. He scoffed somewhat, saying she would probably tell him to pray and go to church and talk to God—but he did not want to go to church because he did not think it would help. The therapist spent some time processing why this exercise had been difficult for him and he reiterated how ashamed he felt and that it was impossible to face her. He engaged in another brief grounding exercise and was provided with homework to write about the costs and benefits of not forgiving himself as well as reflect upon what it would mean if he did forgive himself.

Stew cancelled his session the next week, stating that he was ill. When he returned to treatment for Session 4 the following week, he expressed that he had been feeling very stressed about school. He had also been overwhelmed by the emotional impact of the previous session and wanted to avoid having that experience again. The therapist validated his experience but explained to him that even though it was unpleasant, his strong engagement with his emotions was evidence that he was moving toward healing instead of suppressing his experience. He was reminded that it is common to feel worse before feeling better, but that working through his emotions is the process through which healing comes.

At that point, the therapist asked him about his homework and was pleasantly surprised to find that he had completed it. He said he took a long time to reflect upon the costs and benefits of not forgiving himself and wrote the following:

> *Benefits*: protection against doing more bad things and keeps me ready
> *Costs*: preventing myself from moving forward, holding on to pain and hurt, goes against personal beliefs, prevents me from having friends, makes me feel bad around my family

After reading it aloud, he was surprised at how "costly" it was to maintain the belief that he was unforgivable. Similarly, even though he perceived the benefit as useful, he could see why it might be important to move away from it. In fact, his response to the question of what it would mean to forgive was also indicative of this realization: "I guess it would mean moving forward and understanding that it was a bad time during war and some bad choices were made." The therapist communicated that his insight was impressive and he was clearly internalizing a more adaptive, balanced perspective.

Stew's narrative during this session was very vivid and he engaged with it deeply:

> The guy was a haji wearing a man dress…we are dragging him like a folded mattress… he has dirty feet with mud caked on them…looks like he's had blood poured on him… gurgling, making weird noises…doc shoved a tube down his throat, he is gagging and I'm watching him fight for breath...seems like he will never stop bleeding and I don't care, let him die.

He described again how he felt afterward, "dirty, gross, stained," and what it was like to walk into the chow hall with everyone staring and whispering. His shame mounted once more.

Following the narrative, the conversation continued to focus on alternative explanations as to why he may have chosen not to help. In doing so, a few vulnerabilities were touched upon. First, Stew revealed that he had not been present when some of his buddies were killed while on patrol, and he carried a lot of unresolved grief and anger; as such, in that moment, allowing this man to suffer may have been a way for him to avenge their deaths. Still, he continued to remark that on some level, it was not entirely an active choice but a rather surreal moment where he found himself frozen and helpless. He was asked to think deeply about the man and what attributes may have triggered something in him. Stew paused and returned to the image of his hands and feet, how rough and cold they were. He said he was reminded of how his father's hands and feet had felt when his father was having heart surgery. Even though Stew had a difficult relationship with his father due to his alcoholism and abuse, he remembered being in the hospital at his bedside, feeling a sense of helplessness that his father was ill and there was nothing he could do. He recognized that he felt a similar feeling when facing the Iraqi man; the difference, however, was that while the man was in a vulnerable state, as Stew's father had been, he also represented the face of the enemy and this dissonance may have led to Stew's paralysis in acting on the man's behalf. This was a very powerful connection for him and he sat with it for a moment before reiterating his belief that somehow this will come back to haunt him and "something bad will happen."

For the experiential exercise, it seemed like Stew would benefit from having the opportunity to be in a more assertive role. As such, he was instructed to imagine talking to a junior Marine who came to him struggling with a similar problem. He closed his eyes, sat up straight, and instantly transformed into a strong, powerful Marine. This was very impactful. He imagined the junior Marine telling him that he had done something terrible and he was not a hero. And Stew responded solidly, "You should be compassionate toward yourself, understand what happens in war, and seek the help you need. You served your country. You're a hero to someone." When he was finished, Stew realized he was telling the junior Marine what he needed to tell himself and it had sunk in a little more. Still, the therapist discussed that it would be important for him to revisit speaking with his grandmother and that he might do better if he were to spend some time preparing for it beforehand.

Stew appeared very depressed at the next session. He expressed that although he felt the conversation had been worthwhile and revealed a lot of truth about his situation, it was easier to give advice than to take it himself. Nevertheless, he had completed his homework to prepare for the conversation with his grandmother and indicated that he felt ready to do the exercise again. He went through the trauma narrative and more details emerged—dialogue with his captain, the tactile sensation of the man's skin, warm and swollen…*why are we out here? I haven't called my family in months. I'm not gonna help this haji.* Although clearly still painful, he was gaining a facility with retelling that was very evident as well.

After some comments about the experience with the narrative, the therapist moved him into the experiential exercise: *Imagine that Grandma is here. What would you tell her about what happened?* This time, he told her.

> I'm not a bad person, Grandma, but I made a bad choice. Grandma, I know I didn't do the right thing, I let an enemy die when I could have helped him. I don't feel bad for the Iraqis that died, I lost close friends because of them. I'm not sorry for not helping but I am sorry that my hate toward Iraqis has caused me to break my morals.

When asked how she would respond, he imagined her responding with care and kindness, with words of reassurance that God would forgive him, that he could make himself better if he allowed himself to be open to God and forgiveness, and that despite what happened, she still loved him and was proud of him. The therapist discussed his ambivalence and what it would mean for him to take steps to forgive himself. For homework, he was asked to think deeply about when his suffering would be enough for him and what it would take for him to make amends.

Stew did not return to treatment for a number of weeks following this session because he received devastating news that his cousin had been murdered and he needed to go home to South Dakota. When he did come again, he spoke about the pain of the loss and how hard it was to be around his family because he felt as though he had to be strong for them, rather than tend to his own grief. However, being in the presence of his grandmother and knowing what he had said to her during the previous session brought him strength and made him continue to think about ways to reengage in his life. Moreover, he had taken it upon himself to speak to an Afghani classmate at school and it went better than he had expected. This represented significant progress. In addition, Stew discussed in his homework how sadness and guilt may always be present in his life but "time and acceptance" will help him forgive himself. He wrote about wanting to have a career where he can help others or express himself in some way, channeling his anger, sadness, and depression into something more meaningful.

Stew's trauma narrative continued to go more in depth and included additional detail about the relationship with his captain. During the processing, the therapist reviewed some of the themes with him that had previously been uncovered—the impact of extreme fatigue, the desire to avenge the deaths of his buddies, the connection to helplessness previously experienced with his father—yet the guilt about violating his morals remained very prominent.

At this point, it seemed as though it might be useful for him to confront the Iraqi man through the experiential exercise. When presented with this, Stew responded with some dread. He could not imagine what he would say to the man or what the man would say to him. His concerns were validated but the therapist explained that while the scenario may seem far-fetched, this man was continuing to haunt his life in significant ways and addressing him directly could lead to more resolution. He reluctantly agreed to continue and moved forward with the exercise. The therapist had him imagine the Iraqi man sitting in the room and asked Stew to describe him again. Stew was then asked what he would say to the man about how he was affecting Stew's life. And he said the following:

> I was there when we picked you up and I did not help you. You were bleeding and vomiting and I did nothing. I kept thinking that our Marines would not have returned fire if they had not received fire first and that somehow maybe it was your own fault. But I still should have helped and I am sorry. Since then, I have been thinking about how I will be punished for this and all the terrible things that will happen to me. I can't stop thinking about you and how I lost myself with you. It's changed everything for me. If everyone knew what I had done, they would not call me a hero.

It was hard for Stew to imagine how the man might respond. He was doubtful that he would be sympathetic or forgiving so the therapist suggested that perhaps the man might say something like the following, *This is war. If the roles were reversed, I would not help you so why are you letting me ruin your life?* Stew paused and said he never thought about it that way. He responded with anger, *That's true. You wouldn't help me. It's kill or be killed and I'm glad it was you and not me. I didn't even kill you! I just didn't help you while you were dying. I'm not proud but it will make me a better person in the end. You can't ruin my life*. After the exercise, Stew reported that it was somewhat of a relief to imagine the man in that way and that maybe it was okay to be slightly angry with him. For homework, he was encouraged to continue reflecting upon his anger as well as allow himself to fully experience the sadness of his cousin's death rather than suppress the grief, as was his tendency.

Stew arrived for Session 7 the following week and reported feeling "lighter and less mopey." He said he had been looking at photographs of friends who had been lost, as well as miscellaneous Iraqi people, and it had been restorative to him. He also reported keeping connected with his family as they mourned his cousin. In his homework, he continued to express themes of anger and regret, which had been discussed following the experiential exercise with the Iraqi man, and indicated that it had been helpful for him to address those themes while still recognizing what he could do to be a better person.

Session 7 of adaptive disclosure involves the final retelling of the trauma narrative. It also includes the final experiential exercise, typically involving some element of the patient's future life with the goal of looking ahead and moving forward. Interestingly, Stew's narrative had many visual images that reflected a deeper sense of the man's vulnerability in those moments with him. He described the "gurgling noise" the man made as he choked on his blood. He continued:

> I'm staring at him head to toe, blood drying on his beard like water drops on a baby's bib, flies landing on him, dirt encrusted on his feet, like a farmer's foot, seeing under his mandress, parts of his legs, his genitals, squishy skin, Doc yelling at me, you have to help, you're gonna get in trouble but I don't care…back at the chow hall, we come in like we're video game warriors. Posers.

During the processing, although the event was clearly still distressing to him (he reported his distress at 85 following the narrative), he talked about feeling more resolved in terms of letting go of anger and shame. He expressed a deep sense of redemption and forgiveness.

At that point, the therapist took some time for Stew to discuss how he would imagine his future life. He was feeling more upbeat overall and expressed how he had gotten closer with his girlfriend, sharing things and allowing himself to be more vulnerable with her. He spoke about wanting to have a family someday and, in particular, he really wanted to have a daughter. He described what he would want to teach her and the kind of father he aspired to be: caring, attentive, playful. The tenderness with which he spoke about his future child led to the suggestion that he include her in the final experiential exercise. He agreed. The therapist asked him to imagine what she would look like; initially he laughed and said he hoped she would not look like him but then he quietly said that he hoped she would resemble his grandmother. Then he was instructed to close his eyes and talk to her. *Tell her about being in the Marine Corps*. He began:

> Daddy used to be a Marine which was a very hard job because I had to go far away and fight bad people. I decided to be a Marine because I wanted a better life for myself so I could prepare to have you. It forced me to be brave and have courage and sometimes make difficult choices.

Then the therapist said, "Tell her what was hard and what you learned." He continued:

> I saw some terrible things when I was fighting the bad people and did things that made me feel ashamed. I didn't help someone who needed help. And I didn't want to ever talk about it but it kept bothering me so I had to do something. I had to talk to someone.

The therapist asked him to imagine how she might respond. He shifted to her, *Daddy, that sounds scary. I'm so glad you're okay. You are so brave*. He was told to respond and offer words of wisdom, to share how he had begun to heal himself.

> Sometimes I don't feel brave. Sometimes I still feel scared. But I know it's important to talk about things so you can feel better. It helps me know I'm still a good person who has made mistakes but it's okay to make mistakes if you're willing to ask forgiveness. And I think about your great-Grandma, my Grandma, and how strong she is and that makes me feel strong too.

His words were so poignant and heartfelt, and he became choked up as he continued:

> And I want you to know that you can always talk to me about things that bother you. I don't want you to feel scared alone. I love you and I am here for you. I fought to be here for you.

He was asked how she would respond and he said, *Thank you, Daddy, I love you too*. Then the therapist asked if he had any final words for her and he simply said, *I can't wait to meet you*. And he sat for a moment as tears flowed down his cheeks and he took in what he had just experienced.

Stew's deep emotional engagement was palpable and as the therapist bore witness to it, the emotion was experienced alongside him as they sat together in silent reflection. After a few moments, the therapist shared how moving it was to hear him speak to his future daughter in that way and how beautifully he had expressed himself. He was thanked for being willing to share the dialogue and asked what it had been like for him. He responded that it made him feel "warm and whole," as though what he had done in the Marine Corps mattered, and that if he could learn and grow from his experience with the Iraqi man, and stop punishing himself, he could have meaning in his life and the family he had been dreaming about. The therapist agreed and articulated that he should feel very proud that he allowed himself to be open and vulnerable and that this would ultimately be a path of healing for him. He smiled and said, "I hope so."

For his final written assignment, it seemed appropriate to continue with the theme of envisioning his future so it was suggested that he do some research about course offerings in areas that might interest him. Moreover, in preparation for the last session, he was asked to reflect upon all the previous sessions, how he had benefitted, what he could still work on, and how he would see his life moving forward now that he had gone through the treatment.

23.1.3 Outcome

The final session of adaptive disclosure involves an extensive review of progress over the course of treatment and addressing steps to keep moving forward. Stew's assessments revealed some decrease in symptoms; he had begun treatment with a PTSD checklist [17] score of 60 and at the end of therapy, his score was 50. This score is still high and falls within the clinical range. However, his presentation was markedly different. He was no longer shaky, he maintained eye contact, and he appeared much more deliberate in his actions. He had completed his assignment to research different career avenues and described going through the catalogue of courses at his school and finding a number of areas that interested him. The areas were varied, including photography and nursing, but they all seemed to be consistent with values he had articulated during previous sessions. He said he was planning another trip home to see his family and that his grandmother had been ill but was reportedly doing better. He also reported that his brother would be moving away soon and that this would force him to engage with others in order to have more social outlets. Overall, Stew was in a positive state of mind.

At that point, specific areas of progress were reviewed. These included his gaining a much better understanding of his actions within the context of war, for example, the fact that it was unknown whether or not the man was an enemy, the sadness at the loss of his friends, as well as the emotional triggers that were related to past trauma. It also included a shift in his beliefs about himself, reflecting a sense that even though he had failed to do something that he believed he should have done, it did not mean that he was a bad person; he reiterated how he wanted to have a career where he was doing something to help other people. Moreover, progress was noted in terms of his willingness to engage with his Middle Eastern classmate, spend more time going out with his girlfriend, and the fact that he was feeling less depressed and more motivated. The discussion also addressed areas where he would benefit from continued work such as allowing himself to fully experience sadness, particularly around the loss of his cousin, to find ongoing ways to "make peace" with himself, and continue to let go of shame by sharing his experience with others. He said he might even consider having a conversation with his grandmother when he saw her again. In addition, he identified various triggers to be aware of such as wrestling with his brother and having too much time to think about things. Aspects of self-care were discussed; he suggested writing, doing well in school, fishing, going to the gym, and being proactive about his health as examples of ways he could take better care of himself. Finally, in terms of social reengagement, he said he planned to move forward in his relationship with his girlfriend, continue to make future career plans, broaden his social circle, and maintain contact with his family. All of this was written down as a "roadmap" so that he had a record and could refer to it when needed.

As he continued to reflect upon his experience with the various components of the treatment, Stew expressed that he was glad he went through it and could see that it had been very helpful for him, even though he disliked having to tell the story each time and sometimes "it felt weird" talking to himself. The therapist shared that this was fairly normal and it was impressive that he stuck with it even though it was difficult. The therapist expressed pride at all of the effort he put into getting better and working on himself. During the goodbye, the therapist added that Grandma would also be proud and someday when he had his little girl, she would be proud too. He smiled broadly and then he walked out.

23.2 Summary and Final Comments

The conceptual foundation and an overview of change agents for adaptive disclosure, a new psychotherapy designed to help service members and veterans begin the process of healing from diverse psychological war wounds, have been presented along with the case of a new veteran whose principal harm was moral injury complicated by loss. As previously noted, moral injury and loss cause deeply complex challenges across multiple domains—behavioral, biological, cognitive, social, and spiritual—that are phenomenologically different from danger-based harms and can cause chronic demoralization, anomie, disengagement, and self-handicapping, if not frank self-harm [9]. In the case presented, the patient made only modest gains in PTSD symptom severity, yet there were authentic cognitive and behavioral signs of increased agency, proactivity, hopefulness, and vitality. These signs were a clear departure from moral injury and indicated that the goals of treatment were met, particularly in light of his initial presentation. Since adaptive disclosure is a brief therapy and the nature of psychic wounds among veterans is such that they are deeply entrenched and extensive, the goal of the therapy is simply to plant healing seeds and chart a course; the real work of healing is ongoing and occurs over the lifetime. Within this framework, Stew was visibly on the right track and therefore this case is considered to be a success.

Finally, it is important to emphasize that this case was selected because of its *prototypical complexity*, which required that the therapist use varied tactics and strategies while adhering to the main change agents specified in the adaptive disclosure manual. Adaptive disclosure is manualized and replicable but it also embraces the real-world need for clinicians to flexibly make choices that provide the best opportunities for hot-cognitive experiential change within and between sessions. As long as these strategies keep to the conceptual framework provided in the adaptive disclosure therapy model, that is, providing a path forward for the service member, they are both acceptable and expected.

References

1. Kessler RC, Sonnega A, Bromet E, Hughes M, Nelson CB. Posttraumatic stress disorder in the National Comorbidity Survey. Arch Gen Psychiatry. 1995;52:1048–60.
2. Kulka RA, Schlenger WE, Fairbank JA, et al. Trauma and the Vietnam war generation: report of findings from the National Vietnam Veterans Readjustment Study. Philadelphia: Brunner/Mazel; 1990.
3. Santiago PN, Ursano RJ, Gray CL, et al. A systematic review of PTSD prevalence and trajectories in DSM-5 defined trauma exposed populations: intentional and non-intentional traumatic events. PloS ONE. 2013;8(4):e59236. doi:10.1371/journal.pone.0059236.
4. Steenkamp MM, Litz BT. Early interventions with military personnel. In Moore BA, Barnett JE, editors. Military psychologists' desk reference. New York: Oxford University Press; 2013. p. 256–60.
5. Forbes D, Lloyd D, Nixon RD, et al. A multisite randomized controlled effectiveness trial of cognitive processing therapy for military-related posttraumatic stress disorder. J Anxiety Disord. 2012;26(3):442–52.
6. Schnurr PP, Friedman MJ, Engel CC, et al. Cognitive behavioral therapy for posttraumatic stress disorder in women: a randomized controlled trial. JAMA. 2007;297(8):820–30.
7. Bradley R, Greene J, Russ E, Dutra L, Westen D. A multidimensional meta-analysis of psychotherapy for PTSD. Am J Psychiatry. 2005;162(2):214–27.
8. Litz BT, Schorr Y, Delaney E, et al. A randomized controlled trial of an internet-based therapist-assisted indicated preventive intervention for prolonged grief disorder. Behav Res Ther. 2014;61:23–34.
9. Litz BT, Stein N, Delaney E, et al. Moral injury and moral repair in war veterans: a preliminary model and intervention strategy. Clin Psychol Rev. 2009;29(8):695–706.
10. Foa EB, Hembree EA, Rothbaum BO. Prolonged exposure therapy for PTSD: emotional processing of traumatic experiences. New York: Oxford University Press; 2007.
11. Resick PA, Schnicke MK. Cognitive processing therapy for rape victims: a treatment manual. Thousand Oaks: Sage; 1993.
12. Litz BT, Lebowitz L, Gray MJ, Nash W. Adaptive disclosure: An experiential approach to military trauma, loss, and moral injury. New York: Guilford; in press.
13. Gray MJ, Schorr Y, Nash W, et al. Adaptive disclosure: an open trial of a novel exposure-based intervention for service members with combat-related psychological stress injuries. Behav Ther. 2012;43(2):407–15.
14. Steenkamp MM, Litz BT, Gray MJ, et al. A brief exposure-based intervention for service members with PTSD. Cogn Behav Pract. 2011;18(1):98–107.
15. Foa EB, Keane TM, Friedman MJ, Cohen JA, eds. Effective treatments for PTSD: practice guidelines from the International Society for Traumatic Stress Studies. New York: Guilford; 2008.
16. Gortner E-M, Rude SS, Pennbaker JW. Benefits of expressive writing in lowering rumination and depressive symptoms. Behav Ther. 2006;37(3):292–303.
17. Weathers FW, Litz BT, Huska JA, Keane TM. The PTSD checklist—Civilian version (PCLC). Boston: National Center for PTSD; 1994.

Treatment of Conversion Disorder with PTSD

24

Paulette T. Cazares

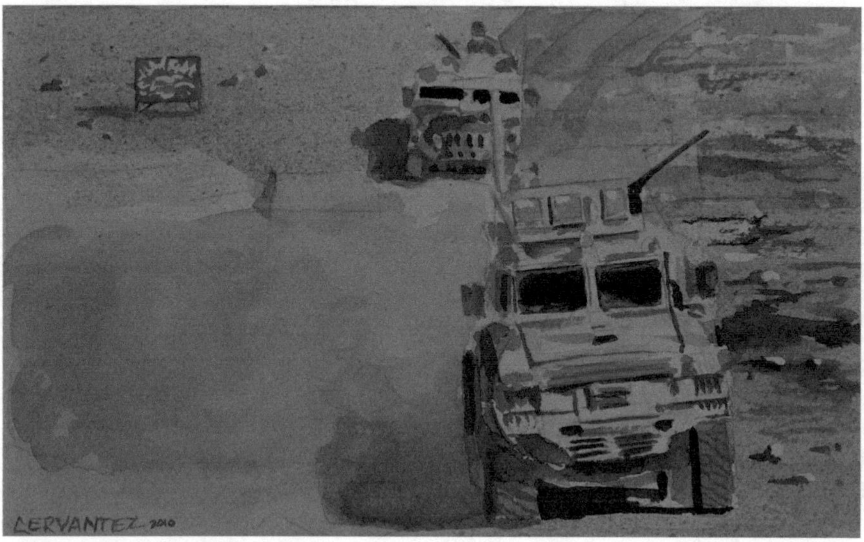

US/Afghan Convoy, by MSG Martin Cervantez, courtesy of the Army Art Collection, US Army Center of Military History.

Some of the most difficult patients to treat are those that require investments of our time, those that challenge our beliefs, and require a review of our countertransference. Patients with somatoform spectrum illness are often categorized as "difficult" patients, because there is no medication that can be prescribed. In the case of conversion disorder, the patient's symptoms are, by definition, unconscious.

P. T. Cazares (✉)
Naval Medical Center, 34800 Bob Wilson Dr, San Diego, CA 92134, USA
e-mail: ptucc76@yahoo.com; Paulette.Cazares@med.navy.mil

E. C. Ritchie (ed.), *Posttraumatic Stress Disorder and Related Diseases in Combat Veterans*, DOI 10.1007/978-3-319-22985-0_24

They are the result of complicated patient history, and very often associated with trauma. What further complicates the treatment of patients with conversion disorder is the dearth of controlled research and the lack of evidence-based treatments [1]. This case describes the course of a female service member who presented with symptoms of seizure-like activity, who was ultimately referred to mental health for treatment after no findings to support epileptiform activity or neurologic illness were discovered.

24.1 Case Report

I met this patient while covering the Consult-Liaison Service one day at our large training hospital. It was a busy afternoon, but not record setting. Prior to my walk to the Emergency Room (ER), I got a call from the outpatient mental health division officer that a female Culinary Specialist Seaman (CSSN) from a local aircraft carrier was waiting to be seen (by rank, this is a junior service member who would work as a cook and provide hotel services (linens, berthing inspections, etc.) at her command.) It was unusual that the call did not come directly from the ER, but I soon learned why this case attracted so much attention, and why division officers were involved.

It turns out that CSSN D (the name used for the patient) had been seen in the ER before. She had been sent there from her ship with escorts when it appeared she was having seizures onboard. She had been admitted at one point for a full evaluation, including consults from internal medicine, neurology, and psychiatry. That being the case, I had multiple records at my avail, and I briefly scanned through everything I could find. Conversion disorder had been deemed the most likely explanation.

Having a special interest in abnormal illness behaviors (contemporarily used to describe the cluster of somatoform spectrum diagnoses) and having some hope I could be helpful, I took an immediate interest in the case. Even more, I had an IDC student (independent duty corpsmen are men and women who are US Navy enlisted personnel trained in a similar capacity as a physician's assistant) with me, and I wanted to teach him the proper way to approach and help patients with somatoform spectrum symptoms and diagnoses. In 5 min or less, we covered rapport, trust building, countertransference and our role as uniformed health-care providers, considering dual agency.

Following our evaluation, I took this patient in my outpatient panel, and I saw the case nearly to the time she was ultimately retired from active duty service.

24.1.1 Presentation/History

CSSN D is a black American single 21-year-old female with approximately 2 years and 3 months active duty as of our initial meeting in August 2014. The patient started to see her ship's psychologist regularly starting in February 2014 following an incident on her ship. She stated that while in ranks, an active duty officer was angrily addressing the group, and punched her on the back of her shoulder. She stated this immediately reminded her of childhood abuse, and soon brought back memories she had suppressed for years.

Over the next 2 months, she saw the psychologist and the ship's medical officer, and took a selective serotonin reuptake inhibitor (SSRI) for anxiety. The record revealed that she endorsed beliefs that her coworkers and chain of command were pursuing information about her in order to make her life worse. At some point, she presented to them with myoclonic jerking, which continued to occur episodically while she was onboard the ship. This was a concern for her and staff, as she worked in the ship's kitchen and was often around knives and hot food. She was admitted to our hospital on 8 April 2014 for a neurology and mental health evaluation. Workups at that time revealed a history consistent with adjustment disorder, present since enlistment, with consideration for posttraumatic stress disorder (PTSD). She was not suicidal in either the inpatient or the outpatient settings, and was discharged from the hospital on 9 April 2014. A brain MRI and EEG were both within normal limits.

Over the course of the early summer months of 2014, the patient's episodes of jerking continued. Episodes persisted and during one, she had reportedly fallen to the floor, but denied alteration or loss of consciousness. She had been evaluated in psychology with psychological testing. Finally, as the ship was preparing for a long underway period, she was sent to the ER in the context of yet another episode in the kitchen, while working with a large pot of boiling water.

When I met CSSN D, she was angry—not upset, not anxious, but grossly angry. The volume of her voice oscillated, and she had a southern accent that was made staccato by her waves of rage. She was agitated. I spent the larger part of an hour establishing rapport and the periods of calm ultimately became longer, the periods of rage, shorter. She felt betrayed by her ship's medical department, stating she had trusted them, but then felt many knew her history (of abuse) that she had kept secret for years. She felt betrayed by the Navy, citing stigma in seeing mental health.

I acknowledged her strength and asked if she had ever described herself as a survivor. It was not smoke and mirrors; she was clearly a woman who had lived through a lot; multiple History & Physical (H&Ps) had already established that fact. Further, in my brief assessment of her educational background, I felt she was not the most prepared or well educated to handle her life's circumstances.

She discussed how when she thinks "bad thoughts," they are very loud in her head and she has to speak loudly so she will not hear the "bad thoughts." She reported feeling unsupported, not cared for, and often lonely. She reported that she cries herself to sleep most nights. She stated that she had been getting 3–4 h of sleep a night, and that it took her approximately an hour to fall asleep due to anxiety. She is woken often by nightmares but is unable to remember them. She denied any change in her eating habits or weight. The patient denied auditory/visual hallucinations or mania. She would not elaborate on her "bad thoughts," but flatly denied suicidal or homicidal ideation and provided her younger sister and God as reasons to live.

A psychiatric review of systems was negative for manic or psychotic symptoms, and she did not complain of significant pain or dysfunction in other organ systems. Labs and radiological scans were negative for pathology.

24.1.2 Past Psychiatric History

She was in therapy as an adolescent while in foster care, which she reported was not helpful. Since that time, she was not in care, until she began to see her ship's medical officer and psychologist. She took Paxil (paroxetine) for approximately 1 month and had been engaging in supportive therapy with the ship's psychologist. She had never attempted suicide.

24.1.3 Family Psychiatric History

Her mother was treated for an unknown diagnosis. Her maternal grandmother was diagnosed with depression. Both biologic parents were diagnosed with substance use disorders.

24.1.4 Social/Developmental History

The patient was born and raised in southern Illinois to an intact family system. She is the oldest child, and has one brother, 17 years old, and one sister, 12 years old who currently reside with their parents. She reported that as a result of her father's infidelity, her mother became physically and emotionally abusive, as well as neglectful when the patient was 7 years old. Eventually, both parents became abusive, and the patient perceived that she needed to withstand the abuse to protect her siblings, although they occasionally were also emotionally and physically abused. The patient reported that after a particularly intense event in which she was whipped by her father with a belt and threatened with a knife, she fled to a neighbor's house and called the police. She reported that she was placed in foster care, first living with her aunts for 1 year, and then with her best friend's family until awkward interactions with her friend's father led her to leave the home to join the US Navy. (She would not elaborate on these interactions and when questioned, denied sexual abuse.)

The patient denied any learning or disciplinary problems while in school and graduated on time with a 3.0 GPA. She went on to attain 25 credits of college prior to US Navy service, and was subsequently able to enter the service as an E-2. The patient worked in the fast food industry and as a cyber-lounge librarian. She denied any military or civilian legal issues.

She reported that she felt chronically guilty for escaping her home environment and leaving her siblings with her parents. The patient does not maintain a relationship with either of her parents and has not spoken to them since she was removed from the home.

The patient is single, never married, and does not have children. She noted that her last romantic involvement was in "A" School (Naval trade school for enlisted members). She reports that she feels unable to trust others enough to develop an emotional relationship.

24.1.4.1 Religion/Spirituality

The patient identified with the Lutheran Christian faith group. She was raised in a religious home. She endorsed that she is a part of the church and often relies on her "church mother" for financial and emotional support.

24.1.4.2 Substance History

- Alcohol: rare (once–twice per month).
- She denied use of tobacco, excessive caffeine, or supplements. She denied illicit drug use as well as OTC medication use.

24.1.4.3 Military History/Legal History

At the time of evaluation, the patient had 2 years of continuous active duty and no deployments. She had no military or civilian legal concerns.

24.1.4.4 Allergies

The patient reported allergies to Penicillin (PCN) and shellfish.

24.1.5 Past Medical History

Noncontributory; she denied chronic pain. The HIV status was up to date (negative). She denied a history of blast exposure as well as Traumatic Brain Injury (TBI).

24.1.5.1 Mental Status Exam

August 2014: thin-appearing well-nourished, well-developed female in no acute distress but visually anxious. She was reluctantly cooperative; a tenuous rapport was established. She had impaired military bearing and disheveled hair; eye contact was often directed at objects around the room other than the provider. Speech varied from normal rate, rhythm to loud and staccato, all the while accented. Intermittent truncal, neck, or upper extremity jerking motions noted. Patient's mood was "stressed" with congruent angry, anxious, unpredictable affect. Thought process was non-linear and minimally goal-directed. Thought content was without Suicidal Ideation/Homicidal Ideation (SI/HI)/plans/intent or auditory or visual hallucinations (AH/VH). No impairment of concentration or memory noted. Judgment: fair, impulse control: adequate, insight: fair.

24.1.6 Diagnosis/Assessment

At the time of initial assessment, she was deemed to have diagnoses that included non-epileptiform motor activity (by history) and Anxiety Not Otherwise Specified (NOS), with a rule-out diagnosis of PTSD. Despite reports of a strong GPA and some college work, I had an additional concern for borderline intellectual functioning. This was based on her spotty description of her academics, rudimentary vocabulary, and frequent derailment in conversation. Over time, this concern resolved and the latter two observations were deemed secondary to anxiety.

24.1.6.1 Personality Functioning

Prior to my meeting with her, psychologic testing had been completed. Her Minnesota Multiphasic Personality Inventory-2 Restructured Form (MMPI-2 RF) showed she over-endorsed items when compared to normative populations. She reported a high level of concern regarding fatigue and neurological symptoms. She also endorsed a high level of concern regarding family problems, and residual symptoms from her childhood trauma experience. The patient reported that she has a high level of anxiety, with intrusive thoughts and nightmares. There were no indications of disordered thinking or maladaptive externalizing behaviors.

Although routine objective scales were performed throughout treatment (e.g., PCL and Patient Health Questionnaire-9 (PHQ-9)), they were deemed unreliable. Responses were often marked all absent or all severe.

24.1.7 Treatment/Management

We quickly established a standing weekly visit in the outpatient setting. She was moved off her ship and assigned to an administrative position at the hospital. This is an administrative assignment, commonly seen when a patient is placed in a "Limited Duty" status, allowing treatment to be their primary responsibility. The idea is to move the patient to a less demanding position while they engage in treatment and continued assessments, and to allow commands to fill billets that require sailors deemed fit for full duty. In the visits that followed, minimal additional history was gathered, and the majority of time I continued to focus on rapport building, safety, and crisis plan development. As has been suggested by literature on the treatment of somatoform spectrum disorders, the establishment of a strong relationship is critical and great time was spent establishing trust. Although not initially interested in medications, the patient did soon accept prazosin and trazodone, both off label for the treatment of nightmares and insomnia, respectively.

She came to reveal great difficulty expressing her emotional needs to nearly anyone, from family, to her command, to her religious support system. She cited a recent disagreement with her "church mother" and even intimated that the woman had asked her for money. She had considerable worry at baseline about her younger sister, which would intermittently peak, based on information she would hear from the extended family. She also reported great financial stress due to assistance she gave to her grandmother.

Visits often started with her detailing her most recent life crisis, and frequently this occurred simultaneously with displays of truncal jerks, as well as varied upper extremity movements and jerks of the neck. It would not be unusual to find her suffering from these movements in the clinic waiting room. She was always conscious through these moments, engaged in conversation while they occurred, and responded to varied forms of relaxation, displaying decreased intensity and frequency of movements during the intervention. There was one visit during which she suddenly and angrily left my office, furious with rage, demanding help from the Navy with finances. She reported back the next week, and while she did not apologize for her behavior, she acknowledged she was "stressed" when she left.

She accepted the idea of symptom substitution and we practiced this in the office. She reported over subsequent sessions that she had practiced the idea with some, but limited success. In her case, symptom substitution consisted of a tapping of her index finger on her knee or thumb. Interestingly, this patient never asked for additional nonpsychiatric evaluations or neurologic testing. She never claimed her motor activity was due to a tumor, neurologic illness, or yet undiagnosed disease. Despite her limited ability to express her internal anxiety and anger, she had sufficient insight to appreciate that psychological stress was the source of her symptoms. I referred her for group therapy to a women's trauma group (related to her childhood abuse), but her continued truncal and extremity movements were disruptive to the group, as was her quickness to anger, and she was soon disenrolled back to individual sessions with me.

Although she initially denied certain symptoms of PTSD, it became clear over time that CSSN D did indeed display all the cardinal pillars of PTSD, chronic. She had exposure to significant childhood physical abuse and endorsed daytime flashbacks and avoidance of news stories or movies describing physical abuse or foster care. She had significant and impairing emotional detachment from others, a sense of foreshortened future (a minimal-vague idea of what she will do in the future), chronic insomnia, and severe hypervigilance.

Although her alcohol use was initially rare, with continued questioning, she did report increased intake over the course of treatment despite my education and warnings. She reported specifically using alcohol for the treatment of anxiety and insomnia. Subsequently, her meds were adjusted to specifically target these symptoms, including breakthrough anxiety, and she did report a decrease in alcohol use. She displayed no evidence of physiologic dependence.

Despite attempts at remission of symptoms with psychopharmacology and supportive therapy, non-epileptiform symptoms continued, notably, while she was away from any significant operational or social stressors. Her continued decompensations made it clear that she would not be fit for full duty in any Navy rate, and a referral for a medical retirement Physical Evaluation Board (PEB) was initiated.

24.1.8 Outcomes/Case Resolution

Since initial presentation to the Fleet Mental Health clinic in San Diego in May 2014, the patient took medications and participated in therapy. Although descriptions of conversion disorder have existed for centuries, treatment protocols are rare [2]. However, the idea that the therapeutic relationship can form the basis for resolution of symptoms is well understood. In this case, I framed her treatment on the idea that I would give her the utmost support I could, hoping our work would draw on and magnify some resilience.

She was unwilling to see a psychologist, but did tolerate grounding techniques and incremental attempts at psychotherapy with me. With weekly outpatient visits, ER visits ceased completely. Over time, she reported that episodes of involuntary movements and severe anxiety decreased in frequency and intensity. She identified that these episodes were related to psychologic stress, and although she made appropriate interventions to decrease these symptoms, including symptom substitution, they continued to occur in both occupational and personal settings. She would additionally wake from sleep with panic symptoms including sweating, trembling, palpitations, and rapid breathing. Daytime intrusive thoughts of her trauma were decreased from her initial intake, but still continued, and she displayed strong hypervigilance. She was easily prone to anger, often verbally arguing with herself or engaging in long, loud verbal rants while in public, almost always with difficulty slowing her thought process and physically relaxing.

Prescribed medications included:

- Prazosin off-label for the treatment of nightmares
- Effexor XR (venlafaxine)
- Inderal (propranolol) as needed for the treatment of breakthrough anxiety
- Seroquel (quetiapine) off-label for the treatment of insomnia and anxiety

Overall, the patient did improve, but then she had a significant setback upon learning her youngest sibling was placed in foster care. This triggered memories of her time in foster care, and she felt unable to assist her family in any meaningful way.

Diagnoses included those below. In addition to PTSD, and given a thorough neurologic workup to rule out seizure disorder, conversion disorder with seizures appeared to be the most accurate description of her motor symptoms. Finally, a diagnosis of Alcohol Use Disorder was made. I soon switched jobs and after my transfer of the case to a new provider, her alcohol use reportedly increased again, at which time she was referred to her command Drug and Alcohol Prevention Advisor (DAPA) for a formal substance use screen.

24.1.9 Diagnoses

PTSD, chronic, existed prior to enlistment, service-aggravated
Conversion disorder with seizures, DNEPTE
Alcohol use disorder, mild
Occupational problems, family problems, financial problems

24.2 Summary/Clinical Pearls

1. Conversion disorder is not an uncommon comorbidity with PTSD.

This case displayed for me a not uncommon experience in which patients with high anxiety display neurologic motor symptoms without associated known neurologic pathology. In her case, the anxiety was secondary to PTSD associated with childhood abuse.

2. There is a long history of observations of conversion disorder in the military.
3. Theories of the origin of conversion disorder focus on unconscious conflicts.

Symptoms of abnormal illness behavior (AIB) are certainly not new and have been featured in clinical casebooks for centuries, as well as more recently in the media and in a popular film (*Hollywood Ending,* Woody Allen, 2002 and *Persona,* Ingmar Bergman, 1966).

It is worth noting that over the years, the term conversion disorder has developed a significant stigma. As a result of the stigma for patients, and because many cases are often later diagnosed with a neurologic illness, the term AIB has emerged. This term often includes conversion disorder as well as other illnesses associated with secondary gain, including hypochondriasis, somatization, pain disorder, factitious disorder, and malingering [3]. With the exception of factitious disorder and malingering, it is important to note that these are *unconscious* processes and as here, the patient felt absolutely no control over the onset or duration of her symptoms.

With regard to developmental explanations for symptoms of AIB, a 2014 *Lancet* article points out that "Individuals deprived of nurturing attachments early in life might experience recurrent states of emotional dysregulation and will enact behaviours addressing unmet emotional needs" [4].

4. Treatment is energy intensive but not complex.

Therapy is considered the most essential piece of treatment, and must be consistent and regular. Success hinges on establishing a steady therapeutic relationship with good boundaries. Appointments should be frequent but time limited. It seems critical to acknowledge there is an underlying emotional or psychological deficit, as there is no goal for symptoms of AIB if they are not observed by others [4]. However, in conjunction with that, the provider must also work to help the patient recognize their strengths. These symptoms essentially represent the patient's helplessness and their perceived lack of self-control. The therapist can make great gains with clear affirmations.

In the treatment of children with AIB, one pediatric group noted they aim "to improve children's safety, physical wellbeing, functional ability to engage in standard activities, and capacity to regulate their bodies, and to improve the emotional functioning of each child and family as a whole" [5]. This is the same treatment goal with adults, with particular focus on their need for a sense of control. In this case, symptom substitution served to give her some sense that she was in control of her body, and thus the sense that she could help stop the symptoms once started, even if she felt unable to stop their onset.

5. Beware of countertransference.

Patients like the one I describe here typically evoke feelings of frustration on the part of the provider. That can limit our ability to be effective. On the other hand, sympathetic connections with patients will delude boundaries and decrease effectiveness. My patient was clearly disabled by her symptoms, and she had no significant support system that would otherwise help her psychologically. Even support from her "church mother" appeared to be questionable. I found myself wondering where she would go once she left the Navy and, where she would end up. How would a patient, so impaired, find housing, file for assistance, or find social support?

Another impression bothered me and as I thought about the case over time, I may have been clouded by unconscious racist views regarding my concerns for her intelligence and resourcefulness. I thought about this extensively and as I came to know her more deeply, I realized her frequent derailment was secondary to anxiety and her vocabulary mere southern slang. I ruled out my initial concern for borderline intellectual functioning. Cultural considerations must always be noted, but this is especially true when there are significant differences between the provider and patient [6]. In this case, she was black, I was white; she was from the South and I was from the North. Further, she was enlisted and I was an officer. The case was an important reminder, especially in the military context, of the need to remain open to differences and open to the idea there may be no diagnosis where we initially believe one exists.

24.3 Conclusion

Overall, I personally found this to be a sad case. I know I provided good care, but the patient's experience, both acute and chronic, evoked significant empathy in me, as well as an internal and likely projected sense of my own lack of control in the therapeutic relationship. She did improve initially, but then began to develop symptoms of an alcohol use disorder.

As providers, we all judge ourselves from time to time by our ability to "help" our patients. I am not sure I did here, but I believe the system worked. Had she continued on active duty in a shipboard environment, I believe she would have likely inadvertently harmed herself or a shipmate.

She did have insight into the effect her past had on her psyche, both psychiatrically and psychologically, and she believed and projected the sense that she was powerless. I made attempts to help her portray herself as a survivor, but she was not ready to receive that message. Ultimately, with regard to her fitness for duty, she clearly was unfit. Outside the military, her prognosis is deemed guarded to fair.

I submitted her case to the Physical Evaluation Board for disability evaluation, and she continued individual medication management with me until I transferred positions in early Fall 2014. She was assigned to a different psychiatrist at that time and was to be followed until discharged from the Navy. I recommended a close follow-up with the VA.

References

1. Rosebush PI, Mazurek MF. Treatment of conversion disorder in the 21st century: have we moved beyond the couch? Curr Treat Options Neurol. 2011;13(3):255–66.
2. Stonnington CM, Barry JJ, Fisher RS. Conversion disorder. Am J Psychiatry. 2006;163:1510–7.
3. Schmidt RF, Willis WD, editors. Encyclopedia of pain. New York: Springer; 2007.
4. Kozlowska K. Abnormal illness behaviours: a developmental perspective. Lancet. 2014;383(9926):1368–9.
5. Kozlowska K, Foley S, Savage B. Fabricated illness: working within the family system to find a pathway to health. Fam Process. 2012;51:570–87.
6. Schwartz A, Calhoun A, Eschbach C, Seeling B. Treatment of conversion disorder in an African American Christian woman: cultural and social considerations. Am J Psychiatry. 2001;158(9):1385–91.

Intimate Relationship Distress and Combat-related Posttraumatic Stress Disorder

25

Nicholas A. Tamoria, Miguel M. Alampay
and Patcho N. Santiago

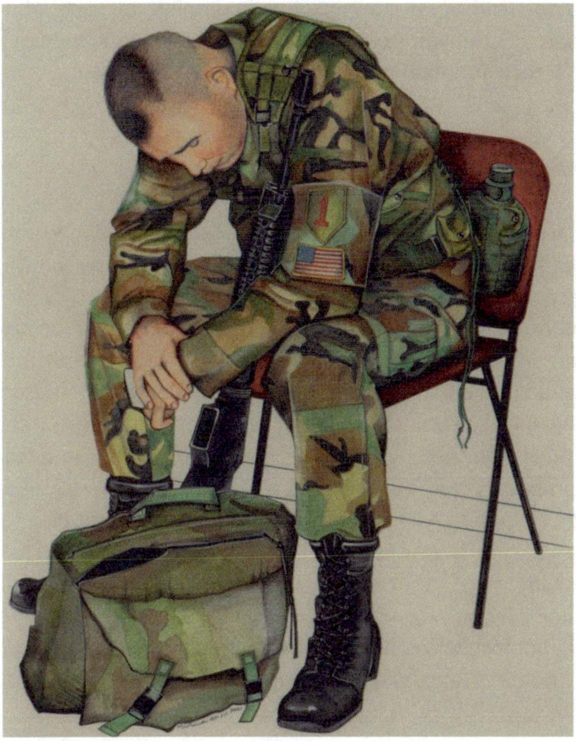

Waiting to Phone Home, MSG Henrietta Snowden, courtesy of the Army Art Collection, US Army Center of Military History.

M. M. Alampay (✉)
Medical Corps United States Navy, Walter Reed National Military Medical Center,
Bethesda, MD, USA
e-mail: Miguel.M.Alampay.mil@mail.mil

E. C. Ritchie (ed.), *Posttraumatic Stress Disorder and Related Diseases in Combat Veterans,* DOI 10.1007/978-3-319-22985-0_25

Decades of research spanning generations of war have firmly established that veterans with posttraumatic stress disorder (PTSD) and their romantic partners suffer significant relationship and psychological distress compared to civilian and veteran populations without PTSD [1]. World War II prisoners of war with PTSD reported more adjustment, communication, and intimacy problems in their relationships compared to prisoners of war without PTSD [2]. Similarly, Vietnam War veterans with PTSD, compared to Vietnam veterans without PTSD, were more likely to report marital and family adjustment problems, parenting difficulty, violence [3], significant relationship distress, intimacy problems, and thoughts or actions toward separation or divorce [4].

Several studies have shown that veterans from Operation Enduring Freedom and Operation Iraqi Freedom (OIF) have significant mental health risk and intimate relationship discord. Soldiers deployed to Iraq are at significant risk of developing PTSD [5] and reported a fourfold increase in interpersonal problems [6]. Developing a greater understanding of the impact and complex interplay of combat-related PTSD on intimate relationships can be of great benefit to the mental health providers, the veterans, their intimate partners, and the family system.

25.1 Case Presentation

Julia is a 28-year-old female spouse of a veteran who presented to a military behavioral health clinic for an urgent walk-in. Her chief complaint was "My husband is driving me crazy and I can't take it anymore!"

She reported being upset and overwhelmed almost daily in the context of worsening problems with her husband. He is a combat veteran with multiple deployments to Iraq and had been diagnosed with PTSD. He was a different person after his deployments and their marriage had become more difficult to the point where she is now thinking of divorcing him. She was more irritable with the children, had difficulty sleeping, reported being angry with him, and felt sad that their family was dissolving before her eyes. She even admitted to fleeting and passive suicidal thoughts but never with any intention or plan.

She was extremely dissatisfied in the marriage and felt her husband's PTSD was to blame. She knew he had seen combat but she did not know the details. He would not talk to her about his deployments, in fact, he did not communicate at all. He was like a stranger in their home and frequently isolated himself in the basement from

N. A. Tamoria
Department of Psychiatry, Walter Reed National Military Medical Center, 8901 Wisconsin Ave, Building 19, 6th fl, Rm. 6407, Bethesda, MD 20889, USA
e-mail: Nicholas.A.Tamoria.mil@mail.mil

P. N. Santiago
National Capital Consortium Psychiatry Residency, Walter Reed National Military Medical Center, 8901 Wisconsin Ave, Bethesda, MD 20889, USA
e-mail: Patcho.N.Santiago.mil@mail.mil

her and the kids. When she tried to talk to him about his experiences he just brushed her off. She felt so lonely in the marriage. She could not remember the last time they had been intimate. She wondered what was wrong with her that he did not trust her or could not let her in.

Besides the emotional and physical distance, he was always on edge. When they did talk, more often than not he would explode with unpredictable anger, triggered by everyday stressors. In response to his anger, sometimes she would get angry and it escalated quickly. He had destroyed furniture and punched holes in the walls. He had never hurt her or the kids but there were times when she was afraid he could. More recently she simply avoided him.

He did not sleep much. When he did, he thrashed about while dreaming, yelling and kicking. One night he jumped on top of her and started to choke her in a crazed state. She slapped him awake and he appeared mortified. After that he preferred to sleep on the living room couch. He liked it because he could "have a visual on all the doors, windows, and rooms." Sometimes he even slept with his firearm because "I have to be ready just in case." Some of these behaviors made sense to her because "It was like he was still in Iraq."

His insomnia and mood swings had affected his work performance. He had been counseled several times by his employer for tardiness and irritable behavior. At home he was often too overwhelmed or withdrawn to manage the kids. He had difficulty with other general household tasks. Julia had to assume responsibility for childcare, chores, home maintenance, and finances. In addition, she had to make sure he attended his medical appointments and took his medications. She felt extremely burdened with all these responsibilities which added to her loneliness, frustration, and hopelessness. Lately, she had been so overwhelmed that she was having more difficulty organizing and managing the household. Ironically, she felt the family worked better when he was deployed.

This was Julia's first behavioral health treatment. She had wanted to seek care earlier but was afraid that if she saw behavioral health it might have a negative effect on her husband's career. He had been initially resistant to seeing a psychiatrist because he did not want his friends or coworkers to think he was "weak or crazy" but she eventually persuaded him. She had no family history or previous personal history of mental illness, depression, anxiety, psychosis, or mania. She denied substance use or medical problems.

Julia was raised by a loving family in a small town in the Pacific Northwest. She met all her developmental milestones. She denied abuse. She excelled in academics and sports. She met her husband when they were in high school. He enlisted in the Army after graduation and she went to college for prelaw. He proposed when she was a junior and she gave up her dream to go to law school to be a stay-at-home wife and mother. Together, they have two young school-age children. They have some financial debt but no legal problems. They attend a Christian church on the weekends.

On exam, Julia was a well-groomed white female who appeared emotionally distressed. She was cooperative, coherent, and articulate. Her speech was at a normal rate but sometimes she raised her voice when upset. She reported some depressive and anxious feelings. Her affect was constricted but appropriate to content. Her thought process was linear and logical. She admitted to rare, passive suicidal thoughts in the past without any intent, plan, or attempt. She denied current suicidal or homicidal ideation. There was no evidence of psychosis or paranoia. She was oriented and appeared to be of above average intelligence. She had good insight and judgment.

25.2 Diagnosis and Assessment

25.2.1 Relationship Distress with Spouse or Intimate Partner (DSM-5)

While the patient presents with mild symptoms of depression, anxiety, and stress, it's clear that the primary problem is relational. Her husband's combat-related PTSD is having a tremendous impact on her own mental health, causing significant psychological distress and functional impairment. In general, partners who perceive greater levels of PTSD symptom severity also report greater individual and marital distress [7]. In this case, Julia's relationship distress is associated with impaired functioning in behavioral, cognitive, and affective domains, specifically reactive to her husband's PTSD symptoms. There is a growing body of research literature examining how the specific symptom clusters of PTSD—intrusions, avoidance, negative alterations of cognition and mood, and hyperarousal—affect the intimate partner. Further, studies are exploring how the behavioral, cognitive, and affective reactions of the intimate partner feedback to the veteran to either alleviate, maintain, or even worsen the PTSD.

Several studies have shown that the degree of relationship distress is particularly correlated with the severity of emotional numbing [2, 4]. In DSM-5, PTSD emotional numbing symptoms have been reorganized primarily into the new negative cognitions and mood cluster. Julia described several ways in which her spouse engaged in these symptoms to include his inability to communicate his experience, both in the present and in the past; his physical withdrawal into the basement, his estrangement from family participation, and marked lack of physical intimacy. In response to these symptoms, Julia developed cognitive, affective, and behavioral reactions. She felt terribly alone in the marriage. Spouses report that loneliness is the hardest thing to cope with while their partners are deployed. Ironically, PTSD reintroduces that loneliness and isolation despite the physical return of their veteran spouse. Julia wondered, "What's wrong with me? Why can't he trust me?"

Using an attributional cognitive model [7], Julia may be misinterpreting her husband's emotional numbing and withdrawal as reflective of her or the relationship itself, instead of being a function of the disorder. She internalized his avoiding behavior and developed reactionary negative cognitions, that is, "Something is wrong with me or he doesn't trust me." This reinforces clinically significant depressive feelings and symptoms. Behaviorally, she initially tried to engage but after being rebuffed so many times she has little option but to reciprocate the emotional withdrawal. The lack of communication and disclosure is inherently isolating to the veteran and their partner, thus feeding back into the couple's relational dysfunction.

Several studies have drawn correlates between the hyperarousal symptoms of PTSD and threat perception, psychological aggression, and physical violence [1]. Julia described several of her husband's hyperarousal symptoms: irritability, anger, hypervigilance, sleep disturbance, and problems with concentration. Hyperarousal symptoms are extremely salient because safety and security become paramount concerns when these symptoms are severe, especially in this military family where both firearms and children are found. Julia has appropriately responded to his hyperarousal symptoms with a combination of anger, fear, and avoidance, all of which significantly increase the inter-relational distress.

Reexperiencing symptoms, in contrast to avoidance or hyperarousal, have been correlated to less individual and marital distress in partners [7]. Returning to an attributional model, partners may be less distressed by these symptoms because they can be clearly linked to the traumatic event instead of the partner or relationship. Julia reported severe nightmares and dissociative symptoms displayed by her husband, yet she was able to reconcile this phenomena with his combat experience and thus found them more understandable.

The socially destructive implications of PTSD are well appreciated in this case. Julia describes a marriage on the brink of divorce: severed relationships with the children and occupational and financial problems. Combat veterans are more likely to separate or divorce [2]. Julia's consideration of divorce signals the severity of the problem and her cognitive landscape where options are limited and dismal. Children of combated-related PTSD veterans are more likely to suffer from psychiatric disorders [8]. In this case, the children are watching both of their parents unravel as individuals and as the parental union. Julia reported feeling overwhelmed with all the responsibility in the household, including the care of her affected veteran spouse. The concept of caregiver burden was coined for those caring for family members with dementia or schizophrenia; however, research has demonstrated that spouses of veterans with PTSD also report high levels of caregiver burden [9]. Caregiver burden and PTSD is not to be underestimated as extant research on the subject has shown high prevalence rates for psychological distress, depression, and suicidal ideation [10].

In addition, there is a significant barrier to care in the form of mental health stigma [5]. Both Julia and her husband struggled with this obstacle, at least initially. They were afraid of being perceived as sick or unstable. For military service members in particular, there is a culture of toughness and resilience which protects individuals against the incredible stresses of war, but acts as a double-edged sword by promoting notions that being traumatized or seeking help for traumatic experiences signals weakness, incompetence, or vulnerability.

25.3 Treatment and Management

In the initial management of PTSD and intimate partner relationships, a thorough safety and risk assessment is preeminent. Suicidal ideation is common when the psychological distress levels become overwhelming for the intimate partner and the veteran. Safety risks are magnified when social supports have been effectively withdrawn from, or when substances such as alcohol become involved. Hyperarousal symptoms increase the risk of aggression and violence to include physical abuse, emotional abuse, and child abuse. An assessment of safety for all family members, including the veteran and children, is critical.

Once safety is addressed, assess whether there is an indication of psychiatric medical management for either the partner or the veteran. An important point to remember here is that the spouse can be an essential facilitator for the veteran to access appropriate care. Considering the stigma toward mental health, spouses and intimate partners are often more willing to seek care for themselves or their veteran partners, making them important in a comprehensive early intervention strategy [6]. Psychiatric medications, typically within the antidepressant class, can biologically reduce symptom severity and frequency. Medications can optimize an individual's cognitive and affective state to improve psychotherapeutic intervention.

Psychotherapy is a critical component of treatment. Assess whether the veteran or the partner has an indication for individual therapy in series or parallel to the couple's therapy. Based on research on veterans, the best evidence supporting efficacy for individual psychopathology and related relationship problems is for behavioral or cognitive-behavioral therapy (CBT) [11]. There are several manualized CBT protocols in the literature. One such protocol is called cognitive-behavioral conjoint therapy for PTSD [11]. This CBT is a three-stage, 15-session intervention consisting of treatment orientation, psychoeducation on PTSD and relational problems, and cognitive interventions aimed to address maladaptive thinking patterns to maintain the conditions. This CBT attempts to address the complex and reciprocal dynamics that PTSD and relational problems create. Another such CBT protocol is called the couple therapy with combat veterans and their partners. This particular intervention is divided into an assessment and treatment phase spread over 12–14 sessions. This CBT attempts to increase social support, decrease interpersonal conflict, and address the experiential avoidance that maintains posttraumatic symptoms [12]. Both programs invest heavily in psychoeducation on trauma and traumatic reactions to provide a foundation of knowledge to participants in order to understand the dynamics they are living in.

An assessment of psychosocial services and referral to supportive programs can be extremely helpful to the veteran and the family. PTSD can incur a variety of medical and mental health, substance abuse, and legal, financial, academic, and occupational problems. There are many organizations and services available to families affected by PTSD. Consider the following online resources as portals to the spectrum of extant programs.

- www.va.gov: This is the website of the Department of Veterans Affairs. There are links to a variety of resources available to veterans and their families, including health care, education, training, benefits, employment, housing, etc.
- www.tricare.mil: TRICARE is the health-care program for military members and their families around the world.
- www.militaryonesource.mil: Military OneSource is a confidential Department of Defense-funded program providing comprehensive information on every aspect of military life at no cost to active duty, National Guard, reserve members, and their families. Information includes counseling, employment, education, parenting, and childhood services.
- www.dcoe.health.mil: The Defense Centers of Excellence (DCoE) for Psychological Health and Traumatic Brain Injury is part of the Military Health System. The DCoE works across the entire continuum of care to promote resilience, rehabilitation, and reintegration for warriors, families, and veterans with psychological health concerns and traumatic brain injuries.

25.4 Outcomes and Case Resolution

A safety assessment of all the family members was completed with reassuring result. Julia engaged in treatment and was seen individually on an ongoing basis. She elected to take an antidepressant to help mitigate her symptom severity, which was effective. Her husband continued to see his psychiatrist. After several individual psychotherapy sessions, she was able to convince her husband to begin a couple-based CBT intervention. A great deal of effort was made to provide psychoeducation on trauma and its psychiatric sequela. She was given information about resources at their local VA and Military OneSource to address their legal and financial problems. With treatment, the relationship distress was eventually reduced and their communication, intimacy, relationship satisfaction, and family functioning improved.

25.5 Conclusion

Combat-related PTSD in veterans has a significant negative impact on intimate partner relationships and families. Understanding the complex interplay between affected intimate partners can help treat the psychiatric and psychosocial sequela of combat-related PTSD. The partner or spouse can be critical to overcome obstacles to care for the veteran. Providers and programs can link resources to spouses for veterans and their families. More research is needed to understand the cognitive, affective, and behavioral variables underlying the PTSD-intimate relationship dyad [1]. Research is also required to understand the role of couple-based CBT interventions and intimate partners as facilitators to access of care.

References

1. Monson CM, et al. Military-related PTSD and intimate relationships: from description to theory-driven research and intervention development. Clin Psychol Rev. 2009;29(8):707–14.
2. Cook JM, et al. Posttraumatic stress disorder and current relationship functioning among World War II ex-prisoners of war. J Fam Psychol. 2004;18(1):36–45.
3. Jordan BM, Marmar CR, Fairbanks JA, Schlenger WE, Kulka RA, Hough RL, Weiss DS. Problems in families of male Vietnam veterans with posttraumatic stress disorder. J Consult Clin Psychol. 1992;60:916–26.
4. Riggs DS, Byrne CA, Weathers FW, Litz BT. The quality of the intimate relationships of male Vietnam veterans: problems associated with posttraumatic stress disorder. J Trauma Stress. 1998;11(1):87–101.
5. Hoge CW, Castro CA, Messer SC, McGurk D, Cotting DI, Koffman RL. Combat duty in Iraq and Afghanistan, mental health problems, and barriers to care. N Engl J Med. 2004;351(1):13–22.
6. Milliken CS, Auchterlonie JL, Hoge CW. Longitudinal assessment of mental health problems among active and reserve component soldiers returning from the Iraq War. JAMA. 2007;298(18):2141–8.
7. Renshaw KD, Caska CM. Relationship distress in partners of combat veterans: the role of partners' perceptions of posttraumatic stress symptoms. Behav Ther. 2012;43(2):416–26.
8. Solomon Z. The effect of combat-related postraumatic stress disorder on the family. Psychiatry. 1988;51:323–9.
9. Beckham JL, Lytle BL, Feldman ME. Caregiver burden in partners of Vietnam War veterans with PTSD. J Consult Clin Psychol. 1996;64:1068–72.
10. Manguno-Mire G, et al. Psychological distress and burden among female partners of combat veterans with PTSD. J Nerv Ment Dis. 2007;195(2):144–51.
11. Monson CM, et al. Cognitive-behavioral conjoint therapy for posttraumatic stress disorder: application to operation enduring and Iraqi freedom veterans. J Clin Psychol. 2008;64(8):958–71.
12. Erbes CR, et al. Couple therapy with combat veterans and their partners. J Clin Psychol. 2008;64(8):972–83.

Index

E. C. Ritchie (ed.), *Posttraumatic Stress Disorder and Related Diseases in Combat Veterans,* DOI 10.1007/978-3-319-22985-0

G

M

N

O

P

Made in the USA
Monee, IL
29 June 2026

55992273R10216